Thieme

Robotic Head and Neck Surgery
The Essential Guide

J. Scott Magnuson, MD, FACS
Professor of Otolaryngology–Head and Neck Surgery, University of Central Florida College of Medicine
Chief Medical Officer, Florida Hospital Celebration Health
Medical Director, Head and Neck Surgery, Celebration Health
Director, Robotic Head and Neck Surgery, Florida Hospital Nicholson Center for Robotic Surgery
Florida Hospital Nicholson Center Global Faculty Board Member
Orlando, Florida

Eric M. Genden, MD, FACS
Professor and Chairman
Department of Otolaryngology–Head and Neck Surgery
Icahn School of Medicine at Mount Sinai
New York, New York

Ronald B. Kuppersmith, MD, FACS
Professor of Surgery
Texas A&M Health Science Center College of Medicine
Bryan, Texas
Texas ENT and Allergy
College Station, Texas

Thieme
New York • Stuttgart • Delhi • Rio de Janeiro

Thieme Medical Publishers, Inc.
333 Seventh Avenue
New York, New York 10001

Executive Editor: Timothy Y. Hiscock
Managing Editor: J. Owen Zurhellen IV
Director, Editorial Services: Mary Jo Casey
Production Editor: Heidi Grauel
International Production Director: Andreas Schabert
Vice President, Editorial and E-Product
Development: Vera Spillner
International Marketing Director: Fiona Henderson
International Sales Director: Louisa Turrell
Director of Sales, North America: Mike Roseman
Senior Vice President and Chief Operating
Officer: Sarah Vanderbilt
President: Brian D. Scanlan
Printer: Replika Press

Library of Congress Cataloging-in-Publication Data

Robotic head and neck surgery : the essential guide / [edited by] J. Scott Magnuson, Eric M. Genden, Ronald B. Kuppersmith.
p. ; cm.
Includes bibliographical references and index.
ISBN 978-1-60406-919-8 — ISBN 978-1-60406-921-1
I. Magnuson, J. Scott, editor. II. Genden, Eric M., editor. III. Kuppersmith, Ronald B., editor.
[DNLM: 1. Otorhinolaryngologic Surgical Procedures—methods. 2. Head—surgery. 3. Neck—surgery.
4. Robotic Surgical Procedures—methods. WV 168]
RF51
617.5'1059—dc23

Thieme Publishers New York
333 Seventh Avenue, New York, NY 10001 USA, 1-800-782-3488
customerservice@thieme.com

Thieme Publishers Stuttgart
Rüdigerstrasse 14, 70469 Stuttgart, Germany, +49 [0]711 8931 421
customerservice@thieme.de

Thieme Publishers Delhi
A-12, Second Floor, Sector -2, NOIDA -201301, Uttar Pradesh, India, +91 120 45 566 00
customerservice@thieme.in

Thieme Publishers Rio de Janeiro, Thieme Publicações Ltda.
Argentina Building 16th floor, Ala A, 228 Praia do Botafogo Rio de Janeiro 22250-040 Brazil, +55 21 3736-3631

Printed in India

5 4 3 2 1

ISBN 978-1-60406-919-8

Also available as an e-book:
eISBN 978-1-60406-921-1

Dedications

To my head and neck cancer patients who bless me with their trust and gratefulness.
– JSM

I dedicate this work to my mother and father, for their love and support. This book is also dedicated to my educators like Tom Farmen, Louis Magnoli, and John Fredrickson, and Bruce Haughey, whose guidance and mentorship have been the cornerstone of my education.
– EMG

To my teachers, family, and patients, for setting high expectations and inspiring the relentless pursuit of excellence.
– RBK

Contents

Menu of Accompanying Videos

Video 5.1 TORS lateral oropharyngectomy for a T3N2b squamous cell carcinoma of the tonsil.

Video 5.2 TORS base of tongue resection for a T3N2b base of tongue squamous cell carcinoma.

Video 6.1 The preoperative findings of a patient with a tongue base cancer, demonstrating the surgical resection and remucosalization that occurs six weeks after surgery.

Video 6.2 Surgical resection of a tonsil cancer using robotic laser technique, demonstrating the use of local pharyngeal flap reconstruction of the defect.

Video 10.1 TORS supraglottic laryngectomy for a T2N0M0 squamous cell carcinoma using the Omniguide CO_2 laser.

Video 10.2 TORS selective supraglottic laryngectomy for an infrahyoid T1N0M0 squamous cell carcinoma.

Video 10.3 A salvage TORS supraglottic laryngectomy for a T2N0M0 squamous cell carcinoma of the supraglottis.

Video 10.4 TORS total laryngectomy for a recurrent T2N0M0 posterior commissure spindle cell carcinoma.

Video 11.1 Transoral robotic resection of hypopharyngeal squamous cell carcinoma.

Video 14.1 Robot-assisted modified radical neck dissection including level I-V via retroauricular approach for a T2N2aM0 oral tongue squamous cell carcinoma.

Preface

Head and neck surgery for benign and malignant disease is undergoing an exciting transformation with the introduction of new technologies. One of the most recently developed technologies is the surgical robot. First used in cardiac and urological surgery, other areas of surgery now employ the use of a surgical robot. Robot assistance in otolaryngology–head and neck surgery is relatively new, but has already demonstrated the potential to change treatment paradigms. Surgical robotics allows the surgeon to approach the complex anatomy of the head and neck from new perspectives, which can potentially reduce surgical morbidity. Additionally, this new technology affords the potential of the development of new procedures not currently performed in head and neck surgery.

Robotic Head and Neck Surgery: The Essential Guide is a collaborative effort of international experts describing the current state of the art of robot-assisted surgery of structures within the head and neck. The text provides a practical approach to robot-assisted techniques starting with the basics of training and education, ethical considerations, room set-up and instrumentation, and avoidance of complications. Specific surgical sites are also discussed, including approaches to malignancies of the oropharynx, larynx, hypopharynx, parapharyngeal space, thyroid, neck, and skull base. There are also chapters on robotic approaches for sleep apnea.

This book is intended for surgeons who may be interested in adopting these techniques into practice. Practitioners who are looking for insight on how to determine and improve their patient selection, understand the surgical approach for a variety of head and neck procedures, and want to incorporate this information in developing a robotic surgery program, will find this book invaluable. Additionally, other specialists, such as medical and radiation oncologists, who treat patients with head and neck illnesses will find this book a useful resource.

As surgeons who have been involved in the introduction of robot-assisted surgery in otolaryngology, we are optimistic about the possibilities that this technology may have for improved patient outcomes. We understand that further innovation and refinement of surgical robotics will be forthcoming, and it is our hope that this synthesis of the current state of robotic surgery of the head and neck can serve as a foundation and inspiration for the development of even less invasive and safer approaches for our patients.

Acknowledgment

We thank all our contributors for their labors on this book.

Contributors

Ahmed Yassin Bahgat, MBBCh, MSc ORL, EBE-ORL
Assistant Lecturer of Otorhinolaryngology
Faculty of Medicine
Alexandria University
Alexandria, Egypt
Clinical and Research Fellow of Prof. Claudio Vicini
G.B. Morgagni–L. Pierantoni Hospital
University of Pavia at Forli'
Forlì, Italy
Clinical and Research Fellow of Prof. Frédéric Chabolle
Foch Hospital
University of Versailles
Paris, France
Research Fellow and Clinical Observer of
Prof. J Scott Magnuson
Florida Hospital Celebration Health
University of Central Florida
Orlando, Florida

Hyung Kwon Byeon, MD
Clinical Assistant Professor
Department of Otorhinolaryngology
Yonsei University College of Medicine
Gangnam Severance Hospital
Seoul, South Korea

Woong Youn Chung, MD, PhD
Department of Surgery
Yonsei University College of Medicine
Seoul, South Korea

Julia A. Crawford, MBBS, FRACS
Advanced Head and Neck Surgery Fellow
Celebration Health, Florida Hospital
Orlando, Florida

Mohamed Eesa, MSc, FEBORL-HNS
Assistant Lecturer
Department of Otolaryngology–Head and Neck Surgery
Sister City, Zigazag. School of Medicine
Zagazig, Egypt

Eric M. Genden, MD, FACS
Professor and Chairman
Department of Otolaryngology–Head and Neck Surgery
Icahn School of Medicine at Mount Sinai
New York, New York

Ehab Y. Hanna, MD, FACS
Director of Skull Base Surgery
Professor and Vice Chairman
Department of Head and Neck Surgery
Medical Director, Head and Neck Center
University of Texas MD Anderson Cancer Center
Houston, Texas

Ehsan Hendawy, MSc, FEBORL-HNS
Assistant Lecturer
Department of Otolaryngology–Head and Neck Surgery
Zagazig School of Medicine
Zagazig, Egypt

Jason I. Kass, MD, PhD
Microvascular Head and Neck Fellow
Department of Otolaryngology-Head and Neck Surgery
Icahn School of Medicine at Mount Sinai
New York, New York

Yoon Woo Koh, MD, PhD
General Secretary
Korean Society of Thyroid–Head and Neck Surgery
Professor
Department of Otorhinolaryngology
Yonsei Head and Neck Cancer Center
Yonsei University College of Medicine
Seoul, South Korea

Suren Krishnan, OAM, FRACS
Associate Professor and Chairman
Department of Otolaryngology–Head and Neck Surgery
Royal Adelaide Hospital
Adelaide, South Australia, Australia

Michael E. Kupferman, MD, FACS
Associate Professor
Department of Head and Neck Surgery
University of Texas MD Anderson Cancer Center
Houston, Texas

Ronald B. Kuppersmith, MD, FACS
Professor of Surgery
Texas A&M Health Science Center College of Medicine
Bryan, Texas
Texas ENT and Allergy
College Station, Texas

Jandee Lee, MD, PhD
Department of Surgery
Yonsei University College of Medicine
Seoul, South Korea

J. Scott Magnuson, MD, FACS
Professor of Otolaryngology–Head and Neck Surgery
University of Central Florida College of Medicine
Chief Medical Officer, Florida Hospital Celebration Health
Medical Director, Head and Neck Surgery, Celebration Health
Director, Robotic Head and Neck Surgery
Florida Hospital Nicholson Center for Robotic Surgery
Florida Hospital Nicholson Center Global Faculty Board Member
Orlando, Florida

Giuseppe Meccariello, MD
Department of Otorhinolaryngology–Head and
Neck Surgery & Stomatology
G.B. Morgagni–L. Pierantoni Hospital
Forlì, Italy

Brett A. Miles, MD, DDS, FACS
Associate Professor of Otolaryngology–Head and Neck Surgery
Co-Chief, Division of Head and Neck Oncology
Department of Otolaryngology–Head and Neck Surgery
Icahn School of Medicine at Mount Sinai
New York, New York

Mara C. Modest, MD
Resident Physician
Department of Otorhinolaryngology–Head and Neck Surgery
The Mayo School of Graduate Medical Education
Rochester, Minnesota

Filippo Montevecchi, MD
Consultant of Otolaryngology–Head and Neck Surgery
University of Pavia in Forlì
G.B. Morgagni–L. Pierantoni Hospital
Forlì, Italy

Eric J. Moore, MD
Professor
Department of Otolaryngology–Head and Neck Surgery
Mayo Clinic
Rochester, Minnesota

Susan K. Sebastian, MS
Head, Department of Otorhinolaryngology
St. Stephen's Hospital
New Delhi, India

Richard V. Smith, MD, FACS
Professor and Vice-Chair
Department of Otorhinolaryngology–Head and Neck Surgery
Montefiore Medical Center
Albert Einstein College of Medicine
Bronx, New York

Roger Smith, PhD
Chief Technology Officer
Florida Hospital Nicholson Center
Professor of Medical Education
University of Central Florida College of Medicine
Graduate Faculty Scholar, UCF Modeling and Simulation Program
Orlando, Florida

Claudio A. Vicini, MD
Chairman
Department of Otolaryngology–Head and Neck Surgery & Oral Surgery
Professor of Sleep Disordered Breathing
School of Medicine of Pavia at G.B. Morgagni–L. Pierantoni Hospital
ASL Romagna
Forlì, Italy

Hilliary N. White, MD
Otolaryngology–Head and Neck Surgery Celebration
Florida Hospital Celebration Health
Associate Professor
University of Central Florida College of Medicine
Orlando, Florida

1 The Contemporary History of Robotic Surgery

Jason I. Kass and Eric M. Genden

Introduction

Robotics in surgery is the modern product of over a century of industrialization. The robotic surgery movement is part of a larger technological movement that has impacted nearly every aspect of life in the United States and other advanced nations. From communications to transportation, robotic technology has been advancing at an exponential pace. The advances in robotic surgery have impacted some specialties more than others and yet many areas remain unexplored. The word "robot" has come to mean something very different than its original intention. The term was coined by the Czech playwright Karl Capek in his dark 1921 play, *Rossom's Universal Robots*, based on the Czech-language word for forced labor, "robota." In the play, robots are manufactured as slaves; however, their artificial intelligence and lifelike appearance allowed them to be mistaken for human beings. The robots ultimately rebel and lead to the extinction of the human race. Though the current version of the surgical robot is far from Capek's vision, the term still evokes both fascination and fear.

Beginnings

The year 1985 saw use of the first surgical robot, called Puma 560—a motorized arm that could perform precisely targeted brain biopsies.[1] This same robot was used 3 years later in urological procedures to perform a transurethral prostatectomy.[2] Limitations of this robotic arm in urology were addressed in the next iteration of the device, the PROBOT, which was specifically designed for prostatectomy.[3] Orthopedic surgeons then began using their own robot, ROBODOC, the first robot approved by the U.S. Food and Drug Administration (FDA) for femur repair during hip surgery.[4] These early robots provided precision and visualization, but had limited range of motion and could perform only a fixed set of limited tasks.

During this time period of the 1980s, scientists at the National Air and Space Administration (NASA) became interested in performing remote surgery, whether for patients in space or on the battlefield; they called it "telepresence surgery."[5] Through collaboration between NASA and researchers at the Stanford Research Institute (SRI), they developed a robotic hand called the telemanipulator (**Fig. 1.1**). This device mimicked the motion of the wrist, thumb, and forefinger and allowed the surgeon to move his or her hands in a more natural fashion to drive a robotic arm. This provided the feeling that the surgeon was operating on the patient, despite being far away. Additional funding from the U.S. Army allowed further development using the telemanipulator as part of a mobile advanced surgical hospital (MASH) with the expectation that advanced care could be provided on the battlefield. Although these MASH units have only been validated with animal models and not been put into field practice, the idea that the surgeon and the robot could be in separate physical spaces is a key element of modern robotic-assisted surgery.

Several commercial enterprises were developed based on the telemanipulator and MASH units. AESOP, the Automatic Endoscopic System for Optimal Positioning, used voice-activated commands to drive a robotic camera.[6] Intuitive Surgical Inc., the company that developed the current da Vinci surgical system, licensed their original system from the SRI telepresence surgery system.

Robotic technology is now routinely applied to perform a variety of minimally invasive procedures in surgical specialties including urologic surgery,[2] gynecology,[7] orthopedic surgery,[8] thoracic surgery,[9] general surgery,[10] cardiothoracic surgery,[11] and most recently otolaryngology–head and neck surgery.

Transoral Robotic Surgery

As demonstrated by our introduction of transoral lasers, advanced optics, and transnasal endoscopy, otolaryngologists–head and neck surgeons are generally considered early adopters of new technology among physicians. In contrast, otolaryngologists are relative latecomers to the use of robotic surgery. The feasibility of head and neck applications of robotic technology was first introduced by Haus et al in 2003 using a porcine model.[12] In their study they performed a submandibular gland excision, selective neck dissection, superficial parotidectomy, and thymectomy using the da Vinci robot (Intuitive Surgical Inc.). In 2005, McLeod and Melder applied the technology clinically and brought the robot into the operating room. They performed the first transoral robotic surgery (TORS), resecting a vallecular cyst.[13]

Hockstein et al expanded on this work and applied TORS for microsurgery of the larynx.[14,15] With the use of an airway mannequin, Hockstein et al were able to position the large robotic cart and arms at the head of the operating room table and then gain wide exposure to the larynx by using a variety of laryngoscopes and mouth gags coupled with the robotic arms. Hockstein et al noted the following advantages: the robot provides three-dimensional (3D) images through a dual endoscope mechanism; robotic instrumentation provides a wide range of motions unavailable with traditional endoscopic instruments; scaling of movement allows large movements of the hands to produce only small movements in the robotic instruments; and the robot dampens hand tremors. Because of the maneuverability of the

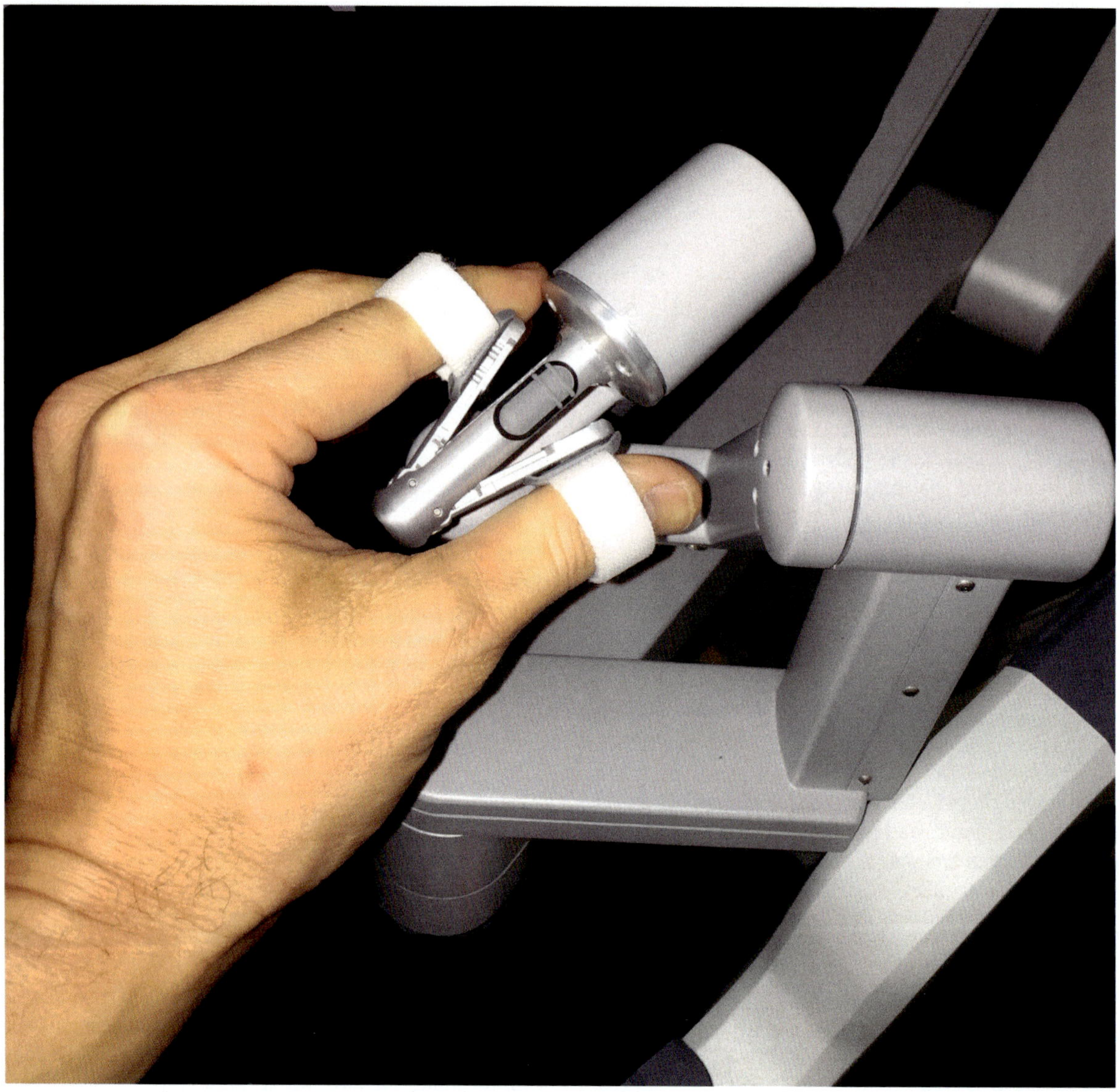

Fig. 1.1 The robotic telemanipulator helps the surgeon to operate the robotic instrumentation.

robotic arms, TORS has a significant benefit over transoral laser surgery, which is limited by the laser's line of sight. Moreover, en bloc resection can be performed rather than the piecemeal or cutting procedures performed using a laser.

In subsequent preclinical investigations the group at the University of Pennsylvania[16] evaluated pharyngeal and laryngeal procedures on human cadavers and the canine model and reported a safety profile for TORS suitable for use in human patients.[17] In 2005, the first human patients were enrolled in a prospective clinical trial established to evaluate the safety and efficacy of TORS. In 2006, the first series of three patients who had undergone TORS was reported by O'Malley et al, which showed the safety, feasibility, and basic efficacy of performing surgical resection in patients with squamous cell carcinoma of the tongue base.[18] Subsequent reports by Weinstein et al from this prospective human trial at the University of Pennsylvania demonstrated the safety, feasibility, and early success of performing supraglottic laryngectomy, radical tonsillectomy, and partial pharyngectomy procedures in head and neck cancer patients. Recently the role of TORS has also expanded to address unknown primary tumors of the head and neck.[19] In a small case series by Mehta et al robotic excision of the tongue base following failure to localize the primary tumor by conventional means identified the tumor in 9 of 10 cases.

Transaxillary, Transcervical, and Transnasal Approaches

The drive for minimal access surgery has led otolaryngologists and general surgeons to use the long robotic arms to reach head and neck structures through small, cosmetically favorable incisions. First popularized in South Korea and Japan, development of a transaxillary approach to the thyroid gland for robotic

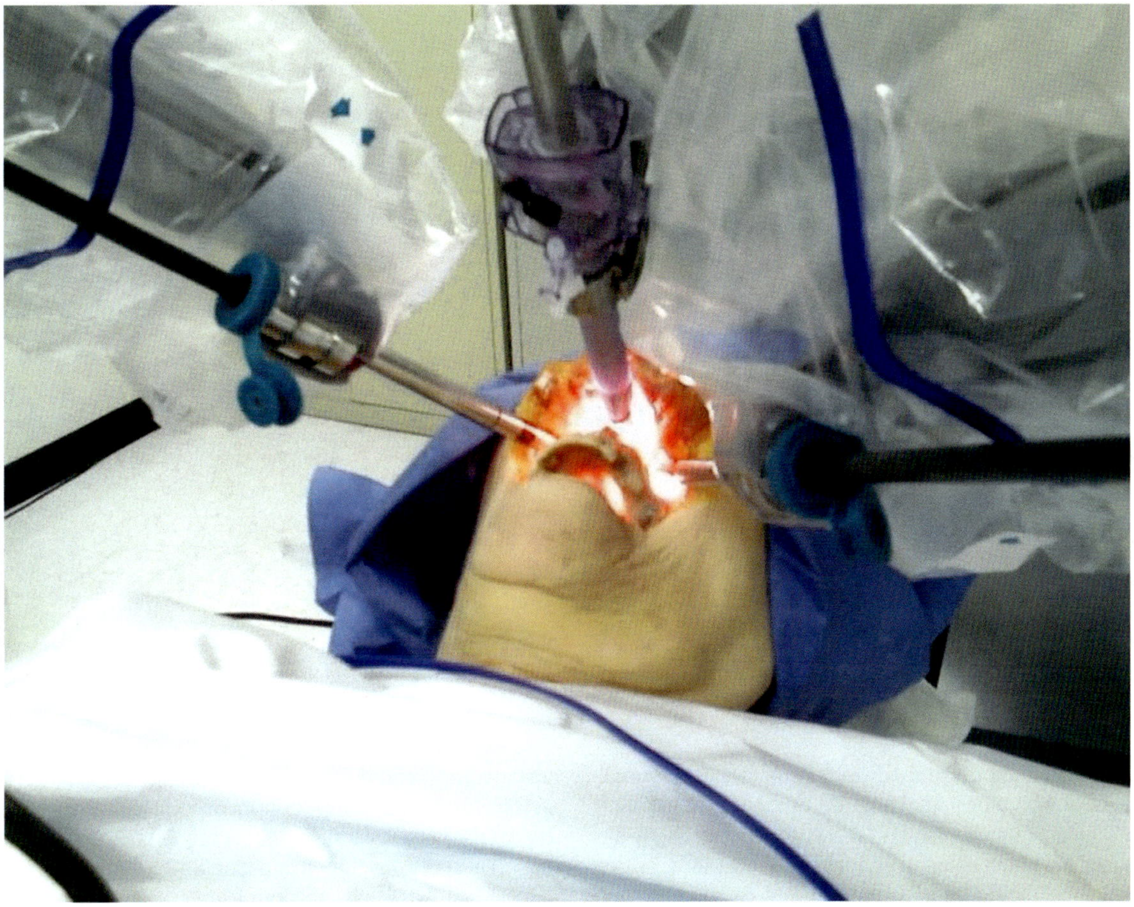

Fig. 1.2 Access to the skull base using a sublabial robotic approach may provide improved visualization and control.

thyroidectomy has been performed at several centers in the United States.[20] As with each new approach there are associated surgical risks. Risks unique to transaxillary approaches include axillary skin flap perforation and unintended brachial plexus injuries from traction.[21] Recently several groups have reported on preclinical and early experiences with robotic-assisted neck dissections via either a combined transaxillary/retroauricular (TARA) incision[22] or pre-/post-auricular incisions.[23] The robot facilitates dissection of the nodal basins lower in the neck, via hidden hairline incisions.

Development in endonasal and skull base surgery has been dominated by endoscopic techniques since the late 1980s. Minimally invasive access via the nasal corridor[24] and most recently via the orbit[25] has enabled radical surgery to the anterior skull base without facial incisions (**Fig. 1.2**). Early investigations are now ongoing to delineate the role for robotic approaches to the skull base. Early cadaver experiences have demonstrated feasibility using composite approaches to the skull base.[26]

■ Nononcologic Application of Robotic Technology

As otolaryngologists have become more comfortable with the improved exposure of the oral cavity and oropharynx afforded by TORS, we have expanded the use robotic-assisted approaches to manage nononcologic surgical indications. Sleep surgery for tongue base reduction lends itself to TORS.[27] In properly selected patients, tongue base reduction with or with a robotic-assisted supraglottoplasty has been shown to be safe[28] and effective,[29] albeit in nonrandomized studies. In the largest series of patients to date, there have been no fatalities associated with this approach, and complications have been limited to transient hypogeusia (18%), pharyngeal edema (3%), and late self-limited bleeding (2.5%).[30]

■ Robotic-Assisted Reconstruction

One of the many benefits of TORS is that reconstruction is not usually required. Cases where open approaches would have caused a pharyngotomy requiring reconstruction can often be robotically resected without risk of fistula. In many cases, patients are sent home after a few days and, postoperatively, resume oral intake immediately. In cases where there are exposed vessels, a pharyngotomy, significant tissue loss in the soft palate or base of tongue, or poor residual tissue quality, primary reconstruction should be considered. The robot has proven to be equally important in reconstruction as ablation when accessing challenging regions deep in the oropharynx. Robotic-assisted

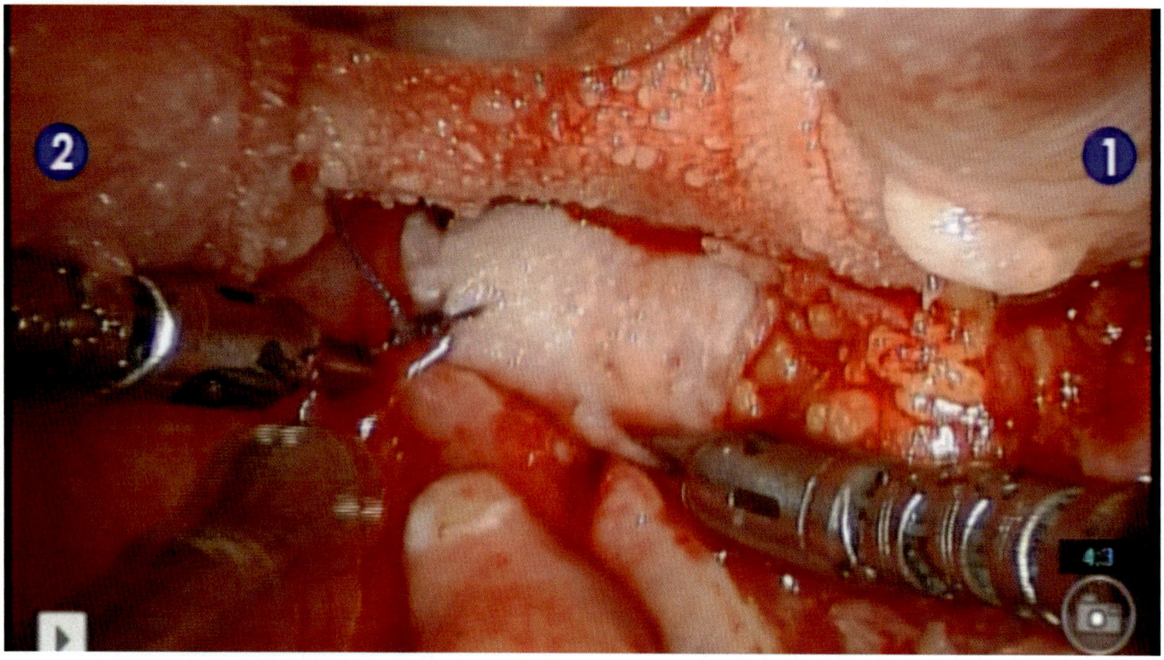

Fig. 1.3 The robot provides the unique opportunity to suture free flaps into the oropharynx. This photo demonstrates a free flap inset.

reconstruction offers the same advantages as ablation: small, wristed instrumentation in confined spaces with high-definition 3D visualization. An initial classification system has been proposed for when reconstruction with either local or free tissues should be considered (**Fig. 1.3**).[31] The da Vinci system has needle holders for sewing in flaps, and the robot has been evaluated for microvascular anastomosis in animal models.[32,33]

Future Directions

Fully automated robotic surgery currently remains science fiction. Additionally the robotic technology used in otolaryngology–head and neck surgery has so far been adapted from robots designed for straight line of sight visualization in the abdomen, pelvis, or thoracic cavity. Despite these limitations, our current robotic-assisted approaches to the head and neck are remarkably effective, accomplishing tasks that are difficult to reach with minimally invasive surgical access. Our field is committed to embracing disruptive surgical innovations, and the theories driving the future of robotics are addressed by Dr. Roger Smith in Chapter 16; however, incremental improvements in both manufacturing and computing are already in development. These include flexible instrumentation, single port access, and computer-driven algorithms making automated intraoperative decisions.

Flexible Robot

In the United States, the da Vinci system remains the dominant surgical robot that is commercially available and FDA approved. The current da Vinci system uses multiple arms, holding straight instruments. Given the natural curvature of the oral cavity, the biggest challenge with robotic cases is the visualization and positioning of the instruments. There are ongoing efforts to develop robotic instruments that can contour to the oral cavity. One such robot, the Flex System (Medrobotics Corp.) initially developed at Carnegie Mellon University, utilizes a robotically driven high-definition endoscope to snake its way into the oral cavity. Early experiences with cadavers have been reported,[34] and the first oropharyngeal and laryngeal cases have been completed in Belgium.[35]

Single Port Surgery

Intuitive Surgical Inc. has recently developed a single port adaptation for the da Vinci robot with the goal of single incision surgery. This system currently uses a 24-mm port with a single rigid arm that deploys two flexible instruments and a flexible endoscope. It received FDA approval in April 2015, but has not been used in otolaryngology.

Automated Intraoperative Decision Making

Artificial intelligence is one key aspect that distinguishes the science of actual robotic surgery from science fiction. While most surgeons are not ready to transfer intraoperative decision making to a robot, computer-aided design has made significant improvements in preoperative surgical planning of complex head and neck reconstruction,[36] skull base,[37] and sleep surgery.[38] With current 3D imaging, registration, and modeling technology, it is not difficult to imagine a robot that could dock itself and position the instruments in preparation for the procedure. Additionally, preoperative identification of critical "No-Go" structures, including large arteries or nerves, could prevent catastrophic injuries by the novice robotic surgeon.

References

1. Kwoh YS, Hou J, Jonckheere EA, Hayati S. A robot with improved absolute positioning accuracy for CT guided stereotactic brain surgery. IEEE Trans Biomed Eng 1988;35(2):153–160
2. Davies BL, Hibberd RD, Ng WS, Timoney AG, Wickham JE. The development of a surgeon robot for prostatectomies. Proc Inst Mech Eng H 1991;205:35–38
3. Harris SJ, Arambula-Cosio F, Mei Q, Hibberd RD, Davies BL, Wickham JE, et al. The Probot—an active robot for prostate resection. Proc Inst Mech Eng H 1997;211:317–325
4. Bargar WL, Bauer A, Börner M. Primary and revision total hip replacement using the Robodoc system. Clin Orthop Relat Res 1998;(354):82–91
5. Satava RM. Surgical robotics: the early chronicles: a personal historical perspective. Surg Laparosc Endosc Percutan Tech 2002;12:6–16
6. Pugin F, Bucher P, Morel P. History of robotic surgery: from AESOP and ZEUS to da Vinci. J Visc Surg 2011;148:e3–8
7. Advincula AP, Song A. The role of robotic surgery in gynecology. Curr Opin Obstet Gynecol 2007;19:331–336
8. Lang JE, Mannava S, Floyd AJ, Goddard MS, Smith BP, Mofidi A, et al. Robotic systems in orthopaedic surgery. J Bone Joint Surg Br 2011;93:1296–1299
9. Weissenbacher A, Bodner J. Robotic surgery of the mediastinum. Thorac Surg Clin 2010;20(2):331–339
10. Fourman MM, Saber A. Robotic bariatric surgery: a systematic review. Surg Obes Relat Dis 2012;8:483–488
11. Diodato MD, Damiano RJ. Robotic cardiac surgery: overview. Surg Clin North Am 2003;83(6):1351–1367
12. Haus BM, Kambham N, Le D, Moll FM, Gourin C, Terris DJ. Surgical robotic applications in otolaryngology. Laryngoscope 2003;113:1139–1144
13. McLeod IK, Melder PC. Da Vinci robot-assisted excision of a vallecular cyst: a case report. Ear Nose Throat J 2005;84:170–172.
14. Hockstein NG, Nolan JP, O'Malley BW, Woo YJ. Robotic microlaryngeal surgery: a technical feasibility study using the da Vinci surgical robot and an airway mannequin. Laryngoscope 2005;115(May):780–785
15. Hockstein NG, Nolan JP, O'Malley BW, Woo YJ. Robot-assisted pharyngeal and laryngeal microsurgery: results of robotic cadaver dissections. Laryngoscope 2005;115(June):1003–1008
16. O'Malley BW, Weinstein GS, Hockstein NG. Transoral robotic surgery (TORS): glottic microsurgery in a canine model. J Voice 2006;20:263–268
17. Hockstein NG, O'Malley BW, Weinstein GS. Assessment of intraoperative safety in transoral robotic surgery. Laryngoscope 2006;116(February):165–168
18. O'Malley BW, Weinstein GS, Snyder W, Hockstein NG. Transoral robotic surgery (TORS) for base of tongue neoplasms. Laryngoscope 2006;116(8):1465–1472
19. Mehta V, Johnson P, Tassler A, Kim S, Ferris RL, Nance M, et al. A new paradigm for the diagnosis and management of unknown primary tumors of the head and neck: a role for transoral robotic surgery. Laryngoscope 2013;123:146–151
20. Kang S-W, Jeong JJ, Yun J-S, Sung TY, Lee SC, Lee YS, et al. Robot-assisted endoscopic surgery for thyroid cancer: experience with the first 100 patients. Surg Endosc 2009;23:2399–2406
21. Ban EJ, Yoo JY, Kim WW, Son HY, Park S, Lee SH, et al. Surgical complications after robotic thyroidectomy for thyroid carcinoma: a single center experience with 3,000 patients. Surg Endosc 2014;28(9):2555–2563
22. Kim WS, Lee HS, Kang SM, Hong HJ, Koh YW, Lee HY, et al. Feasibility of robot-assisted neck dissections via a transaxillary and retroauricular ("TARA") approach in head and neck cancer: preliminary results. Ann Surg Oncol 2012;19:1009–1017
23. Blanco RGF, Ha PK, Califano JA, Fakry C, Richmon J, Saunders JM. Robotic-assisted neck dissection through a pre- and post-auricular hairline incision: preclinical study. J Laparoendosc Adv Surg Tech 2012;22(8):791–796
24. Snyderman CH, Pant H, Carrau RL, Prevedello D, Gardner P, Kassam AB. What are the limits of endoscopic sinus surgery? The expanded endonasal approach to the skull base. Keio J Med 2009;58:152–160
25. Moe KS, Bergeron CM, Ellenbogen RG. Transorbital neuroendoscopic surgery. Neurosurgery 2010;67(September):16–28
26. Carrau RL, Prevedello DM, De Lara D, Durmus K, Ozer E. Combined transoral robotic surgery and endoscopic endonasal approach for the resection of extensive malignancies of the skull base. Head Neck 2013;35(November):691–696
27. Vicini C, Dallan I, Canzi P, Frassineti S, La Pietra MG, Montevecchi F. Transoral robotic tongue base resection in obstructive sleep apnoea-hypopnoea syndrome: a preliminary report. ORL J Otorhinolaryngol Relat Spec 2010;72:22–27
28. Vicini C, Montevecchi F, Pang K, Bahgat A, Dallan I, Frassineti S, et al. Combined transoral robotic tongue base surgery and palate surgery in obstructive sleep apnea-hypopnea syndrome: expansion sphincter pharyngoplasty versus uvulopalatopharyngoplasty. Head Neck 2014;36(January):77–83
29. Hoff PT, D'Agostino MA, Thaler ER. Transoral robotic surgery in benign diseases including obstructive sleep apnea: safety and feasibility. Laryngoscope 2015;125(5):1249–1253
30. Crawford JA, Montevechi F, Vicini C, Magnuson JS. Transoral robotic sleep surgery. Otolaryngol Clin North Am 2014;47(3):397–406
31. De Almeida JR, Park RCW, Genden EM. Reconstruction of transoral robotic surgery defects: principles and techniques. J Reconstr Microsurg 2012 Sep;28(7):465–472
32. Karamanoukian RL, Finley DS, Evans GRD, Karamanoukian HL. Feasibility of robotic-assisted microvascular anastomoses in plastic surgery. J Reconstr Microsurg 2006;22(212):429–431
33. Lee JY, Mattar T, Parisi TJ, Carlsen BT, Bishop AT, Shin AY. Learning curve of robotic-assisted microvascular anastomosis in the rat. J Reconstr Microsurg 2012;28(212):451–456
34. Rivera-Serrano CM, Johnson P, Zubiate B, Kuenzler R, Choset H, Zenati M, et al. A transoral highly flexible robot: novel technology and application. Laryngoscope 2012;122(May):1067–1071
35. Remacle M, MN Prasad V, Lawson G, Plisson L, Bachy V, Van der Vorst S. Transoral robotic surgery (TORS) with the Medrobotics Flex System: first surgical application on humans. Eur Arch Otorhinolaryngol 2015;272:1451–1455
36. Rodby KA, Turin S, Jacobs RJ, Cruz JF, Hassid VJ, Kolokythas A, et al. Advances in oncologic head and neck reconstruction: systematic review and future considerations of virtual surgical planning and computer aided design/computer aided modeling. J Plast Reconstr Aesthetic Surg 2014;67(9):1171–1185
37. Haerle SK, Daly MJ, Chan HHL, Vescan A, Kucharczyk W, Irish JC. Virtual surgical planning in endoscopic skull base surgery. Laryngoscope 2013;123:2935–2939
38. Barrera JE. Virtual surgical planning improves surgical outcome measures in obstructive sleep apnea surgery. Laryngoscope 2014;124(May):1259–1266

2 Training and Education for Robotic Surgery

Julia A. Crawford and J. Scott Magnuson

Introduction

As mentioned in Chapter 1, the first documented use of a robot-assisted surgical procedure occurred in 1985 when the PUMA 560 robotic surgical arm was used in a neurosurgical procedure.[1] From this beginning, there was rapid expansion of the surgical robot into general, urological, pediatric, and gynecological surgery. The surgical robot was seen to increase dexterity and visualization as well as improve hand–eye coordination and ergonomic positioning. In addition, these systems were able to perform surgeries that had previously been technically difficult or unfeasible.[2]

These advances in the available technology led to modifications in established procedures as well as the introduction of entirely new procedures. However, with the introduction of any new procedure or technology into surgical practice, adequate steps must be taken to ensure that patients are not placed at undue risks.[3] One of these steps is ensuring that surgeons are adequately trained and credentialed in this new technology before applying it in practice. It was to this end that a consensus statement on robotic surgery, including guidelines for training and credentialing, from the Society of American Gastrointestinal and Endoscopic Surgeons (SAGES) and the Minimally Invasive Robotic Association (MIRA) was formulated in 2008.[4] This consensus statement aimed to answer the questions of how training in robotic surgery should be accomplished and what the appropriate process for credentialing robotic surgeons was. This training was broken down into two main categories: technical training and capability, and the use of the robot for specific operations.

In regard to the first category, the surgeon must have both a knowledge base and a practical working familiarity with the complexities of the surgical robot prior to clinical use. In addition to standard operating procedures, the surgeon should be familiar with how to safely and rapidly remove the device in the event of an emergency, what to do if the system stops responding, and what actions to take if the system makes movements that could potentially harm the patient.

The second aspect of training relates to applying surgical technology to specific operations. This is simplest when an already fully trained surgeon utilizes previously learned skills but adapts them to incorporate the use of the surgical robot. What is more challenging is a training surgeon who does not yet have established skills learning both the basic steps or tenets of surgery in addition to the complexities of the surgical robot. In developing a curriculum or training manual for any robotic surgery, it is important to address the different needs of these two groups.

There is currently no standardized or validated training program available for robotic surgery. The Fundamental Skills of Robotic Surgery (FSRS) curriculum was developed to allow the novice surgeon to master the basic functions of the surgical console and psychomotor skills necessary to perform robotic surgery.[5] While this provides a fundamental platform from which to begin robotic training, there is no specialty-specific or procedure-based component to the training as yet. It is important to establish a formal training program that makes allowances for both novice surgeons and those who already have significant experience.

This chapter represents a summary of the consensus report of the American Academy of Otolaryngology–Head and Neck Surgery (AAO-HNS) Robotic Surgery Taskforce and the American Head and Neck Society (AHNS) Education Committee whose combined members included J. Scott Magnuson, Eric M. Genden, Neil D. Gross, F. Christopher Holsinger, Umamaheswar Duvvuri, Tamer A. Ghanem, David Goldenberg, Alan M. Miller, Eric J. Moore, Christopher G. Morris, James L. Netterville, Gregory S. Weinstein, and Jeremy Richmon.

Robotics in Otolaryngology–Head and Neck Surgery

With a surgical history of less than a decade at the time of writing, the application of robotic surgery in the otolaryngological field is newer in comparison to other fields of surgery. The first robotic procedure on a patient to excise a vallecular cyst was carried out in 2005 by McLeod and Melder.[6] This showed that the application of robotic surgery to otolaryngology was possible. The intraoperative safety was assessed in a fresh human cadaver study by Hockstein et al in 2006. This study concluded that the da Vinci surgical system demonstrated a safety profile similar to conventional transoral surgery.[7] Since these first studies, the role of robotic surgery has rapidly expanded to include excision of oropharyngeal, hypopharyngeal, and supraglottic malignancies as well as being applied to benign disorders such as surgery for obstructive sleep apnea.[8,9,10,11,12,13]

Much of the benefit of robotic surgery in otolaryngology is attributed to its minimally invasive nature and the ability to improve functional outcomes for patients due to these minimally invasive qualities. The shift from open surgery to primary chemoradiotherapy for treatment of upper aerodigestive tract (UAT) malignancies occurred due to the perceived high morbidity of open surgery. While this is true, chemoradiotherapy itself carries significant long-term morbidity risks. Steiner and colleagues in the late 1970s offered an alternative primary treatment in the form of transoral laser microsurgery (TLM) initially starting with treatment of laryngeal carcinoma and then expanding to other subsites.[14,15,16,17] This technique, however, while oncologically and functionally effective, remains technically challenging. Transoral robotic surgery (TORS) may offer significant advantages over TLM as a minimally invasive technique as it provides superior optics, is not limited by line of sight, and has a shorter learning curve.[18]

With the increasing implementation of these robotic techniques, standardization of training and credentialing of otolaryngologists and head and neck surgeons is imperative to standardize patient care and safety.[19] Currently, credentialing and granting privileges to perform robotic surgeries is the responsibility of individual institutions. While there is a move to formulate standard operating procedures or best practices to use in robotic credentialing, there is currently no established formal training pathway in otolaryngology. Several avenues exist for gaining experience in robotic surgery. These include industry and proctor-lead courses for surgeons with an established head and neck practice, fellowship programs, and the increasing implementation of robotic surgery into academic training programs.

■ Approaches from Other Specialties

In establishing a training pathway, it is important to appreciate the steps that have been taken with similar implementation in other subspecialties with a longer robotic surgical history. The Society of Urological Robotic Surgeons (SURS) recommendations for credentialing of robotic-assisted radical prostatectomy are the most well-established and accepted guidelines to date.[20]

The main objective of these recommendations was to establish a certification body as well as an internationally recognized set of standards and guidelines for the safe application of robotic surgery in urology. This certification body was to be free of any industry influence. Furthermore, it would be this body, rather than industry, that identified proctors to supervise the subsequent training of other surgeons. These proctors would have a standardized checklist to evaluate surgeons seeking credentialing. A minimum of three to five cases is required prior to the granting of unrestricted privileges and the proctor should be involved in the informed consent process for these cases. The recommendations also provided for ongoing evaluation of the safety and efficacy of the procedure with a remediation process available for surgeons with substandard performance.

The multidisciplinary statement previously alluded to and developed by the SAGES-MIRA consensus statement in 2008 laid out guidelines in training and credentialing of robotic surgeons.[4] According to these guidelines, surgeons seeking robotic privileges should firstly have an accredited residency specialty training in the field they were applying for. For surgeons who had formal robotic surgery training during residency or fellowship, a log of cases should be provided as well as a letter from the program director outlining the candidate's experience in robotic surgery. For those who did not receive formal robotic surgery training during residency, a structured training program curriculum is required and this should be established by the individual health care institution. Once permanent privileges are granted, the institution should track the outcomes of the surgeon for this procedure and ensure that appropriate medical education, renewal, and denial of privilege policies are in place.

Perrier and colleagues published a consensus statement regarding the safe implementation of robotic thyroidectomy. They identified multiple steps to a safe implementation process starting with evaluating the candidacy of the surgeon; the surgeon should be in a department that is experienced in surgical management of the thyroid gland and they themselves must be experienced in standard thyroid surgery and have a sufficient case load. The initial education process was broken down into gaining understanding about the surgical robot and systems failure preparation, identifying an appropriate robotic team, in-lab robotic training, case observations, creation of a best practice checklist, and finally cadaveric dissection. In the clinical phase of introducing the robot into surgical practice, they recommended the following: establishment of ideal patient selection criteria; open disclosure of risks and numbers of cases performed by the operating surgeon as part of the informed consent process; appropriate data collection of any morbidity and mortality; and proctoring of initial cases by an experienced robotic thyroid surgeon.[21]

■ Training Models for Robotic Surgery

The pathway for robotic surgical training is dependent on the experience level of the surgeon involved. For residents or fellows (surgeons in training), there is the possibility of a graduated exposure program with increasing responsibility for different aspects of a robotic surgical operation as greater experience is gained. For those surgeons who are already in an established practice, this graduated exposure is not possible due to limitations on time, personal and practice finances, hospital resources, and difficulty with ongoing mentorship. Given these two differing training needs, there must be two distinct training protocols to accommodate each training need.

Surgeon In-Training

Much of the available data regarding resident training in surgical robots comes from urological literature. Shah and Hass divided the training process into nonclinical and clinical stages with the nonclinical phase consisting of informational training followed by hands on experience in a lab setting. The clinical phase begins with the trainee working as the assistant surgeon so that they become familiar with the positioning of the patient, surgical access, and docking of the robot.[22]

Preclinical Training and Simulation

The initial introduction to training should be in the form of understanding the mechanics of the robot itself. This can be achieved by undertaking the basic online training modules that are specific for the robotic system in use. They should include an overview of the robotic system components, the basic functioning of the robot, and an understanding of troubleshooting mechanisms. Development of robotic skills may then begin with dry lab practice and with simulators.

The dry lab practice can include the performance of basic tasks using the robot before moving on to cadaveric models. Moles and colleagues published their preliminary work in developing a curriculum for otolaryngology residents which involved participants performing defined exercises accomplishing the following tasks: circular pin transfer, simultaneous bimanual carrying, precision bead drop, needle passing, and suture tying. They found that residents quickly became proficient in these skills with no previous experience on the robot.[23] As DiLorenzo et al found, however, inanimate teaching models do not necessarily reflect the real clinical environment, which can present the surgeon with complications unique to the living model.[24]

Basic robotic skills can also be reinforced through simulation. Currently, there are four robotic surgical simulators available: RoSS, dV-Trainer, SEP Robot, and da Vinci Skills Simulator. Each system is represented in the literature and all possess varying degrees of face, content, and construct validity. Typically, these systems use dual haptic devices and three-dimensional images to train users on the cognitive and motor aspects of robotic surgery. Tasks begin with nonanatomic modules such as moving balls or rings to targets to learn basic orientation and motor skills. As the trainees become comfortable with the basic tasks, complexity increases to individual surgical skills, such as needle handling and basic electrocautery, then to advanced maneuvers such as vessel dissection, which incorporate previously mastered basic skills. Individual performance metrics are recorded and stored for each individual, to be reviewed by the instructor. The main issue for head and neck robotic surgery work is that none of the available simulators have any advanced simulation available in this subspecialty. Additionally, while simulators are advantageous, confirmation of construct and predictive validity of robotic simulators and their reliability as a training tool will be necessary before they are integrated into the surgical credentialing process.[25]

The next step from inanimate object training and simulation should be application of these acquired skills to cadaveric dissection. This component of training should include TORS-specific tasks including positioning and docking of the robotic system and performance of TORS-related procedures. The trainee should be comfortable and proficient with these tasks prior to moving on to the clinical component of training.

Clinical Training

Residents and fellows in an active head and neck robotic practice can gain graduated skills and expertise in robotic surgery as they would for any surgical procedures. This should typically begin with case observation before active involvement in the case as the bedside assistant.

As the bedside assistant, the trainee should gain a greater understanding of the role and function of each member of the robotic surgical team including the anesthetist and surgical technician. The trainee needs to understand the importance of patient positioning and exposure of the tumor with the appropriate retractor, in addition to positioning and docking of the robot. As the bedside assistant, the trainee will become proficient with the steps of the operation and begin to anticipate the moves of the console surgeon. An understanding of how to retract tissue to improve exposure for the operating surgeon, an ability to assist in suctioning and maintaining hemostasis, and troubleshooting by moving the robotic arms to avoid collisions are all critical skills that will make a more competent console surgeon. Once expertise in these areas is sufficient, a step-wise approach from simpler to more complex surgical console tasks should be started with adequate supervision from the expert robotic surgeon. A step-wise approach would be:

1. Simple palatine tonsillectomy
2. Lingual tonsillectomy
3. Limited pharyngectomy
4. Base of tongue resection
5. Supraglottic laryngectomy

Until formal, validated methods of assessment are developed to measure surgeon technical proficiency, it is recommended that the trainee is proctored for each of the above procedures until competence is achieved.

Established Surgeons

Surgeons who wish to introduce robotic surgery into their practice should have, as a minimum, completed an accredited residency or fellowship training program and be board-eligible or board-certified. The performance of equivalent operations via either an open or endoscopic approach should already be in their scope of practice. It is important that the novice robotic surgeon has an appropriate mentor who can provide case observation and experience in addition to serving as a proctor. Ultimately, these proctors should be accredited by a vetting body within the otolaryngology community rather than assigned from within the robotic industry. In a similar vein to the in-training surgeon, established surgeons should go through a preclinical and clinical training phase, although these will ideally be more time sensitive.

Preclinical Training

This will be essentially the same as the in-training surgeon including didactic or online teaching about the basics of the robotic system in addition to basic exercises with the robot to develop dexterity and familiarly with the robotic functions. Ideally, simulator or dry lab exercises would include an assessment of technical proficiency via a validated scoring system. The next step would be cadaveric training: increasing familiarity with patient positioning, tumor exposure, robotic docking, and troubleshooting robotic issues such as clashing of instruments. The cadaveric sessions should include core procedures such as radical tonsillectomy and base of tongue resection. As part of these procedures, the surgeon should become more familiar with the concept of inside-out anatomy and become more accustomed to the position of important vascular and nervous structures.

Clinical Training

Given the time constraints that apply to a surgeon who is already in active practice, training must be compressed into a shorter period than in-training surgeons. The clinical training experience should begin with case observation, specific to the practice the surgeon is undertaking—be that for oncology or sleep apnea purposes. Preferably, the surgeon could also act as the bedside assistant to gain experience in instrument manipulation, retraction, smoke and blood evacuation, placement of surgical clips, and emergency management.

It is also important that not only the surgeon but also the rest of the robotic team is adequately trained and understands their role in the operation. These team members should either accompany the surgeon during case observation for those in a hospital without robotic experience or, in a hospital with an established robotic program, they should receive training from an already experienced team.

The surgeon's initial robotic operations in their home hospital should be supervised by an experienced proctor who continues to mentor the surgeon until the candidate robotic surgeon is safe and capable of operating independently. It is important that a standardized evaluation is formulated that can help indicate that a core level of competency has been obtained.

Maintenance of Privileges

Any adopted training and credentialing model should include provisions for ongoing training and maintenance of skills. Chia et al found in their survey of TORS surgeons in the United States that the risk of complications is significantly less for surgeons who have performed greater than 50 procedures.[26] Richmon et al and Asher et al both found that the risk of postoperative hemorrhage was greatest in inexperienced surgeons.[27,28] As such, it is recommended that newly credentialed robotic surgeons in otolaryngology–head and neck surgery employ a graduated approach to integrating robotic surgery into their practice.

Requirements for maintenance after initial training and credentialing will vary across institutions; however, a suggested approach is:

- Provisional privileges: These may be appropriate for initial robotic surgical experience. The period of time and number of cases before unrestricted privileges may be granted should be determined at an institutional level by the medical staff committee, chief of staff, or appropriate committee.
- Monitoring of privileges: After the initial training and credentialing, clinical performance, surgical volume, and complications should be monitored via appropriate peer review.
- Continuing medical education (CME): Adequate evidence of CME activity including dedicated CME in robotic surgery.

■ Conclusion

The introduction of any new surgical technology must be implemented in such a way that patients are not placed at any undue risk. A centralized, independent training and credentialing committee for TORS formed jointly from AAO-HNS and AHNS would be the ideal situation to ensure that this occurs. The basic premise for training should include a preclinical phase of gaining familiarity with the basic functions of the robotic and cadaveric practice before progressing to clinical modules. It is important to have ongoing support from a robotic mentor surgeon after initial training and to perform a minimum number of robotic cases yearly to maintain the surgical skill set.

References

1. Kwoh YS, Hou J, Jonckheere EA, et al. A robot with improved absolute positioning accuracy for CT guided stereotactic brain surgery. IEEE Trans Biomed Eng 1988;35:153–161
2. Lanfranco AR, Castellanos AE, Desai JP, et al. Robotic surgery: a current perspective. Ann Surg 2004;239(1):14–21
3. Sachdeva AK, Russell TR. Safe introduction of new procedures and emerging technologies in surgery: education, credentialing and privileging. Surg Oncol Clin N Am 2007;16:101–114
4. Herron DM, Marohn M. SAGES-MIRA Robotic Surgery Consensus Group 2008; A consenus document on robotic surgery. Surg Endosc 2008;22:313–325
5. Attalla K, Rasa SJ, Rehman S, et al. Effectiveness of a dedicated robot-assisted surgery training program. Can J Urol 2013;20:7084–7090
6. McLeod IK, Melder PC. Da Vinci robot-assisted excision of a vallecular cyst: a case report. Ear Nose Throat J 2005;84:170–172
7. Hockstein NG, O'Malley BW, Weinstein GS. Assessment of intraoperative safety in transoral robotic surgery. Laryngoscope 2006;116(2):165–168
8. Boudreaux BA, Rosenthal EL, Magnuson JS, et al. Robot-assisted surgery for upper aerodigestive tract neoplasms. Arch Otolaryngol Head Neck Surg 2009;135(4):397–401
9. Moore EJ, Olsen SM, Laborde R, et al. Long-term functional and oncologic results of transoral robotic surgery for oropharyngeal squamous cell carcinoma. Mayo Clin Proc 2012;87(3):219–225
10. O'Malley BW, Weinstein GS, Snyder W, et al. Transoral robotic surgery (TORS) for base of tongue neoplasms. Laryngoscope 2006;116:1465–1472
11. Weinstein GS, O'Malley BW, Magnuson JS, et al. Transoral robotic surgery: a multicenter study to assess feasibility, safety and surgical margins. Laryngoscope 2012;122:1701–1707
12. Park YM, Lee WJ, Lee JG, et al. Transoral robotic surgery (TORS) in laryngeal and hypopharyngeal cancer. J Laparoendosc Adv Surg Tech A 2009;19(3):361–369
13. Vicini C, Dallan I, Canzi P. Transoral robotic surgery of the tongue base in obstructive sleep apnea-hypopnea syndrome: anatomic considerations and clinical experience. Head Neck 2012; 34(1):15–22
14. Steiner W. Experience in endoscopic laser surgery of malignant tumours of the upper aero-digestive tract. Adv Otorhinolaryngol 1988;39:135–144
15. Steiner W. Results of curative laser microsurgery of laryngeal carcinomas. Am J Otolaryngol 1993;14(2):116–121
16. Steiner W, Ambrosch P, Hess CF, Kron M. Organ preservation by transoral laser microsurgery in piriform sinus carcinoma. Otolaryngol Head Neck Surg 2001;124(1):58–67
17. Steiner W, Fierek O, Ambrosch P, Hommerich CP, Kron M. Transoral laser microsurgery for squamous cell carcinoma of the base of the tongue. Arch Otolaryngol Head Neck Surg 2003; 129(1):36–43
18. Li RJ, Richmon JD. Transoral endoscopic surgery: new surgical techniques for oropharyngeal cancer. Otolaryngol Clin North Am 2012:45:823–844
19. Bhayani MK, Holsinger FC, Lai SY. A shifting paradigm for patients with head and neck cancer: transoral robotic surgery (TORS). Oncology 2010;24:1010–1015
20. Zorn KC, Kautam G, Shalhav AL, et al. Training, credentialing, proctoring and medicolegal risks of robotic urological surgery: recommendations of the society of urologic robotic surgeons. J Urol 2009;182:1126–1132
21. Perrier ND, Randolph GW, Inabnet III WB, et al. Robotic thyroidectomy: a framework for new technology assessment and safe implementation. Thyroid 2010;20(12):1327–1332

22. Shah G, Hass G. Teaching daVinci robot surgical system: a new paradigm. J Urol Urogynakol 2006;13:22–23
23. Moles JJ, Connelly PE, Sarti EE, et al. Establishing a training program for residents in robotic surgery. Laryngoscope 2009;119:1927–1931
24. Di Lorenzo N, Coscarella G, Faraci L, et al. Robotic systems and surgical education. JSLS 2005;9:3–12
25. Liss MA, McDougall EM. Robotic surgical simulation. Cancer J 2013;19(2):124–129
26. Chia SH, Gross ND, Richmon JD. Surgeon experience and complications with transoral robotic surgery (TORS). Otolaryngol Head Neck Surg 2013;149(6):885–892
27. Richmon JD, Feng AL, Yang W, et al. Feasibility of rapid discharge after transoral robotic surgery of the oropharynx. Laryngoscope 2014;124(11):2518–2525
28. Asher SA, White HN, Kejner AE, et al. Hemorrhage after transoral robotic-assisted surgery. Otolaryngol Head Neck Surg 2013;149(1):112–117

3 The Ethics of Surgical Innovation

Ronald B. Kuppersmith

■ Introduction

During a surgeon's career, techniques and devices will be introduced to the field with purported benefits that may include improved patient outcomes, lower costs, increased efficiency, or technical superiority. Some of these innovations are significant and become widely adopted. These innovations may go on to become the standard method utilized and may be used for years, benefiting many patients. Other innovations are no longer used within a few years of introduction, or may have even been found to be harmful to patients. As surgical innovation seems to be constantly occurring, it provides challenges for a practicing surgeon.

How does a physician determine whether to incorporate a new technology into their practice? There are many motivations that drive the entry and adoption of new technology. How does one separate marketing hype from reality and truly determine whether a new technology adds value while avoiding harm to patients?

Robotic surgery is clearly a major innovative technology with evolving applications in the head and neck. While the rest of this textbook addresses clinical and technical aspects of specific applications of robotic surgery within the head and neck, this chapter is intended to help surgeons to critically evaluate the ethics of implementing new surgical technology, to better understand the innovation process, and to consider the implications of incorporating new techniques into practice.

■ Ethical Principles

Ethics is the study of the moral principles regulating a person or group's behavior. Numerous organizations and documents address issues related to medical ethics, and several excellent books specifically on surgical ethics have been published.[1,2,3] Discussion about medical ethics extends back into history. Many important reports from the 20th century were in response to atrocities including medical research performed in Nazi Germany or unethical research carried out in our own country such as the Tuskegee Syphilis Study. Some commonly discussed documents addressing medical ethics include the Nuremberg Code, the Declaration of Helsinki, and the Belmont Report. Concerns raised by these groups and others have resulted in the adoption of federal regulations by the Department of Health and Human Services and the U.S. Food and Drug Administration (FDA) governing human subjects research.

While these reports are important, the core ethical principles, which we are all familiar with from medical school, should serve as internal controls and should be considered in patient interactions and clinical decision making:

- **Respect of patient autonomy** means autonomous choice is the right of all patients and is expressed in the doctrine of informed consent.
- **Nonmaleficence** means a physician should refrain from causing harm to a patient.
- **Beneficence** means physicians must act in the best interest of their patients. Or restated, physicians must put the interests of their patients ahead of their own interests or the interests of third parties.
- **Justice** means all patients should be treated equally, and health care services and resources should be distributed evenly and fairly.
- **Confidentiality** dictates medical information must be kept confidential.

Even though these principles have been discussed extensively in most training environments, complex situations may arise particularly in the face of new technology. As an example, in the instance of patient autonomy, a patient's self-determination is jeopardized when they are not given accurate and complete information about the nature of a procedure or the opportunity to choose or reject a specific treatment during the informed consent process. Or in the case of nonmaleficence, "first do no harm," it has been pointed out that "surgery harms before it heals."[1] Since surgical interventions do harm before they heal, the surgeon has great responsibility when deciding whether to add an innovative approach to their armamentarium.

■ Definition of Innovation

Innovation is the creation of a *better* or *more efficient* product, process, service, or technology. In surgery, this may be represented by anything from a new suture material, to a more efficient method to organize the operating room, to a completely new surgical technique to cure a previously untreatable disease. The drive to innovate comes from the ability to obtain better outcomes or help more patients. For the innovator, this can have very positive rewards for their reputation and from a financial standpoint.

Typically innovation comes from an individual or small group who identify what they ***believe*** to be a new solution to a problem. While many new ideas and methods are developed, many never come to fruition. As has been said many times, ideas are cheap. Execution and implementation are required for innovation to really take place.

Innovation occurs in stages. These stages may not always be clearly defined, and may occur at different speeds. Initially, the *innovator(s)* are only a small group of people or an individual working on a solution. If innovators are successful, a group of *early adopters* may start using the technology or process. Based on their experience, modifications may be made; an improved understanding of the limits and possibilities may occur. During this time, a critical point is reached. This is known as the *chasm*. The chasm frequently determines whether the technology will gain acceptance or fail. Many ideas or innovations do not get past this point. If an innovation gets past the chasm, more people may become convinced of its usefulness. Ultimately, it may reach a tipping point where the majority of people use the technology and it becomes the standard method. Eventually the more skeptical may join in. The actual process of moving through these stages may not be linear, but rather chaotic in nature.[4]

While the number of true innovations in surgery is very small, many surgeons have the opportunity to be early adopters of new technology. Frequently, these occasions are driven by the marketing efforts of industry, for which the profit motive is the main driver. As surgeons, it is important to critically evaluate each innovation prior to implementation to determine if a conflict occurs with the ethical responsibility to patients.

■ Innovation in Surgery

In order to understand surgical innovation, there has to be a baseline from which improvements take place. The concept of standard of care, a legal term, is one possible yet imperfect baseline defined as: "the level at which an ordinary, prudent professional having the same training and experience in good standing in the same or a similar community would practice under the same or similar circumstance." At face value it sounds great, but there is a fair amount of subjectivity in determining what is the standard of care. As it is difficult to define the standard, it is also difficult to clearly define what constitutes innovation in surgery.

Several groups have attempted to differentiate levels of surgical innovation. The Society of University Surgeons published a position statement in 2008, called the "Responsible Development and Application of Surgical Innovations," and they classified surgical innovations as follows[6]:

- A *minor modification of an accepted procedure or technique*, which is something like carving your own implants for thyroplasty versus using a commercially available one; or closing the wound with an adhesive glue rather than sutures. Another example would be the availability of a wide range of tympanostomy tubes, which has resulted from many minor modifications being made by different surgeons. These types of modifications would be considered a surgeon's preference, and according to the Society of University Surgeons' position paper, generally do not need to be disclosed.
- An *innovative procedure* would be something very different than the current standard technique. Examples include the transition from the fenestration procedure to stapedectomy, open to endoscopic sinus surgery, or the use of robotics in head and neck surgery. These types of innovations need to be disclosed to the patient as part of the informed consent process. This is especially important when the procedure is first being introduced and before it becomes the standard of care.
- The final category is *surgical research*. This is an innovation performed as part of systematic investigation to contribute to **generalized knowledge not for patient benefit.** This type of activity requires Institutional Review Board (IRB) approval. Several authors point out that if a retrospective review is being considered before patients have even been treated, research is being conducted and IRB approval should be sought whether publication is intended or not.

Just as it is difficult to determine the standard of care, there may be debate among surgeons about what constitutes a minor modification versus an innovative procedure versus surgical research. In the case of robotic surgery of the head and neck, applications probably cross the spectrum of the Society of University Surgeons' classification scheme.

■ Issues Related to Surgical Innovation

Safety and Efficacy

Safety and efficacy must be the top priority in the case of innovative treatments. Unlike medications, which go through rigorous testing by the FDA, new surgical approaches or techniques using standard instrumentation potentially can be performed without any oversight in almost all cases.

At the FDA, the standard for medical devices is much lower than the process for pharmaceuticals. Ninety percent of medical devices are approved through the 510(k) pathway, in which the standard is to prove the device is "substantially equivalent" to a device already approved by the FDA, and **does not necessarily require clinical evidence.** The other 10% of devices have to go through the much more rigorous premarket approval (PMA) process by which clinical evidence of safety and efficacy has to be provided.[6]

Dr. Angelique Reitsma, in her book *Ethical Guidelines for Innovative Surgery*, points out "while the safety of these procedures will eventually be established through routine surgical mechanisms . . . their true effectiveness may never be known, because randomized control trials were never done."[2] Additionally, there is an ethical dilemma and problems surrounding the use of placebo or sham surgery as a control in randomized trials.

Within the field of surgery there are many examples of safety being proven, but efficacy not being completely evaluated, including some of the applications of robotics within the head and neck. Ultimately, who will pay for and perform the trials acceptable to all parties?

In an ideal world, surgeons should not adopt innovative techniques or devices until they are proven to be efficacious, but many adopt them when they are thought to be safe. Not only is determining when to implement new technology a problem, but determining when to abandon a technology can also be problematic for practicing surgeons. Frequently techniques are abandoned long after they have either been proven to be unsafe or shown to be not efficacious, or worse yet, they are abandoned when an even more attractive yet unproven alternative comes along.

Training Issues, Surgical Education, and Learning Curves

Many surgeons in otolaryngology remember the introduction of endoscopic sinus surgery to our specialty and the bad complications that occurred in the early experience including blindness and death. The introduction of laparoscopic cholecystectomy was fraught with similar issues resulting in preventable deaths related to injuries caused by trocar placement. There have been anecdotal reports about bad outcomes with robotic surgery of the head and neck.

While there are well-established and increasingly regulated methods for training residents after medical school, once residency is completed, mechanisms for learning new surgical techniques and verifying surgical competence are not well established or validated. There have been many concerns raised by both the public and by physicians about learning to do surgery at weekend courses sponsored by industry, as well as about the presence of industry representatives in the operating room teaching surgeons how to perform surgery.[7]

The appropriate steps needed in surgical skill acquisition after residency training will vary based on the specific procedure and may not always be known. It is also important to realize that just because a physician is credentialed to perform a procedure does not mean they are competent to perform the procedure. Credentialing standards vary across medical staffs. Often the expertise to evaluate a request for new credentials does not exist and economic conflicts of interest may prevent serious scrutiny from taking place. Ultimately, it is incumbent on the surgeon to determine whether they have taken all of the appropriate steps to acquire the necessary surgical skills prior to performing their first procedure in order to ensure nonmaleficence.

The concept of learning curves in surgery can be confusing, especially for new procedures. The use of learning curves is derived from manufacturing. Most studies involving learning curves look at a specific surgical process measure, such as operative time, blood loss, or technical adequacy, or a specific patient outcome, like length of stay, morbidity, or patient satisfaction.[8] So if the wrong process is being measured, the number of cases to get through the "learning curve'" is irrelevant. The most important thing from a learning curve standpoint is recognize the patient is the one who is vulnerable and it is essential to minimize potential harm to patients while surgeons are learning a new technique. It is also important for surgeons to disclose to patients their personal experience level, especially for new techniques.

Informed Consent Issues

All surgeons are familiar with the concept of obtaining informed consent. When a procedure is new, obtaining true informed consent may be difficult. Due to lack of data, the actual risks and benefits may not be completely known. Long-term consequences of an intervention may not be readily apparent early in the history of a new technology. Additionally, published results may reflect more experienced surgeons' outcomes or may have biases or other flaws. These experiences may not be easily transferred to other surgeons. Additionally, the willingness to utilize new techniques implies the surgeon believes there is a chance a benefit exists and may influence the presentation of information to the patient.

When there is an alternative technique that is safe, efficacious, and well-accepted, it may be difficult to justify an innovative technique with unknown risks. This has been a criticism of robotic thyroid surgery to date with respect to adoption of this technique, as it would require a very large study to prove its equivalence to standard techniques and how this translates to surgeons of different skill levels.

In the case of a patient with a condition without an acceptable standard treatment, ethicists have an easier time with the informed consent process. In this situation, patients can make an informed decision and understand the treatment being considered may not have a benefit at all.

In the case of some innovative technologies, limited information and potential biases on the part of the surgeon can make it difficult for patients to truly make an informed choice. In these situations, all efforts should be made to help patients understand both what is known and the possibility of unforeseen complications and issues.

Is New Better?

Peter Angelos, an endocrine surgeon at University of Chicago, points out we live in a society where new always means better. He points out the marketing phrase "new and improved" indicates they are always linked together. New always means improved. This is deep seated in our culture. He offers the example that computers and smart phones become obsolete within months of purchase.[9,10] Surgeons commonly encounter this phenomenon in practice. How often does a patient come in requesting a treatment they read about online or saw on television?

Many surgeons are known to have a strong desire to be on the cutting edge and use the latest technology. Dr. Angelos fairly states that making an objective assessment of the value of innovative technologies is difficult for both **surgeons** and **patients**. It is the surgeon's responsibility to carefully separate the potential benefits to the patient from the potential benefits to themselves, upholding the principle of beneficence—putting the patient's interests before their own.

Conflicts of Interest

Conflict of interest is another issue that needs to be discussed. Most patients typically have no awareness about these conflicts. Many hospital administrators and physicians are motivated by financial gain and their reputation. Being seen as innovative may attract referrals and is generally perceived as positive by the public and frequently by colleagues regardless of the long-term consequences for patients. Hospital administrators and surgeons frequently do not have the ability to determine the efficacy of innovative new technology. They also may be motivated to adopt a new technology so their competitors do not appear to be getting ahead of them in the marketplace.

Other physicians' professional and reputational interests in the field also may create conflicts affecting the adoption of new technology. There have been situations where beneficial innovations have been stifled by physicians with powerful reputations within the field committed to their existing methods from a reputational or financial standpoint.

Companies that manufacture medical devices are driven to make a profit to provide a return to their shareholders. While in the long run, they will be more profitable if they provide safe and efficacious solutions, not all companies are driven by long run motives, and some companies seem to be increasingly aggressive in their marketing tactics. Additionally, industry needs physician input to help improve their products. Financial relationships between industry and physicians for this input are important and introduce additional issues. These types of arrangements should be separated from relationships purely for marketing purposes, which should be avoided by physicians.

Additionally, it is often difficult for practicing physicians and the public to evaluate and interpret the validity of industry-supported research, speakers, and publications. One recent and well-publicized example in orthopedic surgery involved safety of recombinant human bone morphogenetic protein-2, concerns surrounding industry-sponsored research, the validity of published data, off-label use, and the outsized compensation investigators received from industry.[11]

Many other conflicts of interest may occur including issues related to the interests of patients, family members of the patient, other specialties, insurance companies, the government, or even society at large. This is a very complicated issue. While transparent disclosure in the realm of patient care is essential for informed consent, conflicts of interest insert another layer of complexity to be considered by the surgeon.

Current Oversight

What safeguards are currently in place to ensure patients' rights are respected? Some have argued surgery is an art and every case is different, surgeons can monitor this on their own, and furthermore the surgical culture has developed rituals ensuring surgeons follow ethical principles.

At a local level, there may be a chief of service who sets standards. Conferences such as Morbidity & Mortality exist at some institutions, where difficult cases can be discussed and lessons can be learned. Hospital peer review committees can provide retrospective review and retrospective enforcement. Hospital ethics committees also may be a resource at some institutions. Credentialing committees exist to determine if physicians meet the appropriate criteria to perform a certain service. All of these mechanisms of oversight have their limitations, vary based on the institution, and may have different levels of influence depending on the setting.

The other local-level mechanism is the use of an Institutional Review Board (IRB). In the surgical literature, there have been concerns raised about the slow nature of an IRB, the lack of surgical input/availability/understanding, and the difficultly in determining at what threshold an IRB should be invoked.[1,2] Also, the IRB relies on the surgeon to submit their plans prospectively and is typically underutilized.

Outside of the local hospital, there are many other agencies and institutions with potential oversight roles.

The federal government has influence through the FDA's regulation mechanisms, the National Institutes of Health through the funding and regulation of research, and the Centers for Medicare & Medicaid Services through their payment coverage determinations. State governments set rules and regulations as well and control licensure-related issues. Enforcement efforts are usually retrospective in nature after a complaint has been filed or egregious violations are discovered. The court system also serves as another retrospective mechanism for oversight.

Medical specialty boards, like the American Board of Otolaryngology, aim to assure the public that the physicians they certify have met professional standards of training and knowledge through the board certification and maintenance of certification process.

Medical societies such as the American Medical Association (AMA), American College of Surgeons (ACS), and specialty societies like the American Academy of Otolaryngology–Head and Neck Surgery (AAO-HNS) and American Head and Neck Society (AHNS) help by creating ethical codes. These organizations and their leaders often have their own set of conflicts, including their relationships with industry and their academic reputations.

When physicians under the jurisdiction of medical specialty boards and medical societies start to misbehave, these groups are not particularly motivated to investigate and sanction physicians due the great expense, potential legal exposure, and complexity of evaluating these problems. They typically act retrospectively and only after government-imposed punishments, such as through a criminal conviction or state medical licensing board action.

Potential Solutions

Clearly the current system of oversight is not ideal and has its limitations. But what is a reasonable alternative? Several groups have made suggestions.

The Society of University Surgeons' position statement proposes a solution that includes the development of a new local committee, called an innovative surgical committee. Surgeons would bring their innovations to this committee for an unbiased review. They also propose that surgeons should submit their efforts to a national innovations registry. They also recommend additional informed consent be used for each patient. They have an algorithm that helps determine when these steps should be taken.[5]

Another group convened at Oxford University, called the Balliol Collaboration, came up with what they called the IDEAL recommendations.[12] This group broke innovation down into several stages: Idea or proof of concept, Development, Exploration or learning, Assessment, and Long-term study or surveillance. They describe each stage and make specific recommendations for what should occur in each stage including who should be involved, what type of ethical approval should be sought, and what the expected outcome should be. They recognize the process will not always follow these stages.

■ Conclusion

Should surgeons be innovating on their patients? Should surgeons be early adopters of new technology seen at the meetings or that companies bring to the office? Is what a surgeon is planning to do in the best interest of the patient? "Should we be encouraging more new technology and innovation to help more patients or should we be protecting patients from the unbridled enthusiasm of surgical innovators?"[13]

Many surgeons feel compelled to try or even adopt the newest techniques, sometimes without adequate efficacy data, rather than feel left behind. This creates a challenging situation and makes objective assessment difficult. Surgeons must consider whether a particular innovation is known to be safe and efficacious, and if not, recognize they may be experimenting on their patients. Since this can be considered surgical research, IRB supervision should be sought. If surgeons decide to become early adopters, they need to look for better oversight, not influenced by industry, so outcomes can be accurately measured and quality of care can be assured.

Surgeons need to constantly remind themselves of their ethical and moral duties to patients and carefully separate the potential benefits to the patient from the potential benefits to themselves. Regardless of the external influences and lack of formal oversight mechanisms, ultimately, the responsibility is the surgeon's.

References

1. McCullough LB, Jones JW, Brody BA. Surgical Ethics. Oxford: Oxford University Press; 1998
2. Reitsma AM, Moreno JD. Ethical Guidelines for Innovative Surgery. Hagerstown, MD: University Publishing Group; 2006
3. Jones JW, McCullough LB, Richman BW. The Ethics of Surgical Practice. Oxford: Oxford University Press; 2008
4. Moore GA. Crossing the Chasm: Marketing and Selling High-Tech Products to Mainstream Customers. New York: Harper Collins Publishers; 1999
5. Biffl WL, Spain DA, Reitsma AM, et al. Responsible development and application of surgical innovations: a position statement of the Society of University Surgeons. J Am Coll Surg 2008;206(6):1204–1209
6. Orlandi RR, Marple BF. Developing, regulating, and ethically evaluating new technologies in otolaryngology—head and neck surgery. Otolaryngol Clin North Am 2009;42:739–745
7. Perrier ND, Randolph GW, Inabnet WB, Marple BF, van Heerden J, Kuppersmith RB. Robotic thyroidectomy: a framework for new technology assessment and safe implementation. Thyroid 2010;20(12):1327–1332
8. Hopper AN, Jamison MH, Lewis WG. Learning curves in surgical practice. Postgrad Med J 2007;83(986):777–779
9. Angelos P. The ethical challenges of surgical innovation for patient care. Lancet 2010;376(9746):1046–1047
10. Angelos P. When the evidence isn't there—seeking informed consent for new procedures. Virtual Mentor 2011;13(1):6–9
11. Stanton T. Lessons learned: What the BMP trials controversy has taught us. Available at: http://www.aaos.org/news/aaosnow/mar12/research2.asp. Accessed May 7, 2015
12. McCulloch P, Altman DG, Campbell B, et al. No surgical innovation without evaluation: the IDEAL recommendations. Lancet 2009;374:1105–1112
13. Angelos P. Ethical issues in surgical innovation. Available at: http://associationdatabase.com/aws/ACS/pt/sd/news_article/31920/_PARENT/DC_layout_details/false. Accessed May 7, 2015

4 Room Setup and Instrumentation

Julia A. Crawford, Hilliary N. White, and J. Scott Magnuson

■ Introduction

Advances in robotic technology have allowed increasingly complex medical procedures to be performed via minimally invasive approaches. The most commonly used robotic systems in otolaryngology use the master–slave arrangement with the surgical robotic cart containing multiple manipulation arms that are operated remotely from a console. This chapter reviews currently available robotic surgical technology and explains the operative room setup for transoral robotic surgery and transaxillary robotic thyroid surgery.

■ Present Robotic Systems

There are presently two systems which are approved by the U.S. Food and Drug Administration (FDA) for use in head and neck surgery. These include the daVinci series of robots from Intuitive Surgical, Inc. and the Flex Robotic System from Medrobotics Corp. which received FDA approval in July 2015.

The da Vinci Surgical Robot

The da Vinci robot is manufactured by Intuitive Surgical, Inc. There are several different models of this robot available but all are composed of three individual components: a vision system, bedside cart, and surgeon console. The current models that have FDA approval for use in otolaryngology are the Standard, S, and Si models. The S and Si systems have mostly replaced the Standard system, which was the first model available.

The S model was introduced in 2006 and is superior to the previous Standard model in that it provides enhanced image resolution, redesigned patient-side manipulators, and a shortened set up time. The Si model entered the market in 2009 and further improved visual resolution, redefined the instrument controllers, increased the ergonomics, and was overall more user-friendly. One of the main advantages of the Si system is the availability of a dual console system that allows two surgeons to simultaneously collaborate on one case. The dual console also enhances the training of new robotic surgeons, as the proctor can provide real-time feedback and assistance and they can work in tandem as a team. The Si model is compatible with Intuitive Surgical's Firefly fluorescence imaging system. This technology utilizes integrated fluorescent imaging to provide the surgeon with additional visual information by enabling enhanced visualization of anatomical landmarks and tissue perfusion through near-infrared technology.[1]

The newest available model is the Xi system; however, this does not yet have FDA approval for use in otolaryngology–head and neck surgery. The advantage of the Xi system over the other available models is that it has an overhead instrument architecture with smaller, thinner arms. The joints in these arms are designed to facilitate anatomical access from virtually any position around the patient. This is particularly beneficial in head and neck surgery, as it allows four-arm rather than three-arm access to the surgical site, thereby improving the ability of the surgeon to manipulate and retract tissue during surgery through a single access site. The endoscope itself is also more compact in design with improved visualization and clarity. It can be attached to any robotic arm, which allows for numerous different angles of visualization. One of the potential drawbacks of this newer model for otolaryngology is that there are currently only 8-mm arms available, whereas the other models offer 5-mm instrument arms.

As mentioned above, all da Vinci robotic systems, regardless of model, include the same key basic components:

- The surgeon console (**Fig. 4.1**): Once the robot has been appropriately docked, the remainder of the surgery will be performed with the surgeon seated at the surgeon console. The surgeon console is typically situated at a remote location in the room, several feet away from the patient on the operating table. The viewer provides the surgeon a magnified, three-dimensional (3D) image of the surgical field. While seated at the console, the surgeon manipulates the master controls that are located below the 3D display. The console may be customized to each surgeon's individual settings to enable them to work in the most ergonomically comfortable position possible. The instrument controls enable the surgeon to move within a one cubic foot area of workspace.
- Patient-side cart (**Fig. 4.2**): This component of the system contains the robotic arms and is positioned beside the surgical bed. It consists of two or three instrument arms and one endoscopic camera arm (although in the Xi model these are interchangeable).
- Vision system (**Fig. 4.3**): The vision system allows for the surgical assistant and surgical scrub to have a two-dimensional representation of the surgical field as viewed by the surgeon. In the S model this is via a slave monitor attached to the robot, while in the Si model there is a separate control tower/vision cart.

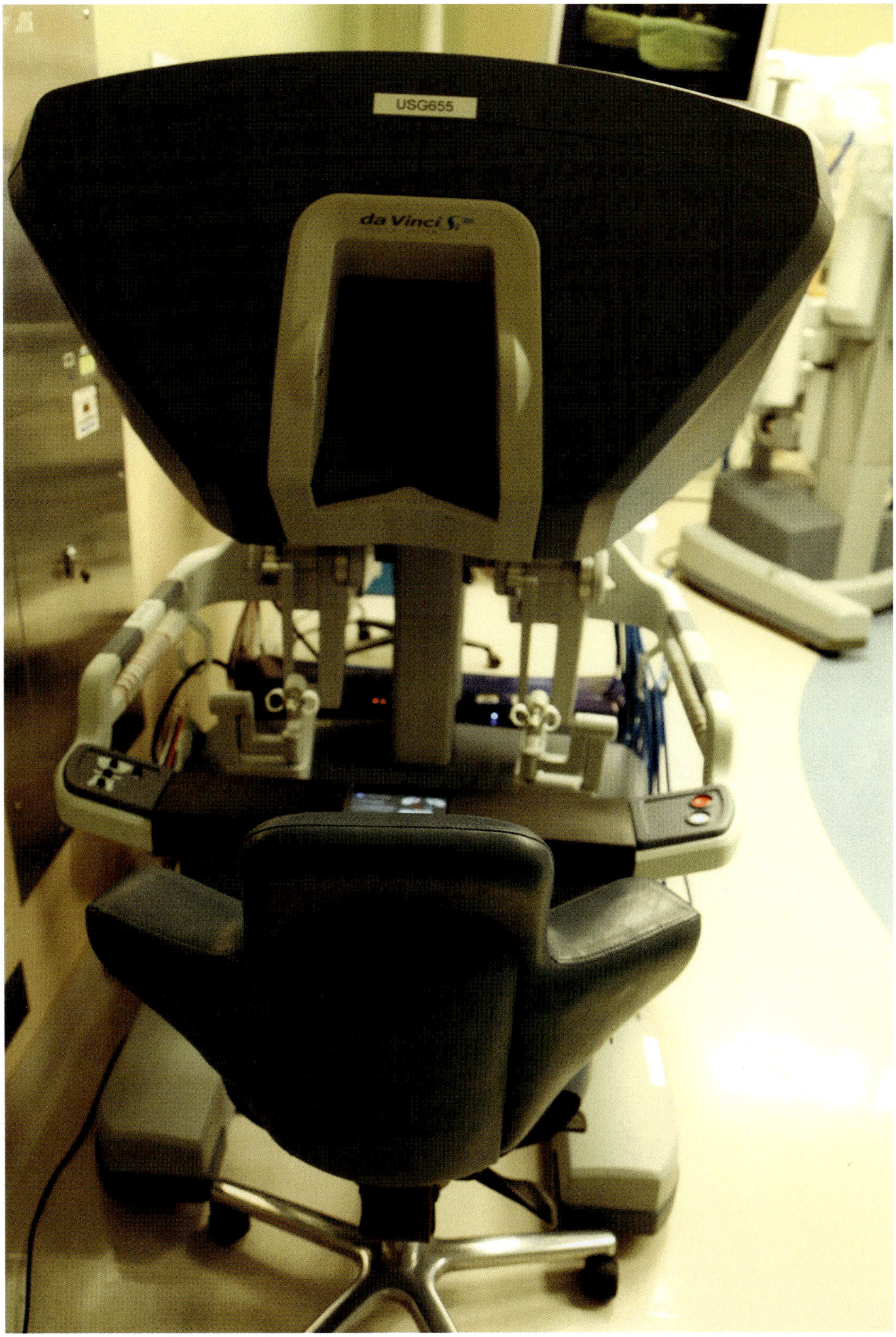

Fig. 4.1 The da Vinci Si surgeon console.

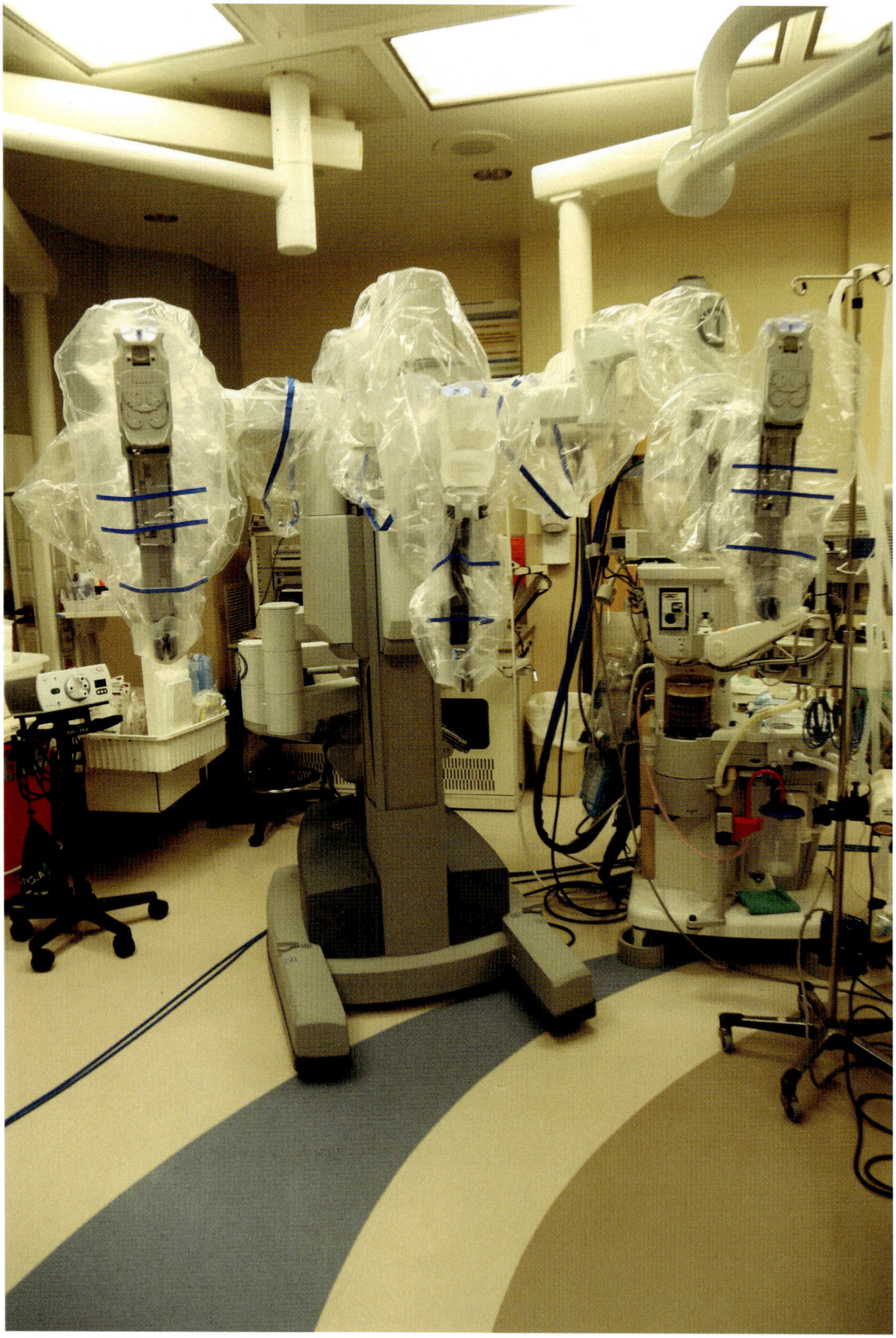

Fig. 4.2 The da Vinci Si patient-side cart.

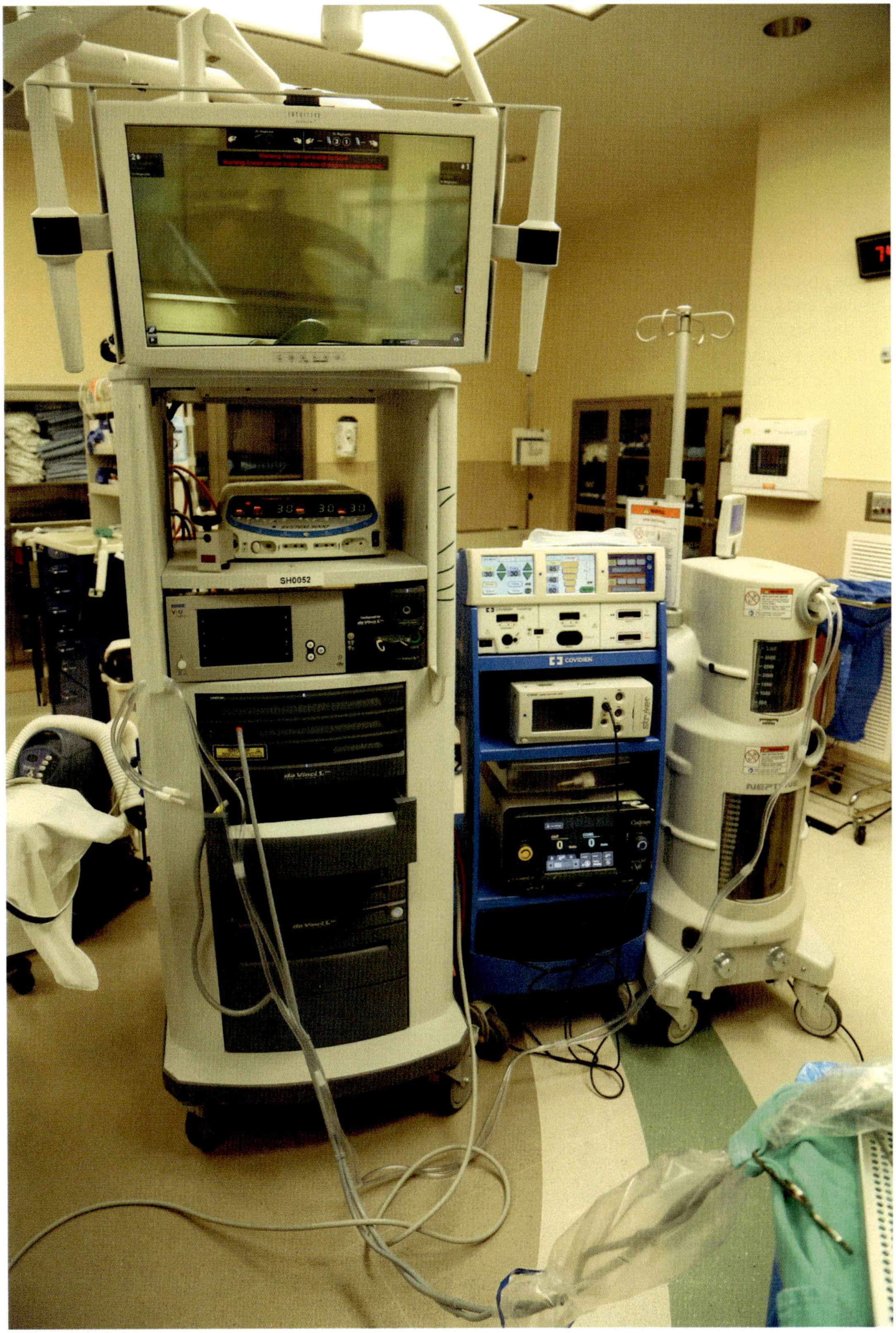

Fig. 4.3 The da Vinci Si vision system.

Flex System

Another system recently introduced is the Flex Robotic System manufactured by Medrobotics Corp (**Fig. 4.4**). This device received the CE mark in March 2014 and FDA clearance in July 2015.

The Flex System robot is a camera device with 102 degrees of freedom and a snakelike advancement mechanism capable of steering a nonlinear, self-supported path. The flexible robot platform provides a chip-on-tip endoscope through nonlinear pathways and also delivers flexible tools that can perform a variety of surgical procedures. The robot is controlled by the surgeon at the Flex console until it reaches the desired site. Once docked in this position, the robot will maintain its nonlinear shape and the surgeon can insert flexible endoscopic instruments into the external accessory channels to perform the planned procedure. The instruments utilized are typically 3.5 mm in diameter and allow for tissue handling and energy delivery. The reported advantage over the da Vinci system is the degree of flexibility it provides for all instruments and camera arms, which will markedly improve access to all surgical sites in head and neck surgery, most notably the larynx and hypopharynx. The disadvantages of the system are two-dimensional visualization and fewer instruments in the operative field—although, with technological advancement these are likely to be addressed. The supporting evidence for use of this device is currently only in cadaveric models, but it suggests that the Flex System is a viable surgical tool for oropharyngeal, hypopharyngeal, and laryngeal surgeries.[2]

■ Room Setup and Instrumentation for Transoral Robotic Surgery

The feasibility of transoral robotic surgery (TORS) in a cadaver model was first demonstrated by Hockstein et al in 2005 at the University of Pennsylvania.[3] This study helped overcome the technical difficulties that had been demonstrated

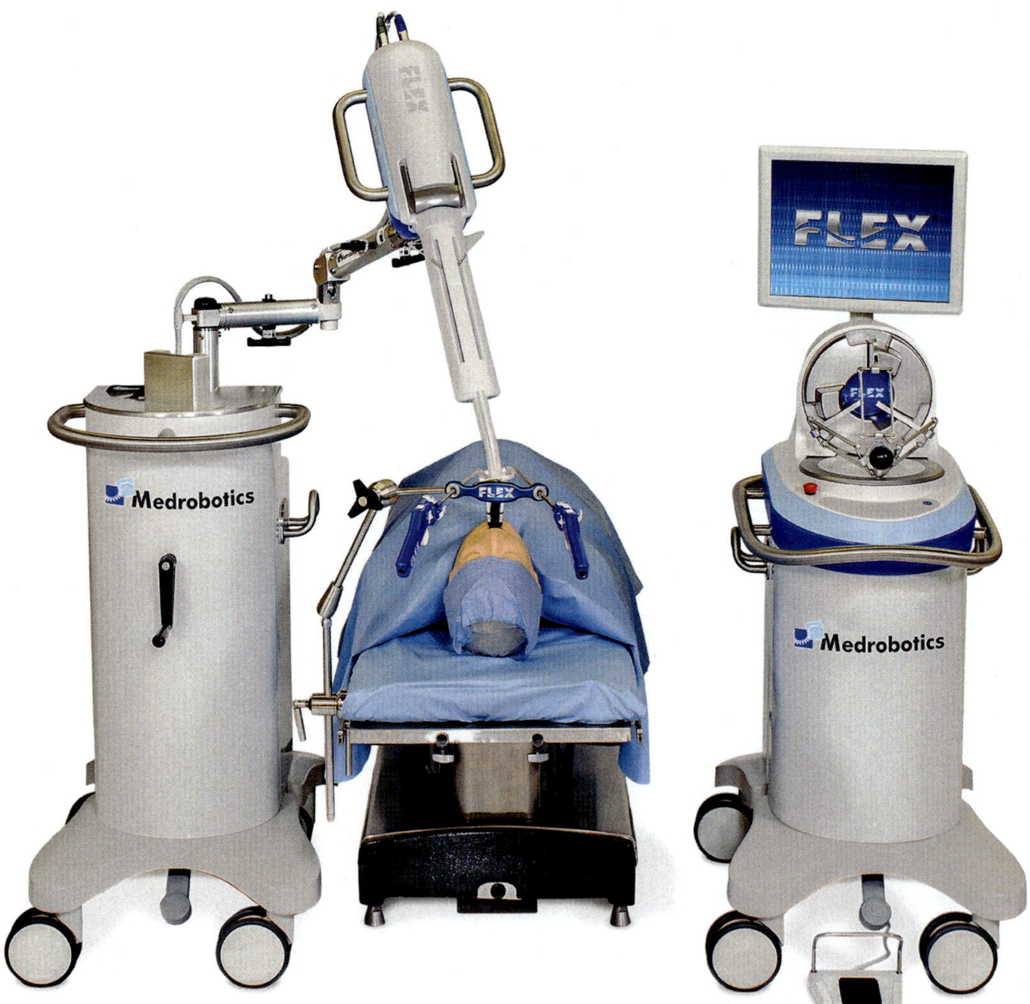

Fig. 4.4 The Flex System. (Courtesy of Medrobotics Corp., Raynham, Massachusetts.)

by McLeod et al in their initial live animal study.[4] The introduction of an ideal robot-to-patient angle of 30 to 45 degrees allowed greater freedom of movement with minimal restriction of movement to the robotic arms.[5] Furthermore, the use of a mouth retractor rather than a traditional laryngoscope allowed greater simultaneous access to the oral cavity with the three robotic arms. Since this initial study, the application of the robot to oropharyngeal surgery has rapidly expanded, and the positioning and surgical setup have been further refined.[6,7,8,9,10,11,12,13,14]

The Robotic Team

The Primary Surgeon

The primary surgeon will be seated at the robotic console. This is typically in close proximity to the operating room table. The console affords a 3D view of the surgical field and allows manipulation of the utilized robotic arms and the camera.

The Surgical Assistant

The role of the surgical assistant is to assist the primary surgeon with retracting tissues, creating a smoke-free environment to work, and suctioning blood to aid visualization. The assistant is typically seated at the patient's head. As needed, the assistant will also be able to assist with adjusting the robotic arms and camera to prevent collisions in addition to assisting with hemostasis with suction diathermy or through the application of vessel clips. There is an integrated microphone-loudspeaker system built in the robotic system that facilitates communication between the primary surgeon and surgical assistant.

The Surgical Technician

The surgical technician is located at the patient's bedside with ready access to all instrumentation and equipment. Their primary role is to pass instruments to the surgical assistant and assist with surgical field setup, but they can also perform similar duties of the surgical assistant if needed. It is imperative that they are familiar with the TORS setup to aid in decreasing both setup and operative time.

Operating Room Configuration

The operating room (OR) is set up to allow for efficient use of space while maximizing access to the patient for the anesthetic and surgical team (**Fig. 4.5**). The operating table is the epicenter of the room with the surgical assistant located at the head and the anesthetic team at the foot. Most importantly, the operating

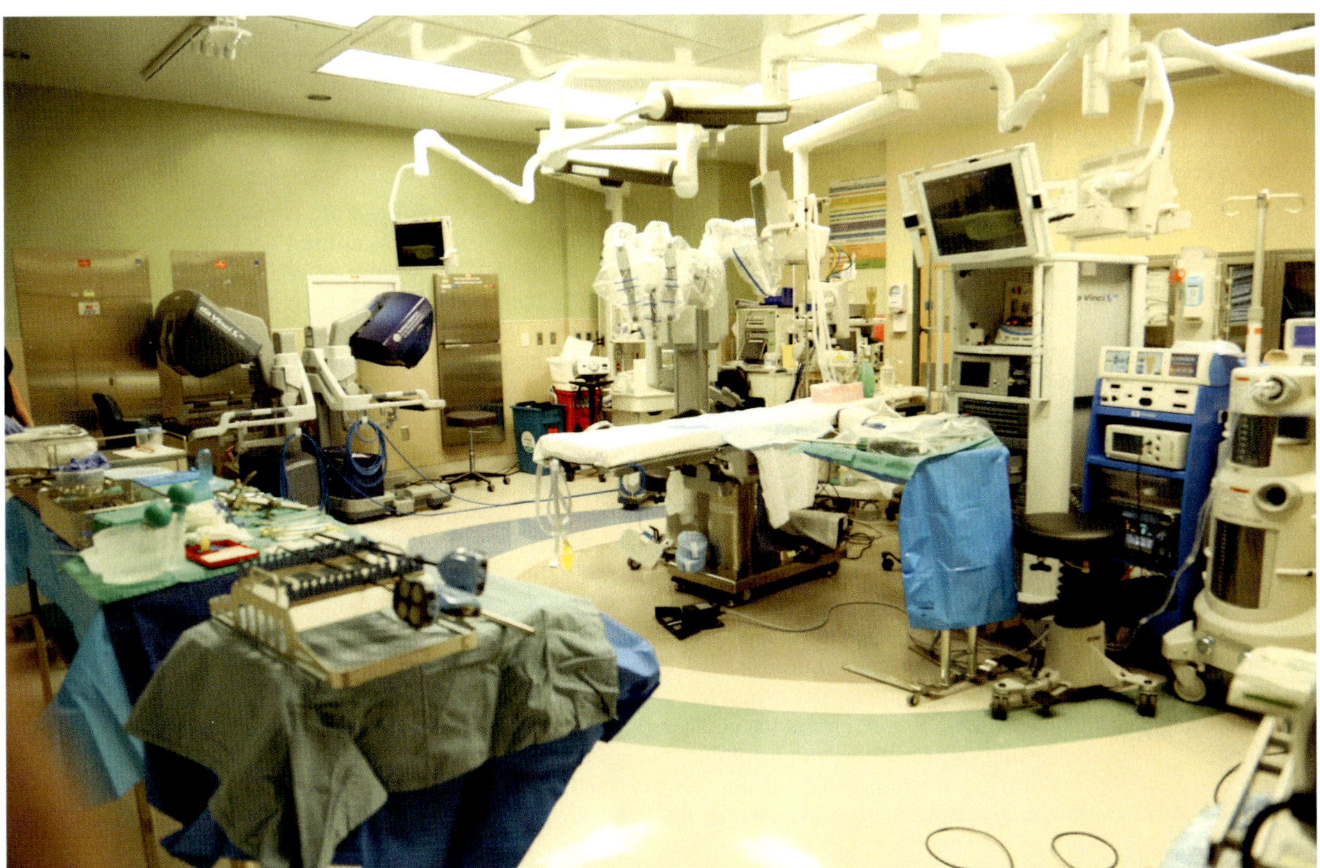

Fig. 4.5 Operating room configuration.

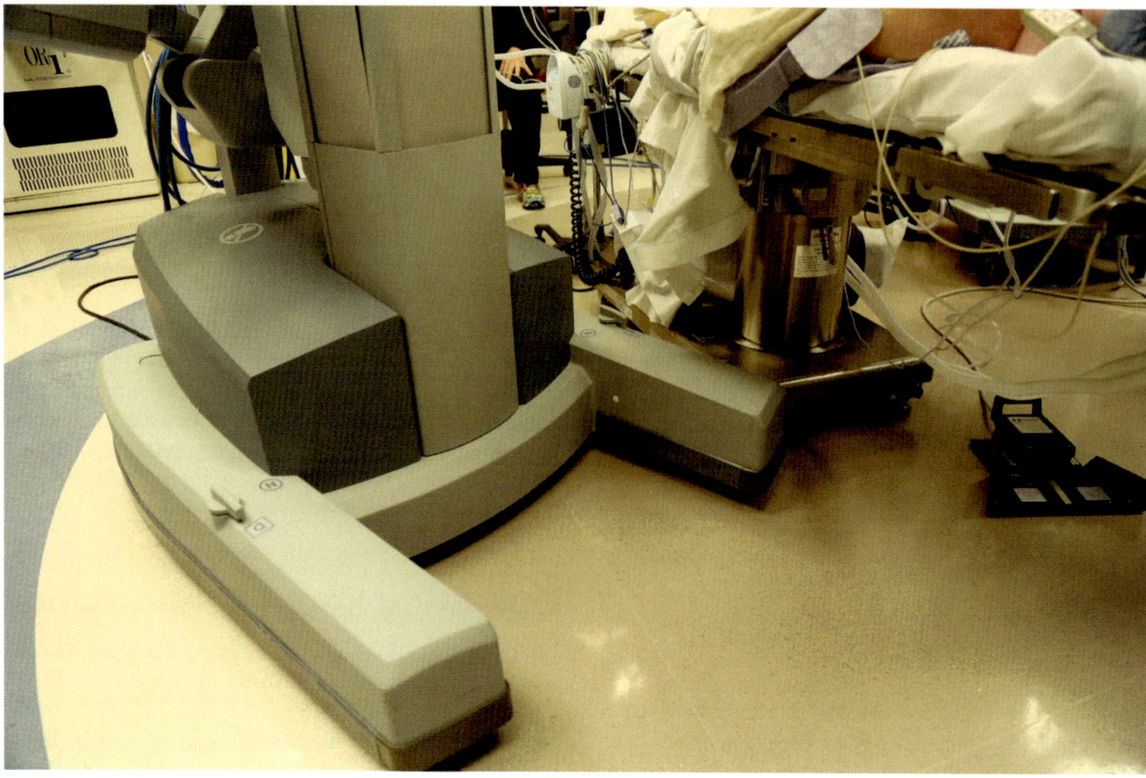

Fig. 4.6 Angle of the patient-side cart in relation to the operating table.

table must be located such that the patient-side cart can be positioned at an angle of approximately 30 degrees, which maximizes the range of deployment of the robotic arms in the Standard, S, and Si models (**Fig. 4.6**).

The surgeon console is located close to the surgical assistant to provide ease of communication. The scrub nurse stands to one side of the operating table and can provide further assistance with suction or retraction as required. The vision system is located so that both the surgical assistant and scrub nurse can ergonomically view the system. The robotic instrumentation and general instruments are located on a rectangular draped operating room table (**Fig. 4.7**).

Instrumentation

General Instrumentation

The general instrumentation that is required to perform transoral robotic surgery is minimal. A head light is needed for the initial mouth gag placement. A needle driver, forceps, and scissors are used to place a nonabsorbable tongue suture at the beginning of the procedure to assist with tongue retraction and mouth gag placement. Multiple suction devices including a Yankauer sucker and a suction cautery device are helpful to provide evacuation of smoke, tissue retraction, and hemostasis as required. A Heard retractor is useful for retraction of tissues, and a vessel clip applier (**Fig. 4.8**) may be required for hemostasis. Depending on hospital and surgeon preference, various hemostatic aids such as Tisseel or FloSeal (Baxter Healthcare Corp.) should be available in the operating room to aid with hemostasis at the end of the case.

Mouth Gags

An increasing number of gags are available for use during TORS. The two most commonly utilized gags are the Davis-Meyer gag and the Feyh-Kastenbauer-Weinstein-O'Malley retractor (**Fig. 4.9**). Both of these systems include multiple tongue blades of different lengths and shapes that allow access to perform a range of surgeries. Their use is determined by surgeon preference and surgical site.

The newer commercially available systems include the LARS (FENTEXmedical) (**Fig. 4.10**) and the FLEX retractor (Medrobotics Corp.) (**Fig. 4.11**). A retractor from Marina Medical Inc. of Sunrise, Florida, will also soon be commercially available (**Fig. 4.12**). After placement of the mouth gag, it is secured directly to the side of the operating bed (preferred) or suspended on a stand placed across the chest of the patient (**Fig. 4.13**).

Robotic Instrumentation

The required da Vinci robotic instrumentation will include the high-definition camera and EndoWrist instruments.

The binocular camera provides magnification of up to 10×, which results in a 3D high-definition image. For TORS, a 12-mm scope is utilized. An 8-mm scope is available but provides no

(text continued on page 28)

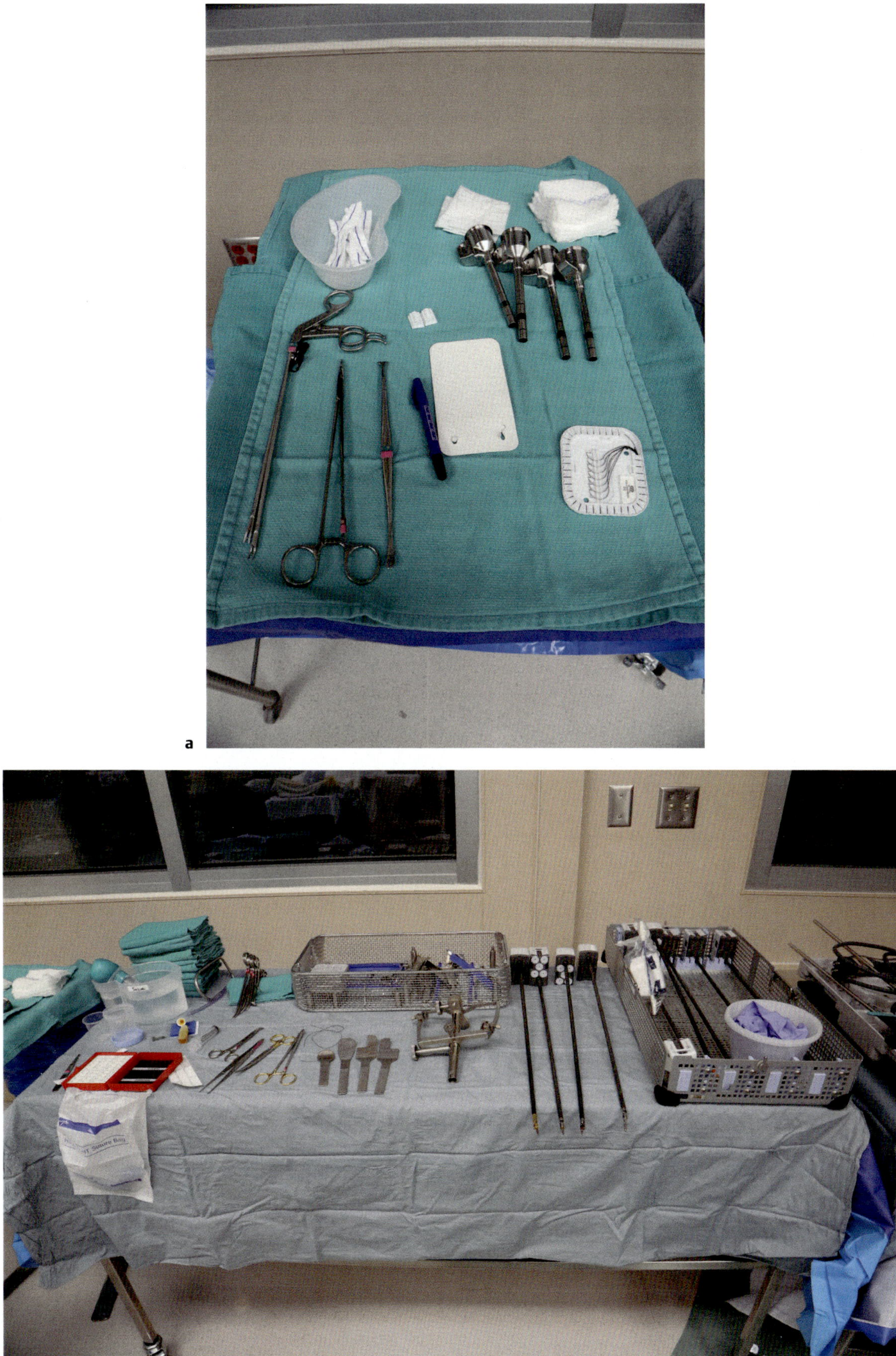

a

b

Fig. 4.7 (a,b) Layout of the instrumentation tables.

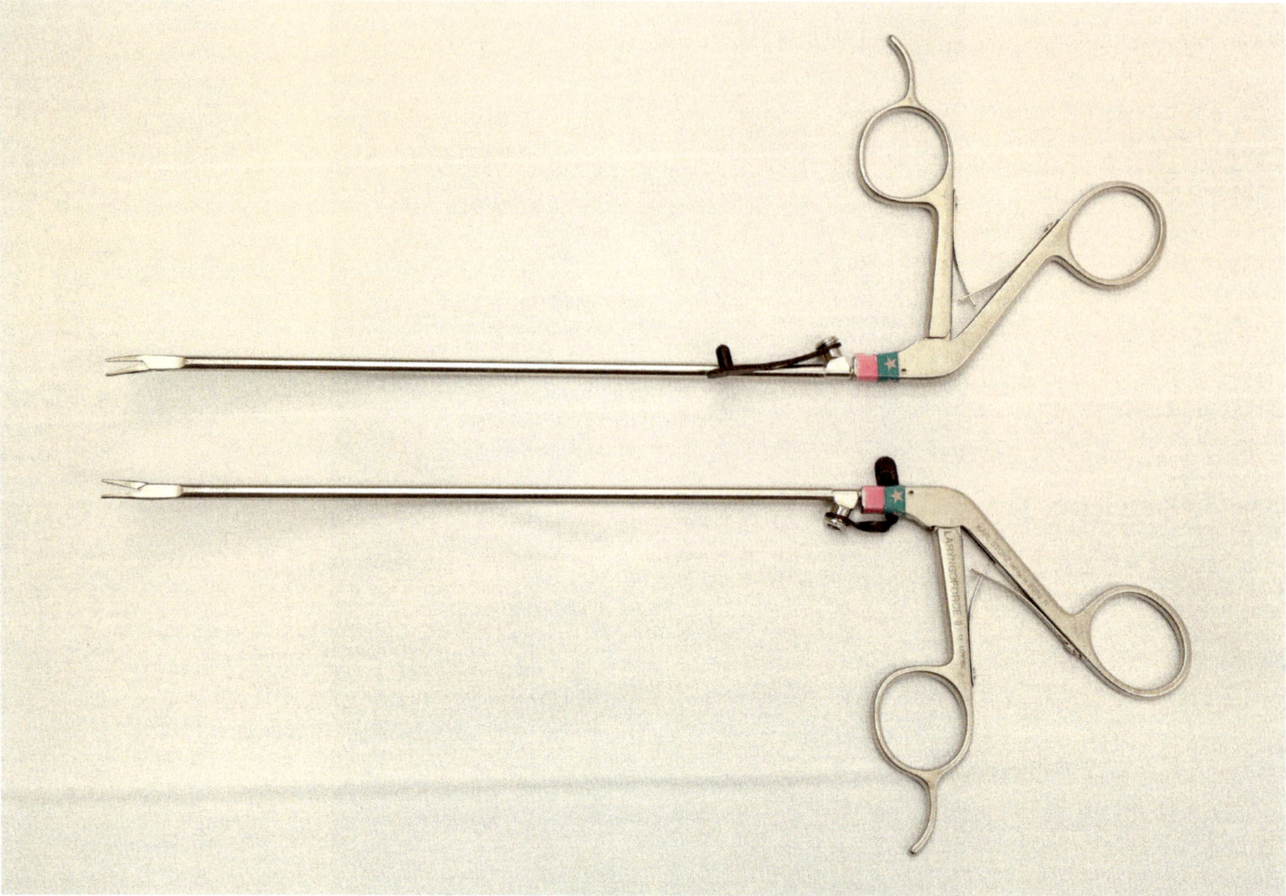

Fig. 4.8 Endoscopic clip applier.

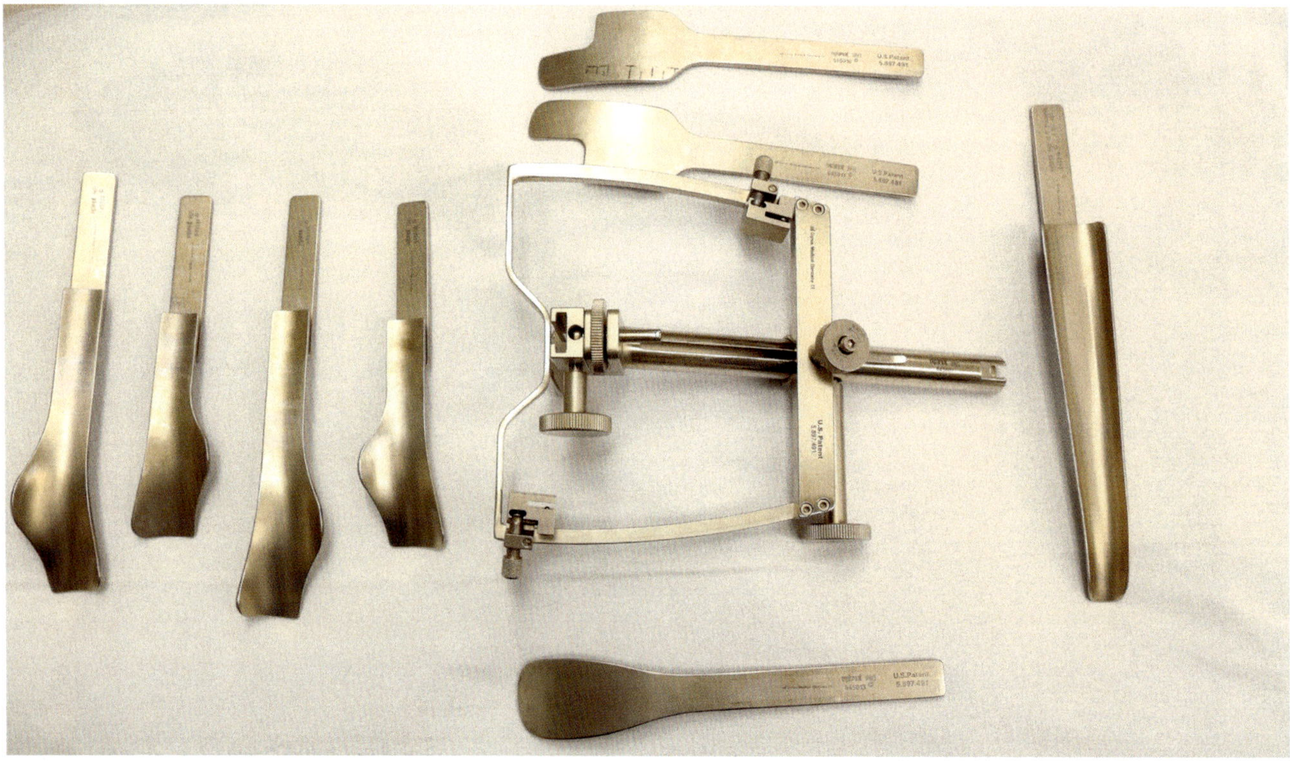

Fig. 4.9 FK-WO mouth retractor.

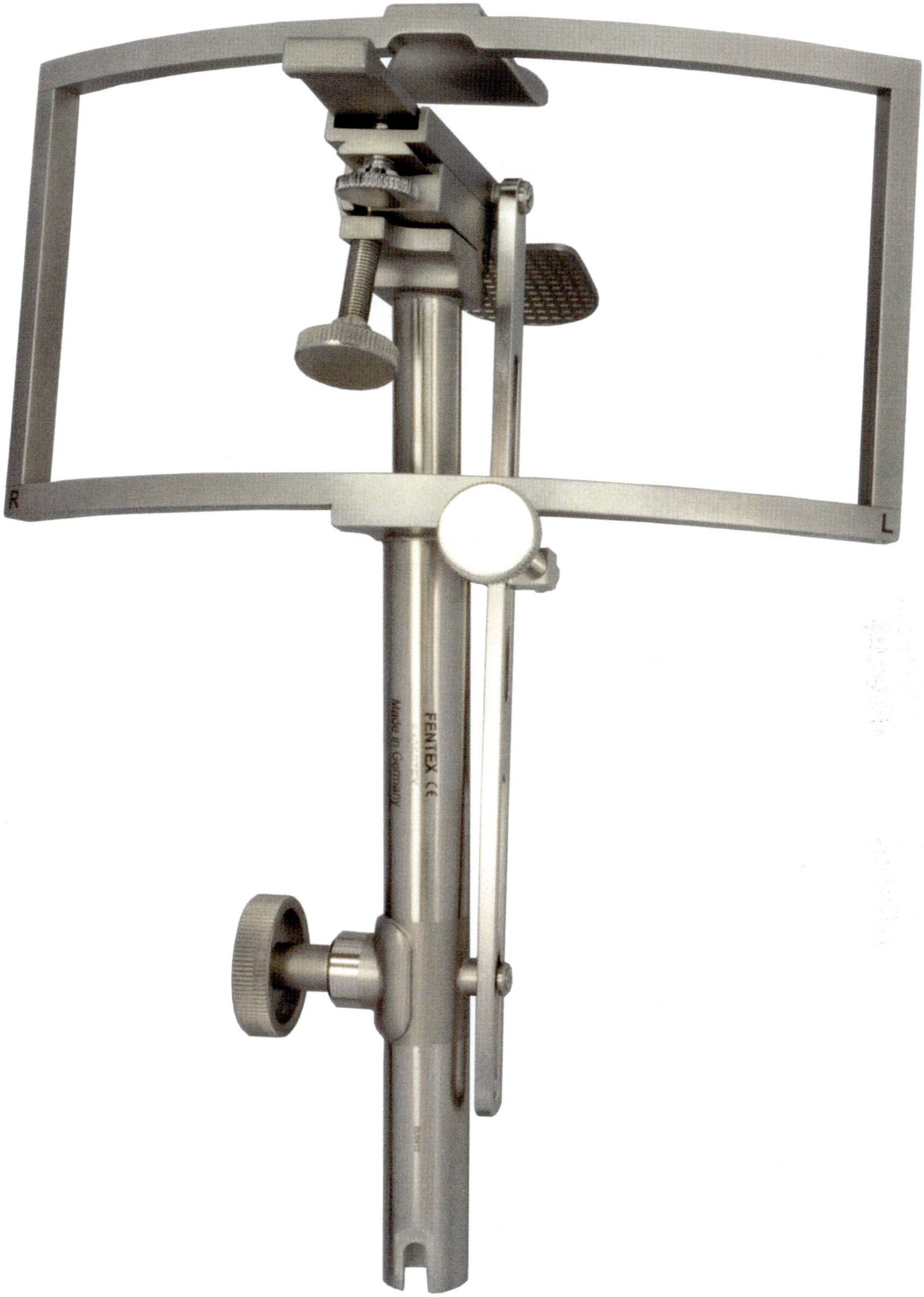

Fig. 4.10 LARS mouth retractor. (Courtesy of Grace Medical Inc., Memphis, Tennessee.)

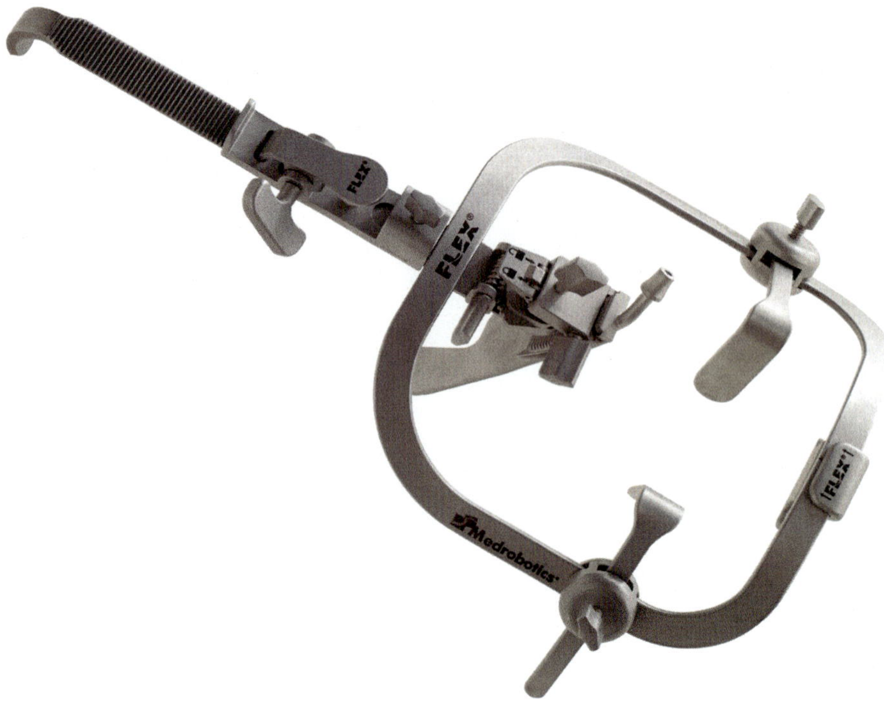

Fig. 4.11 FLEX retractor. (Courtesy of Medrobotics Corp., Raynham, Massachusetts.)

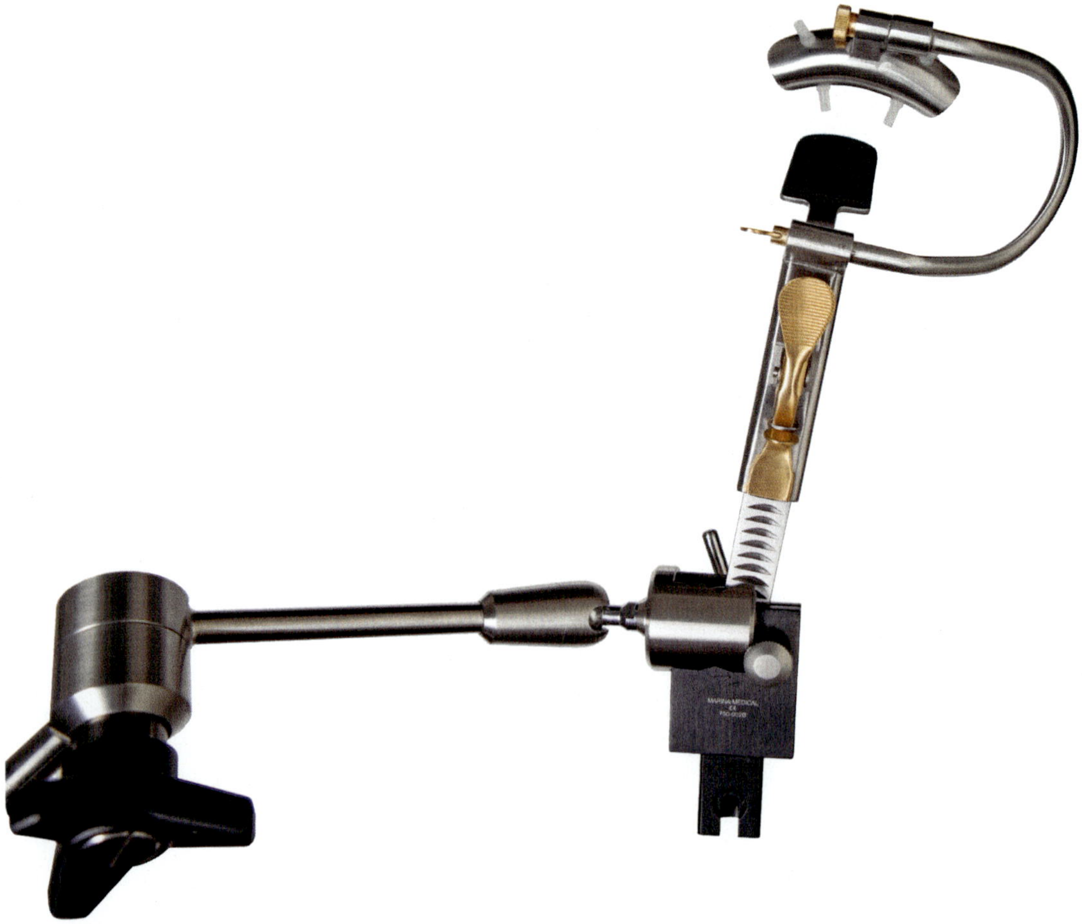

Fig. 4.12 Marina Medical mouth retractor. (Courtesy of Marina Medical Inc., Sunrise, Florida.)

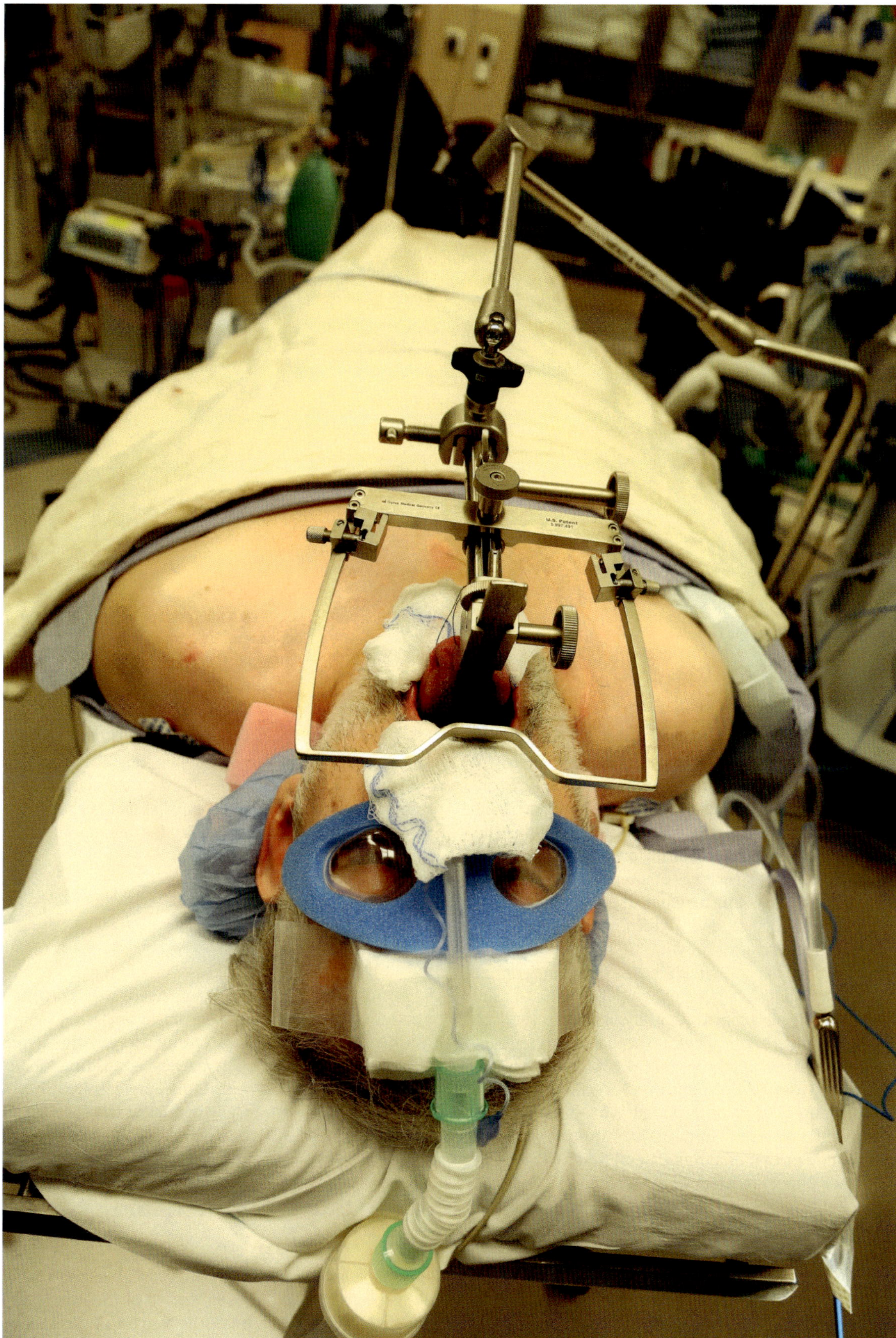

Fig. 4.13 Retractor in suspension using bedside support.

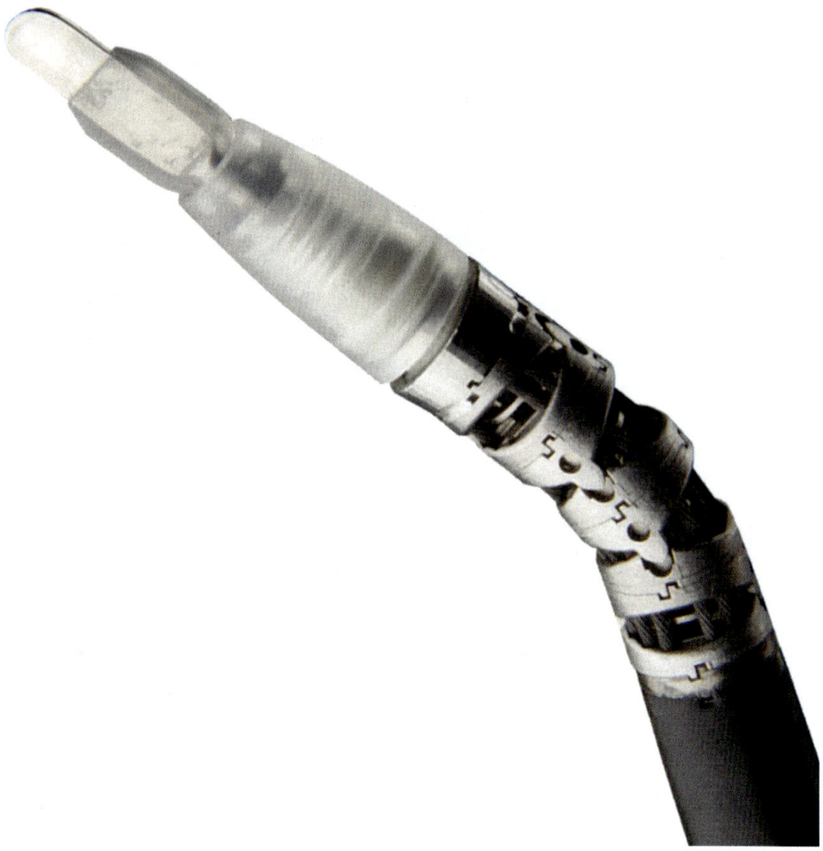

Fig. 4.14 The 5-mm monopolar cautery EndoWrist instrument. (Courtesy of Intuitive Surgical, Inc., Sunnyvale, California.)

added benefit to the procedure. Both 0- and 30-degree scopes must be available for use. For radical tonsillectomy, a 0-degree scope is employed, while for base of tongue, supraglottic, or hypopharyngeal work, a 30-degree scope is required. The 30-degree scope is used in an up slanting orientation, which is dictated by the anatomical structures of interest.

For TORS, typically two 5-mm articulated EndoWrist instrument arms, an energy device, and a grasping instrument are utilized. These instrument arms provide 180 degrees of articulation and 540 degrees of rotation while also providing tremor filtration and amplitude scaling, allowing bimanual tissue manipulation in multiple planes. Typically, a grasper will be placed in one arm and an energy device placed in the other arm.

The spatula tip monopolar cautery (**Fig. 4.14**) is the most frequently used energy device. Depending on surgeon preference, the monopolar cautery may be replaced with a compatible flexible laser fiber.[3,4] Intuitive Surgical, Inc. no longer manufactures an instrument that accommodates a flexible laser, but after-market laser fibers are produced by companies with the intended use for TORS. These include the OmniGuide carbon dioxide laser fiber system (OmniGuide Inc.),[15] thulium:YAG laser,[16] and RevoLix 2 micron Holmium surgical laser (Lisa Laser USA). Harmonic energy and bipolar cautery are not available in 5-mm instruments. Additionally, harmonic energy is not available as a wristed instrument.

A few grasping devices are available for use. Each differs in shape and the aggressiveness of traction (**Fig. 4.15**). While device preference is surgeon dependent, the most commonly used grasping device is the 5-mm Maryland forceps. The resemblance of the Maryland forceps to a hemostat allows for excellent traction as well as ability for dissection.

Operative Setup

Patient Position

The position of the operating table needs to be considered prior to patient placement. The base of the operating table must be positioned such that it does not interfere with the placement of the patient-side cart. The patient is positioned supine and intubated with a nasotracheal tube, preferably through the nares opposite to the tumor. The operating table is then rotated so that the patient's head is 180 degrees from the anesthesia cart.[17]

Mouth Gag Placement and Robot Docking

Under direct visualization, a nonabsorbable stitch (typically 2.0 silk) is placed in the anterior portion of the tongue to assist in retraction and positioning of the tongue. Gauze is then placed over the upper and lower teeth to minimize soft tissue injury and dental trauma during placement of the mouth gag. The

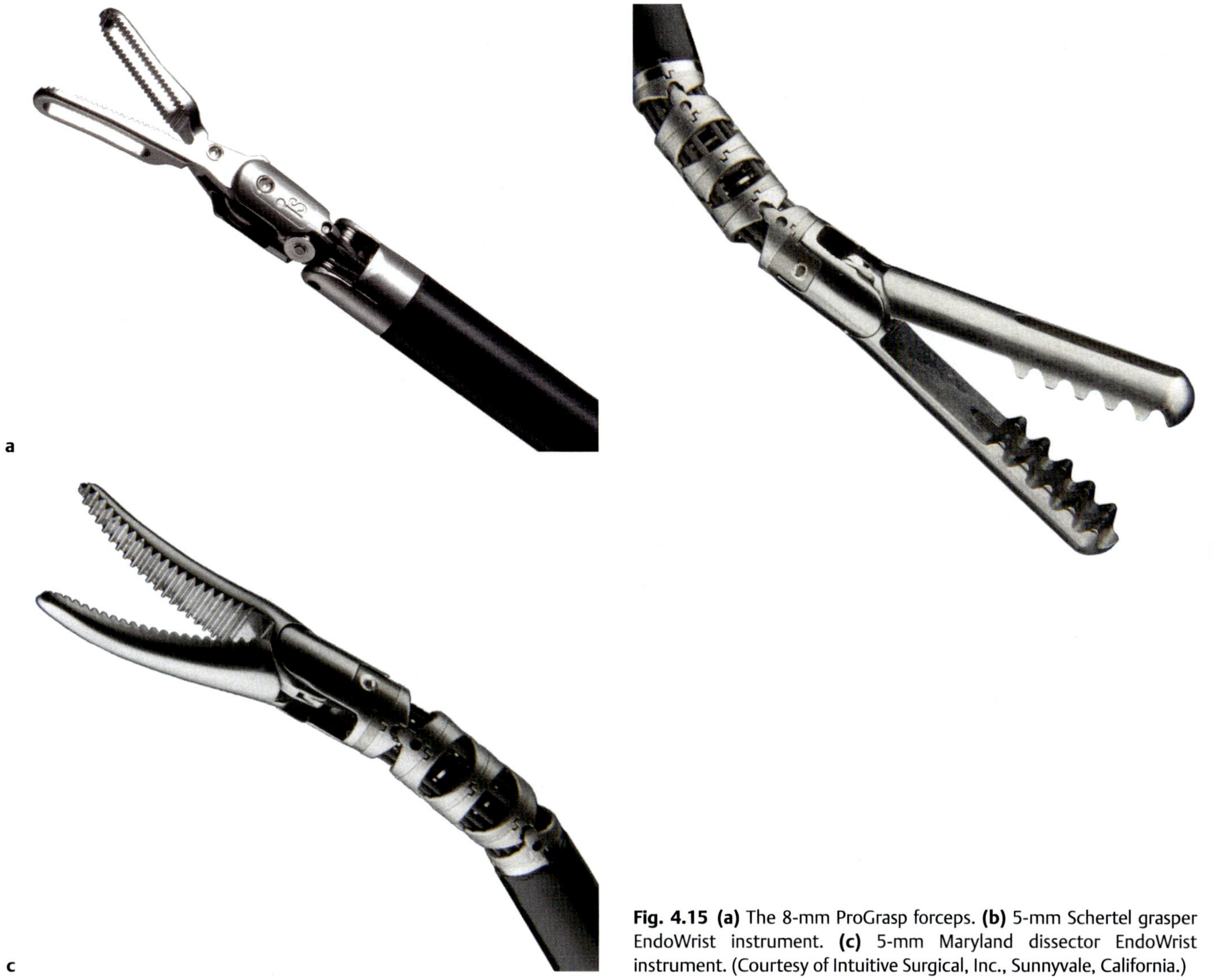

Fig. 4.15 (a) The 8-mm ProGrasp forceps. (b) 5-mm Schertel grasper EndoWrist instrument. (c) 5-mm Maryland dissector EndoWrist instrument. (Courtesy of Intuitive Surgical, Inc., Sunnyvale, California.)

mouth gag is then inserted and positioned to provide adequate exposure of the primary tumor using a surgical head light for visualization. At this point the surgical table is lowered to the lowest position possible. The robotic patient side cart is then wheeled to the bedside toward the patient's head such that the base of the robot is approximately at a 15- to 30-degree angle with the base of the surgical table. The robotic base may be on the patient's left or right side depending on the room setup. This slight angling assists with placement of the robotic instruments intraorally and helps to minimize collisions during the case.

The three robotic arms are aimed toward the patient's mouth and positioned in a triangular format. The camera is placed in the center arm and the grasping instrument and cutting instrument are placed in the side arms. The grasping instrument should be placed on the contralateral side to the tumor. The instruments are inserted into the patient's mouth so that the apex of the instruments meets at the area surrounding the tumor (**Fig. 4.16**). Care should be taken to ensure that the instruments will not clash, their movement will not be impeded by intraoral structures, and they safely move within the patient's oral cavity.

The operation is then performed by the surgeon from the surgeon console. At the completion of the operation, the robotic patient-side cart is removed from the field. At this time, a nasogastric feeding tube may be placed and the mouth gag is removed from the patient. Finally, the patient is extubated per anesthesia protocol.

Conclusion

Robotic surgery for upper aerodigestive pathology and for thyroid removal is rapidly evolving. It is expected that as further experience is gained in the field and more devices and equipment become available the setup and room positioning will be modified to accommodate.

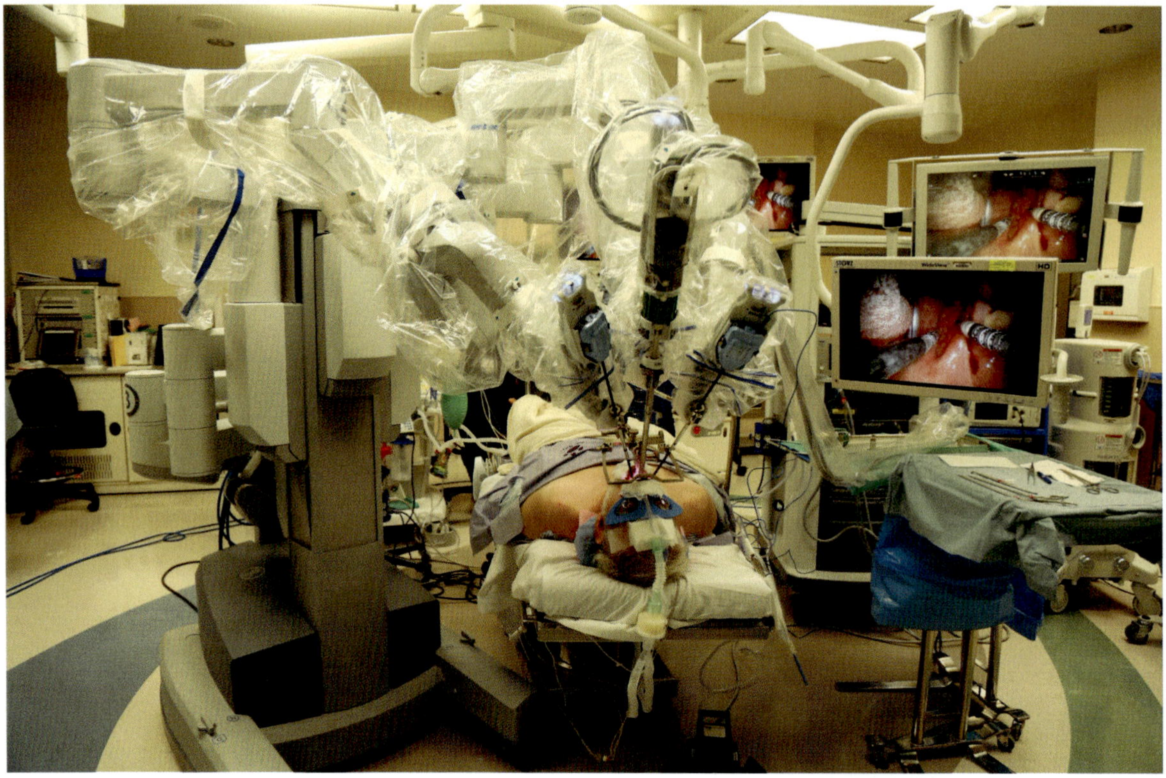

Fig. 4.16 The da Vinci Si robot docked.

References

1. Beasley RA. Medical robots: current systems and research directions. J Robotic Surg 2012;2013:1–14
2. Johnson PJ, Rivera Serrano CM, Castro M, et al. Demonstration of transoral surgery in cadaveric specimens with the medrobotics flex system. Laryngoscope 2013;123:1168–1172
3. Hockstein NG, Nolan M, O'Malley BW. Robotic microlaryngeal surgery: a technical feasibility study using the da Vinci surgical robot and an airway mannequin. Laryngoscope 2005;115:780–785
4. McLeod IK, Mair EA, Melder PC. Potential applications of the Da Vinci minimally invasive surgical robotic system in otolaryngology. Ear Nose Throat J 2005;84:483–487
5. Weinstein G, Abuzeid W, Khan K, et al. Patient positioning and setup utilizing the da Vinci Robotic System. In: Weinstein GS, O'Malley BW, eds. Transoral Robotic Surgery (TORS). San Diego: Plural Publishing Inc; 2012:25
6. Genden E. The role for surgical management of HPV-related oropharyngeal carcinoma. Head Neck Pathol 2012;6:S98–S103
7. Dowthwaite SA, Franklin JH, Plama DA, et al. The role of transoral robotic surgery in the management of oropharyngeal carcinoma: a review of the literature. ISRN Oncol 2012;2012:945162
8. Moore EJ, Hinni ML. Critical review: transoral laser microsurgery and robotic-assisted surgery for oropharynx cancer including human papillomavirus-related cancer. Int J Radiation Oncol Biol Phys 2013;85(5):1163–1167
9. Boudreaux BA, Rosenthal EL, Magnuson JS, et al. Robot-assisted surgery for upper aerodigestive tract neoplasms. Arch Otolaryngol Head Neck Surg 2009;135(4):397–401
10. Weinstein FS, O'Malley BW, Snyder W, et al. Transoral robotic surgery: radical tonsillectomy. Arch Otolaryngol Head Neck Surg 2007;133(12):1220–1226
11. Li RJ, Richmon JD. Transoral endoscopic surgery: new surgical techniques for oropharyngeal cancer. Otolaryngol Clin North Am 2012:45:823–844
12. Moore EJ, Henstrom DK, Olsen KD, et al. Transoral resection of tonsillar squamous cell carcinoma. Laryngoscope 2009;119: 508–515
13. O'Malley BW, Weinstein GS, Snyder W, et al. Transoral robotic surgery (TORS) for base of tongue neoplasms. Laryngoscope 2006;116:1465–1472
14. Weinstein GS, O'Malley BW, Magnuson JS, et al. Transoral robotic surgery: a multicenter study to assess feasibility, safety and surgical margins. Laryngoscope 2012;122:1701–1707
15. Desai SC, Sung CH, Jang DW, et al. Transoral robotic surgery using a carbon dioxide flexible laser for tumors of the upper aerodigestive tract. Laryngoscope 2008;118:2187–2189
16. Van Abel KM, Morrer EJ, Carlson ML, et al. Transoral robotic surgery using the thulium:YAG laser. Arch Otolaryngol Head Neck Surg 2012;138(2):158–166
17. Crawford JA, Montevecchi F, Vicini C, et al. Transoral robotic sleep surgery: the obstructive sleep apnea-hypopnea syndrome. Otolaryngol Clin North Am 2014;47:397–406

5 Robotic Surgery for Management of Oropharyngeal Malignancies

Mara C. Modest and Eric J. Moore

■ Description of the Clinical Problem

Worldwide, head and neck cancer is the sixth most common cancer, with 12% of these occurring within the oropharynx.[1] Oropharyngeal squamous cell carcinoma (OPSCC) is the most common pathology, composing 90% of all oropharyngeal malignancies. Its incidence in the United States has continued to increase, with some predicting that the incidence of oropharyngeal cancers in men will even eclipse that of cervical cancers by 2020.[2] The majority of surgical experience has been with OPSCC, and is the focus of this chapter.

In surgical oncology, the primary goal is to remove disease while maintaining function. This is especially relevant in tumors involving the oropharynx, which plays an important role in speech, swallowing, and respiration. Tumor extirpation in the oropharynx is intrinsically difficult due to the complex anatomy. Thus, historically, access has been limited to open surgical methods such as the suprahyoid pharyngotomy, the pull-through approaches via a visor incision, and the lip-split mandibulotomy, all followed by adjuvant radiation therapy. While these open methods address the goal of removing pathological disease, function is often sacrificed. For this reason there has been a constant push over the past few decades to minimize surgical impact through minimal access techniques and "keyhole" incisions.

This drive toward reducing surgical impact in the treatment of oropharyngeal malignancies led to the development of transoral laser microsurgery (TLM) and the use of transoral robotic surgery (TORS). While the aim of this chapter is to outline the use of TORS in oropharyngeal malignancies, it is imperative that the head and neck surgeon be comfortable with all surgical approaches for this anatomical region. The goal should always be to attain oncologic cure with minimal morbidity and excellent functional outcomes.

■ Current Standard Treatment of Oropharyngeal Malignancies

Open Technique

Classic surgical approaches to the oropharynx consist of en bloc resection of the primary tumor. The three primary open techniques used for oropharyngeal malignancies include lip-split mandibulotomy (mandibular swing), suprahyoid (transhyoid) pharyngotomy, and pull-through techniques using a visor incision. These techniques should be considered for oropharyngeal tumors that are endophytic, nonmobile, and invade deep structures such as the buccopharyngeal fascia where transoral exposure simply does not allow for complete resection of the tumor. Although these techniques provide the surgeon with the greatest access to oropharyngeal malignancies, they are associated with significant morbidities, especially when combined with postoperative radiation. Nonetheless, it is important for the surgeon to be familiar with these techniques, discuss them with their patient, and be prepared to transition to an open approach if transoral excision is inadequate.[3]

Transoral Laser

TORS has its foundation in TLM. The use of TLM for the resection of oropharyngeal tumors was first pioneered in 2003 by Wolfgang Steiner of Goettingen, Germany.[4] By using a distending bivalve laryngoscope for tumor exposure and an operating microscope for operative field visualization, he allowed the surgeon to employ two hands: one for mobilization and retraction of the tumor, and one for operation of the carbon dioxide (CO_2) laser micromanipulator.[4] While this was a significant improvement in transoral surgery, and allowed surgeons the ability to access hard to reach areas of the oropharynx without an open approach, incisions made with the CO_2 laser are "line of site" and therefore can limit the surgeon's ability to make angled cuts around bulky tumors.

To circumvent these restrictions, Steiner began using piecemeal resection. This approach went against the en bloc resection touted by Halsted in the early 20th century. Investigation of this approach revealed comparable oncologic outcomes, with a local control rate of 85% without recurrences in T1 and T2 tumors, and a 20% recurrence rate in T3 and T4 tumors.[5] The argument for the success of piecemeal resection via TLM is that the laser would not carry tumor to adjacent sites and therefore is limiting the potential for tumor seeding.[4] Steiner's data also supported an excellent functional outcome, with 92% of his patients ultimately tolerating a normal diet and none requiring a tracheotomy for a prolonged period.[4] Patients undergoing TLM are less likely to be overtreated for a mis-staged tumor, and are also more likely to maintain a serviceable voice.[4] Therefore, TLM quickly gained wide acceptance as an oncologically and functionally sound transoral option in the management of oropharyngeal cancers. The use of TLM can also be advantageous in patients where the retractor most commonly used for TORS

(Feyh-Kastenbauer, or FK, retractor) does not fit into the mouth and a smaller laryngoscope is required. In addition, if TLM is unsuccessful or the patient recurs, the surgeon can still use an open approach.[4]

Even with its widespread acceptance as a treatment option for oropharyngeal malignancies, TLM is not without limitations. These include difficulty with visualization, tissue manipulation, and ablation, and a more challenging hemostasis.[3] The first two limitations primarily result from the surgeon working through the barrel of a smaller laryngoscope where visualization and manipulation of a bulky tumor can be more challenging. This approach also requires the surgeon to switch between cautery and clips in order to maintain hemostasis. The procedure itself is also technically difficult, requiring specific training as well as considerable experience to reach an acceptable level of competence.

In an effort to take advantage of transoral access, while avoiding the limitations of TLM, surgical oncologists turned to the da Vinci surgical system (Intuitive Surgical, Inc.). TORS provides surgeons exceptional visualization with binocular 0-degree and 30-degree cameras. Seated in an ergonomic operating position, the surgeon has 540 degrees of wristed instrumentation with tremor minimization. However, in its initial stages, the application of TORS was limited by inadequate retraction and the bulky instrumentation. Even with these initial limitations, TORS has made great strides in the management of oropharyngeal malignancies.[3]

■ Transoral Robotic Surgery Technique

The da Vinci system was first introduced into the otolaryngology literature by Neil Hockstein from the University of Pennsylvania in 2005.[6] He adapted the da Vinci robot to be used for transoral access and evaluated the safety and feasibility of TORS in cadavers, and eventually in human patients, which spurred a huge influx of TORS research into the literature. These early clinical studies established that TORS was a feasible option for the treatment of oropharyngeal malignancies and culminated in the U.S. Food and Drug Administration (FDA) granting approval for TORS for select tumors of the head and neck.

Advantages of TORS for the management of oropharyngeal malignancies include its 540 degrees of wrist instrumentation, tremor reduction, and improved accessibility of difficult to reach oropharynx and base of tongue (BOT) lesions while minimizing morbidity. Multiple studies have shown that with proper patient selection, the application of TORS for malignant oropharyngeal processes can result in better swallowing function, lower tracheostomy rates, shorter operative and hospitalization time, and decreased overall morbidity when compared to conventional open techniques.[7,8,9,10]

Disadvantages of the TORS system include the expense of the da Vinci system, the comparatively large size of the robotic arms and instrumentation in relationship to the head and neck, and the additional training required for operative staff. In addition, the surgeon does not have any tactile feedback intraoperatively with the da Vinci. Therefore, we recommend that the surgeon palpate the lesion and establish a mental map of the tumor boundaries before putting the patient into retraction.[7]

Description of Transoral Robotic Surgery Procedure

Transoral Candidacy

Before one can even consider how to use the da Vinci robot for TORS, the question of who this procedure should be used for must be clearly understood. Three categories should be considered when evaluating transoral candidacy: anatomical restrictions, patient comorbidities, and tumor characteristics.[11]

Because transoral surgery uses the oral cavity as the keyhole to the oropharynx, understanding how the anatomy can impair adequate access to the surgical site is imperative. While experience can help the surgeon to correctly identify anatomical constraints preoperatively, it is often necessary to perform an exam under anesthesia before one can truly appreciate the adequacy of transoral access. Specific anatomical restrictions that can limit TORS include:

1. Mandibular width (can use tongue blades to measure): should be wide enough to accommodate the retractor used by the surgeon. If too narrow, once the retractor is put in place the tongue has no space to move laterally and instead is forced posteriorly toward the vallecula and can obstruct the surgeon's view of the lesion.
2. Trismus: mouth opening < 1.5 cm; can also use the Mallampati score to assess mouth opening. Trismus due to pain can be overcome by general anesthesia. However, trismus due to tumor invasion, fibrosis, or scarring from prior interventions will not improve, and can limit transoral access.
3. Retrognathia: a posteriorly positioned mandible can make suspensions and exposure challenging.
4. Cervical spine inflexibility: can prevent adequate extension and proper positioning.

Transoral operations involving the oropharynx can result in significant discomfort for the patient. There is a risk of devastating hemorrhage, difficulty swallowing, difficulty with secretion management and airway protection, and the potential for wound healing issues if there is any communication between the throat and neck. Therefore, it is critical to assess patient comorbidities that increase these risks, resulting in poor TORS candidacy. These include, but are not limited to:

1. Immune suppression (this will lead to difficulty with wound healing by secondary intention)
2. Increased age
3. Coagulopathies
4. Cardiovascular and respiratory health
5. Pulmonary reserve
6. Recurrent oropharyngeal tumor
7. Microvascular disease (e.g., poorly controlled diabetes, atherosclerosis)

Finally, the surgeon must consider the primary goal of the operation, which is to completely remove the tumor, leaving negative margins. Therefore, regardless of anatomical and comorbid candidacy, if the tumor itself cannot be exposed, manipulated, and resected to negative margins, or if doing so would result in significant morbidity, open approaches should be considered. The ideal tumor for transoral resection is easily accessible, mobile, and exophytic. Interestingly, the size of the tumor is less important than these critical factors.[11] Patients with the following tumor characteristics should therefore be considered poor candidates for TORS:

1. Fixation of the tumor to the lateral or posterior pharyngeal wall, indicating deep neck space invasion into the parapharyngeal space.
2. Involved or closely associated with the carotid artery, internal jugular vein, or prevertebral fascia, as supported by imaging or physical examination.
3. Skull base invasion, mandibular invasion, or invasion of the pterygoid musculature as indicated by clinically significant trismus.
4. Distal extension into the hypopharynx.[11]

Anesthesia Considerations

Once the patient and the surgeon decide to proceed with TORS, the first step is always management of the airway. The anatomical location of these tumors directly impacts the anesthesiologist's access to an orotracheal or nasotracheal intubation and can result in a difficult airway. Therefore, communication between surgical and anesthesia teams must be thorough and include discussion of the choice of intubation technique which should be tailored to a patient's specific anatomy, tumor characteristics, and the planned procedure. It is also very important for the surgeon to communicate clearly with the anesthesiologist not only the preferred airway plan, but also a backup plan.[12]

General approaches to securing the airway include intubation under general anesthesia or awake versus sedated intubation. Using either of these approaches, tracheal intubation can be achieved via transoral, transnasal, or transcervical routes. The transoral route can be aided by the use of traditional laryngoscopes or the Glide Scope (Verathon). Fiberoptic intubation is useful for both the transoral and transnasal routes.

The transnasal approach can be useful in the resection of oropharyngeal tumors by moving the endotracheal tube (ETT) out of the oral cavity. Even so, it will pass through the posterior pharynx and thus never be entirely out of the operative field. Also, the placement of armored or laser-proof ETTs is often more difficult transnasally. To bypass the oropharynx, the surgeon may consider a tracheostomy. This approach should be kept in mind for patients in acute airway distress due to upper airway obstruction; those with large, bulky, friable tumors; and those patients who will eventually require a tracheostomy based on the planned operative procedure.[8]

Deciding on the proper ETT to use during a case is another important consideration. One should factor in the position of the tube, the risk for kinking or compression, and what risk there is of airway fire. In TORS, a wire-reinforced[12] or laser-safe ETT[7] is usually used.

Once the ETT has been placed, it can be taped to the contralateral side of the mouth, or sutured to the nasolabial fold and buccal mucosa.[12] Before using cautery or laser, it is important to communicate with the anesthesiologist that the FiO_2 should be below 30% to prevent an airway fire. Throughout the duration of the transoral procedure, paralysis should be used to maximize surgical access. Prophylactic antibiotics with coverage of oropharyngeal organisms should be administered prior to the beginning of the case.

Transoral Surgical Equipment Used in Transoral Robotic Surgery

Before the robotic arms are introduced into the oral cavity, the tumor has to be properly visualized. This is usually done with an oral retractor such as the FK laryngeal retractor (Gyrus ACMI), but a Crowe-Davis or other oral retractor can be utilized.

Many of the instruments commonly used in transoral surgery have been adapted to the robot allowing the surgeon to grasp and cut. These include the EndoWrist 5-mm Shertel grasper, the 5-mm Maryland dissector, and the 5-mm monopolar cautery (Intuitive Surgical, Inc.). Even with these specifically adapted tools it is important to have all the standard transoral instruments available on the back table and accessible to the surgical assistant in order to allow for immediate vascular control, evacuation of smoke, additional suctioning and retraction, and removal of the surgical specimen.[12]

Surgical Approach Using Transoral Robotic Surgery

Once intubation is complete, with the patient lying supine, the operating table is positioned so that the head is turned 90 degrees from the anesthesia team.[13] To the right of the patient's head, with the leading edge slightly overlapping the head of the bed, the side cart or micromanipulator unit is positioned (up to 30 degrees from the operating table). The surgeon's console is located 8 to 10 feet away from the head of the bed (**Fig. 5.1**).[7,13] The patient's eyes must be protected, as well as a head-wrap placed. This can be done as a sterile procedure or clean transoral procedure, depending on whether a neck dissection is being performed before or after. The patient's teeth are protected using custom-molded thermoplastic sheeting (WFR/Aquaplast Corp.) made at the time of surgery.

With the patient properly positioned, the oropharynx is then exposed using an oral retractor. As previously mentioned, the FK laryngeal retractor is frequently used, with another option being the Crowe-Davis. The surgical field should be illuminated using a headlight, and the surgeon should palpate the oropharynx with a gloved finger to establish the palpable extent of the lesion and confirm there is adequate visualization with both retraction and suspension. If there appears to be any fixation of the tumor to the lateral pharynx or skull base, this should dissuade the surgeon from continuing with a transoral approach. Once exposure is satisfactory, the retractor is usually suspended to the left side of the bed using a Storz laryngoscope holder (Karl Storz). At this point the surgical assistant helps with docking the robotic arms. Usually three arms are used for TORS: the first side arm is docked with a tissue manipulator or a grasper, the second side arm is docked with either the cautery or the laser as the cutting instrument, and lastly the middle arm is docked

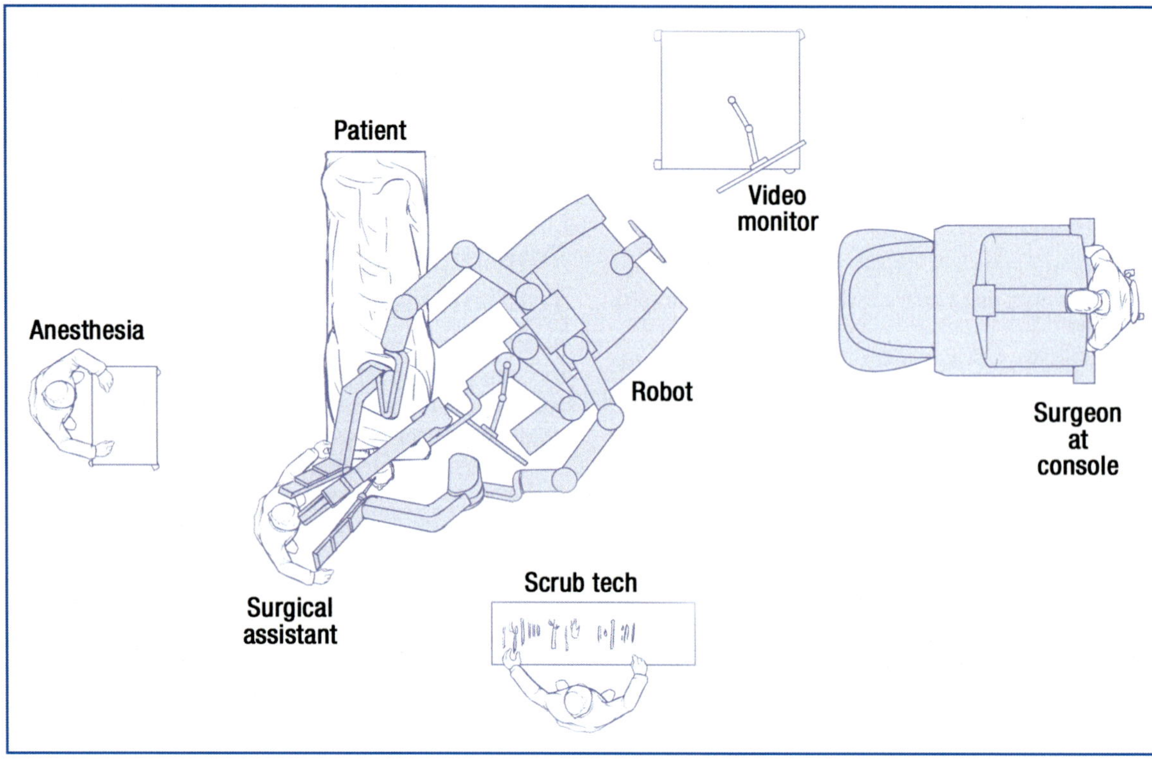

Fig. 5.1 Birds-eye view of the transoral robotic surgery (TORS) setup in the operating room. Note the relationship of the TORS side cart to the edge of the bed, which allows proper positioning of the robotic arms. The surgical assistant sits at the head of the bed, while the surgeon sits at the console. (Courtesy of the Mayo Clinic, Rochester, Minnesota.)

with the binocular endoscope that is either 0 degrees (for tonsillar fossa) or 30 degrees (facing upward, for BOT).[7] With each of the side arms positioned 30 degrees from the middle endoscope, all three arms are advanced intraorally. The head of the bed is where the surgical assistant sits, attended by the surgical technician (**Fig. 5.1**).

The surgical assistant is responsible for having a variety of instruments accessible, including suction cautery, bipolar cautery, tissue manipulators, graspers, surgical clips, and two insulated suctions in the immediate vicinity. Positioning of a monitor should be done so that the assistant, surgical technician, and nurse can all see the operative field on the monitor. In the operating room, it is important that communication between the surgeon and surgical team is audible. Throughout the procedure, repositioning of the surgical arms, endoscope, or retractor may be required. To prevent the endoscope from fogging, and in order to maintain adequate visualization, proper smoke evacuation via suctioning is important.

Lateral Oropharyngectomy (Video 5.1)

Pearl: A difference in lateral oropharyngectomy via TORS versus TLM is the use of blade tip monocautery, where the zone of injury is larger and the aggressiveness of cutting is greater compared to the laser.

The surgical technique for transoral removal of tonsillar tumors has been described by Holsinger et al and Weinstein et al.[12,14] The first step is to expose the oropharynx and the tonsillar region to allow palpation and ensure tumor mobility. Holsinger et al make the recommendation to palpate both the mucosa and the submucosal raphe.[14] Tumor exposure is critical (**Fig. 5.2a**). The initial incision begins with the mucosa at the retromolar trigone, with dissection carried down to the pterygomandibular raphe, which separates the superior pharyngeal constrictor from the buccinator muscle, and runs between the hamulus of the medial pterygoid plate and the mandible (**Fig. 5.2b**).[11,12,15] The pterygomandibular raphe acts as a useful landmark for the surgeon for the proper lateral dissection plane. In order to open the submuscular plane for dissection, the tonsillar tissue is grasped and pulled in the direction of the midline, as this allows the superior constrictor muscle to be drawn medially (**Fig. 5.2c**).[14,15]

At this point, the lateral margin of the specimen is the superior constrictor, palatoglossus, and palatopharyngeus muscles, while the deep plane of dissection is comprised of the buccopharyngeal fascia.[11] Deep to this, the medial pterygoid muscle and the parapharyngeal fat pad can be visualized (**Fig. 5.3**).[12,15] The buccopharyngeal fascia should be kept intact if at all possible, as this preserves the layer of fat in the parapharyngeal space surrounding the carotid artery and also prevents communication between the oropharynx and the neck.[11]

The decision to proceed with surgery cranially to caudally or vice versa depends on the tumor's location and extent. If the tumor is inferiorly based, Holsinger recommends working

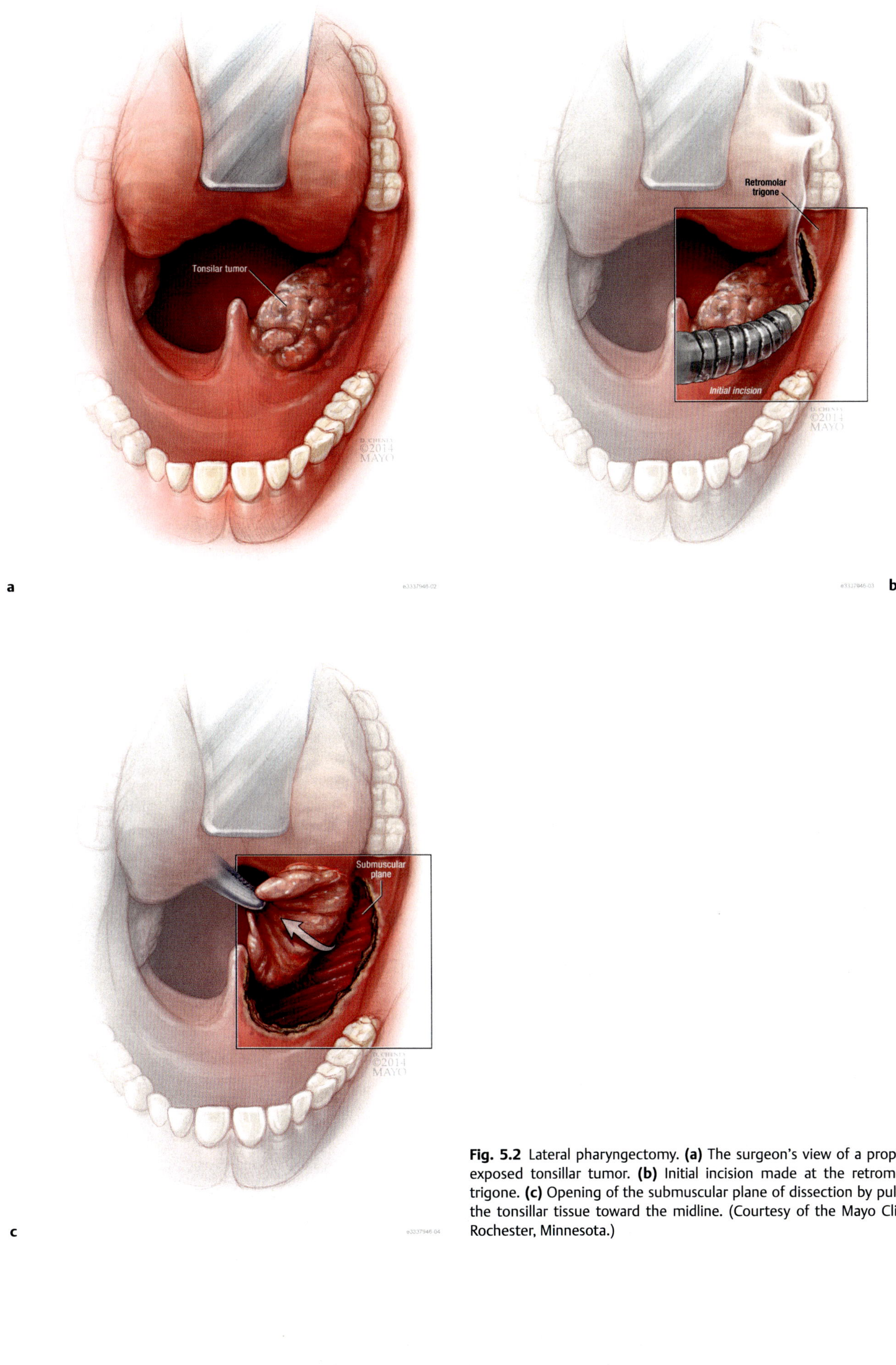

Fig. 5.2 Lateral pharyngectomy. **(a)** The surgeon's view of a properly exposed tonsillar tumor. **(b)** Initial incision made at the retromolar trigone. **(c)** Opening of the submuscular plane of dissection by pulling the tonsillar tissue toward the midline. (Courtesy of the Mayo Clinic, Rochester, Minnesota.)

superiorly to inferiorly, and vice versa with a superiorly based tumor.[14] Throughout the entire procedure it is important to provide countertraction, as it allows for careful dissection between structures. More specifically, medial traction should be applied when possible as it provides a safety margin between planes of dissection and the internal carotid artery (**Fig. 5.3**).[14]

Medial dissection is done via palatal cuts, being careful to avoid the superior extent of the tumor. As long as the tumor does not extend to the midline of the palate the medial palatal cut only needs to extend just medial to the uvula. However, if there is tumor extension beyond the midline, the uvula can be transected. Laterally and inferiorly, dissection should then continue down to the level of the stylopharyngeus and styloglossus muscles. The surgeon should be aware of the glossopharyngeal nerve, as it may be visualized anterolaterally to these two muscles. Throughout this area of dissection are numerous vascular contributions of the lingual, facial, and ascending pharyngeal arteries and veins (**Fig. 5.4**).

These vessels are easily injured, and bleeding should be controlled by additional cautery for smaller vessels, and single clips for small or medium-sized vessels. The facial and lingual arteries should be managed using two to three clips on the patient side. With the lingual artery, if bleeding is encountered, the surgical assistant can apply external pressure to the neck in the area of the greater cornu of the hyoid bone to help slow bleeding, so that the vessel can be identified and clipped.[12,16] Superiorly, cuts that are dependent on tumor extent are made through the anterior and posterior pillars as well as the ipsilateral soft palate.[12] Dissection continues through the constrictor muscle on the posterior pharyngeal wall until the prevertebral fascia is reached. Using blunt dissection, the medial superior pharyngeal constrictor muscle is separated from the prevertebral fascia. Then the styloglossus and stylopharyngeus muscles should be transected inferiorly where they travel between the superior and middle pharyngeal constrictors.[11,14,15] In order to prevent injury to the lingual artery, Weinstein et al advocate starting

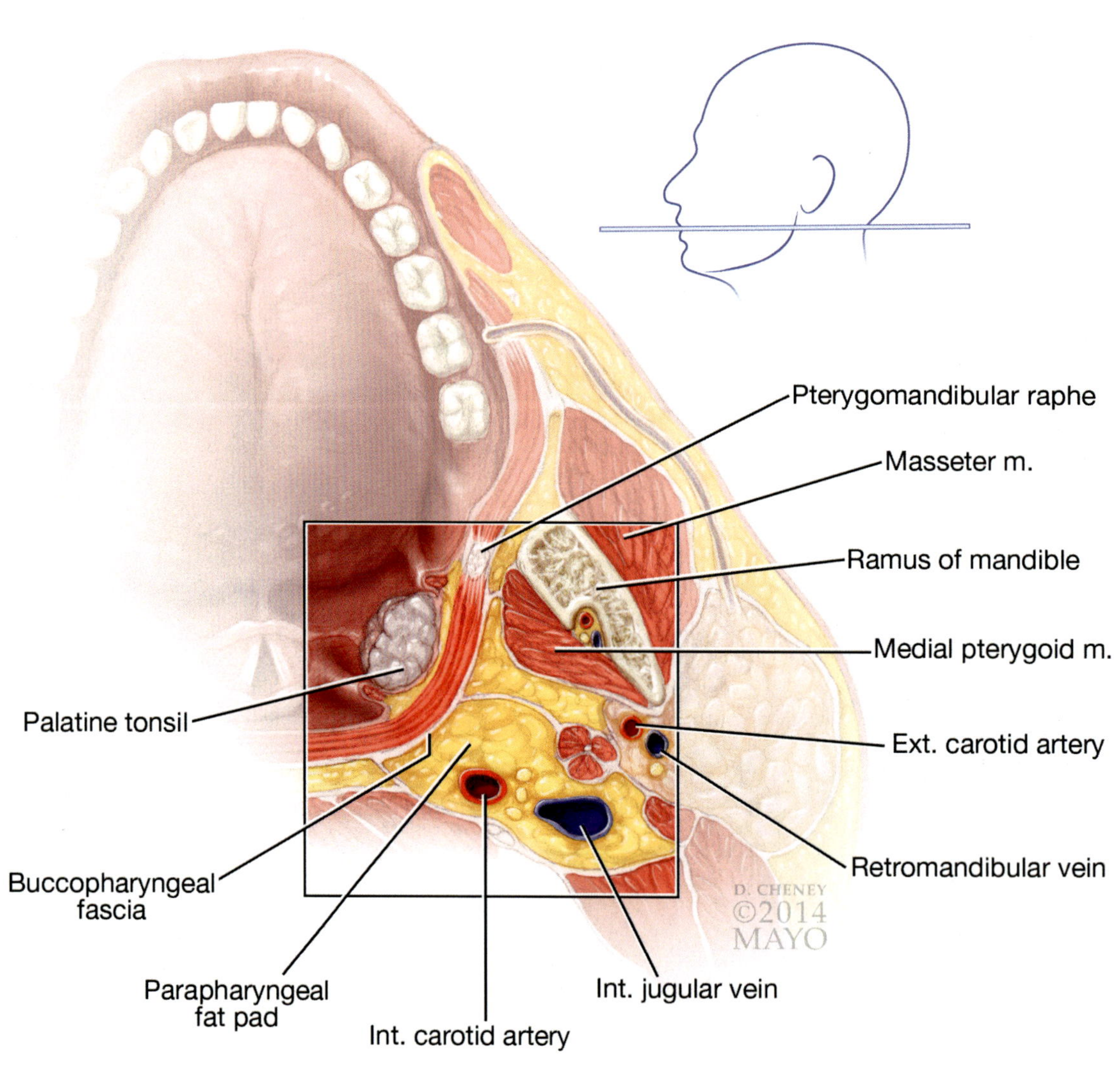

Fig. 5.3 Axial cut showing the important anatomical relationships the head and neck surgeon needs to be aware of as he or she begins to dissect out the tumor. Special attention should be paid to the relationship of the buccopharyngeal fascia, the parapharyngeal fat, and the internal carotid artery. (Courtesy of the Mayo Clinic, Rochester, Minnesota.)

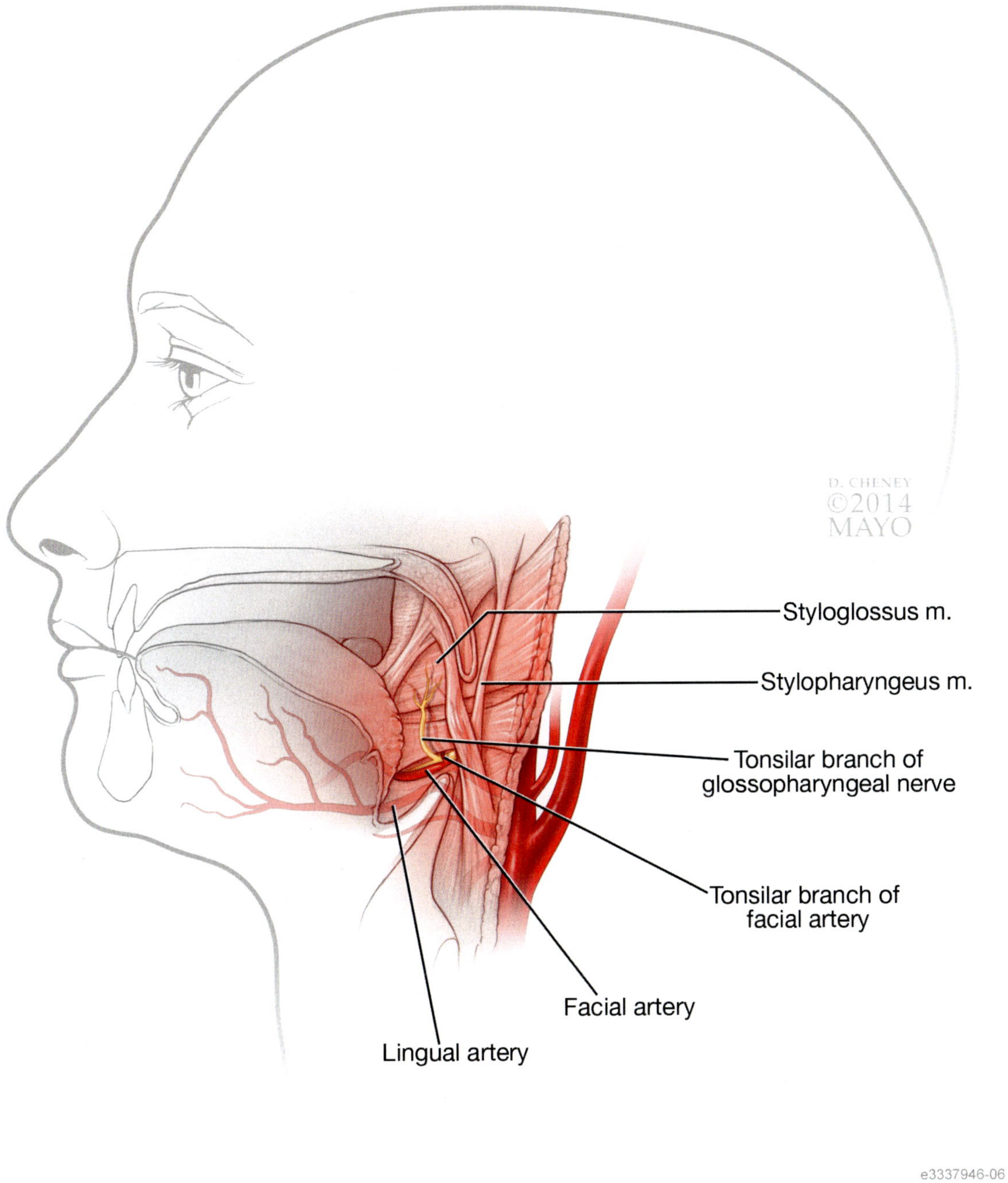

Fig. 5.4 Sagittal view showing the relationship of the stylopharyngeus and styloglossus muscles as compared to the relevant neurovasculature. (Courtesy of the Mayo Clinic, Rochester, Minnesota.)

this with blunt dissection done circumferentially around these two muscles. They also emphasize the importance of reaffirming the location of the internal carotid artery during this time, as seen by pulsations in adjacent fat and soft tissue (**Fig. 5.3**).[12] Dissection continues into the lingual lymphoid tissue until the most inferior extent of the tumor is safely mobilized and the tumor itself is released with a margin of normal tissue. It is important that as the surgeon grasps the tumor and removes it from the mouth, that he or she maintains orientation before preparing it for pathology (**Fig. 5.5**).

Base of Tongue Resection (Video 5.2)

Pearl: The surgeon must be mindful of vasculature, as it is easy to transect dorsal lingual artery branches with cautery and not know it because the vessel can be temporarily sealed. This is not the case when using TLM where brisk bleeding will ensue with accidental transection using the laser.

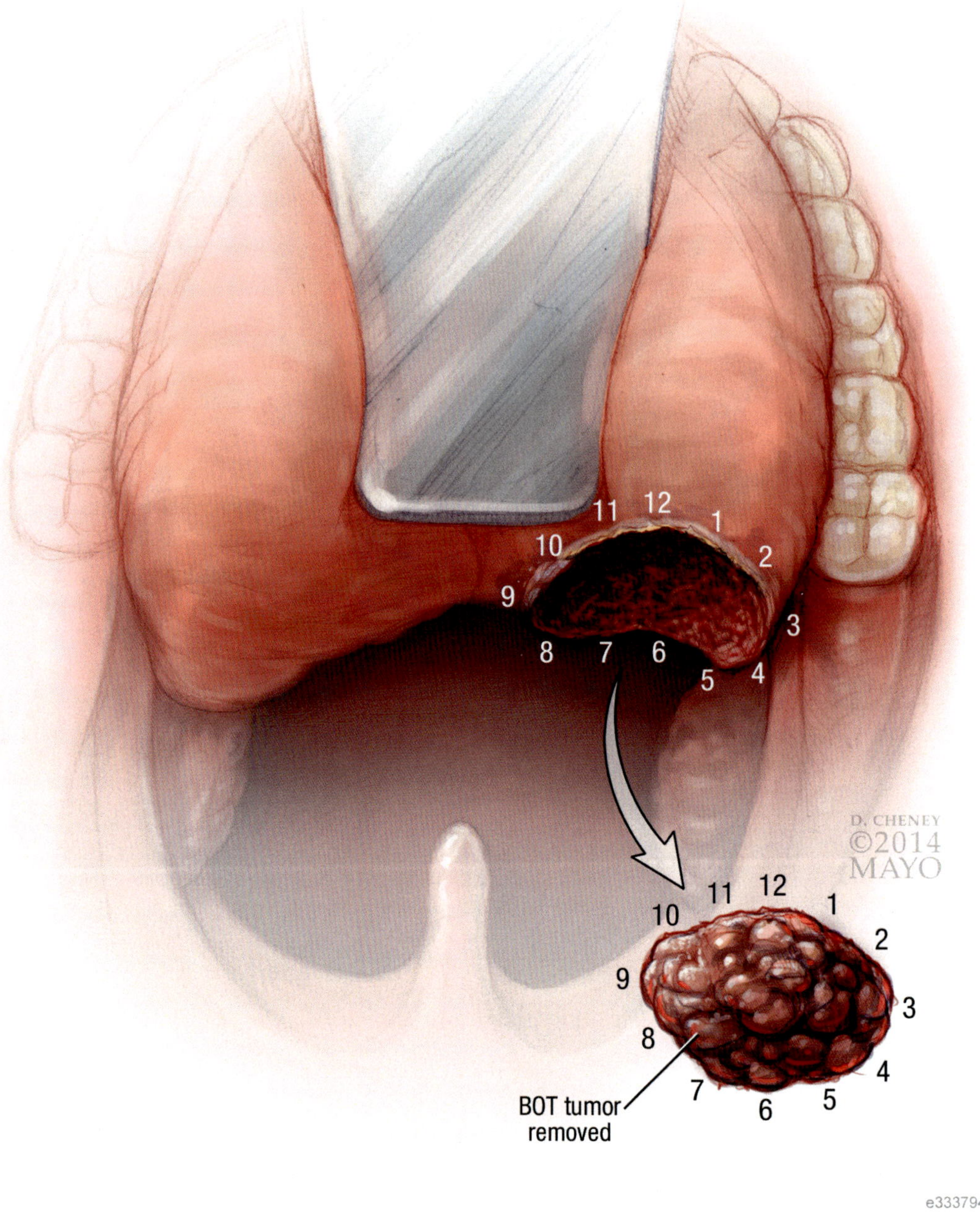

Fig. 5.5 For both tonsillar and base of tongue (BOT) tumors, it is important that the surgeon maintain proper orientation of the specimen as it is passed on to pathology for frozen section. This ensures that any margins that are positive can be accurately re-excised. (Courtesy of the Mayo Clinic, Rochester, Minnesota.)

Pearl: With regard to vessel ligation, it is important to pay attention to the facial, lingual, and superior thyroid artery. If one knows the tumor involves or is intimately associated with a specific vessel, then one should consider ligation during the process of tumor removal.

It is important for the surgeon to perform a careful physical examination of the BOT tumor prior to transoral excision, as it allows the surgeon to create a three-dimensional (3D) image of the tumor and correlate it with preoperative imaging if available, as well as assess the tumor for mobility (**Fig. 5.6**). This should be done before the retractor is placed, as the anatomy of the oropharynx can become distorted. With retractor placement, one should try to provide the widest tumor exposure, as this step is crucial for successful tumor removal. The placement of a tongue stitch or applying tongue retraction with a sponge before mouth gag or laryngoscope insertion can help the surgeon with tongue retraction in order to obtain deeper access. Both the anterior edge and most of the inferior extent of the

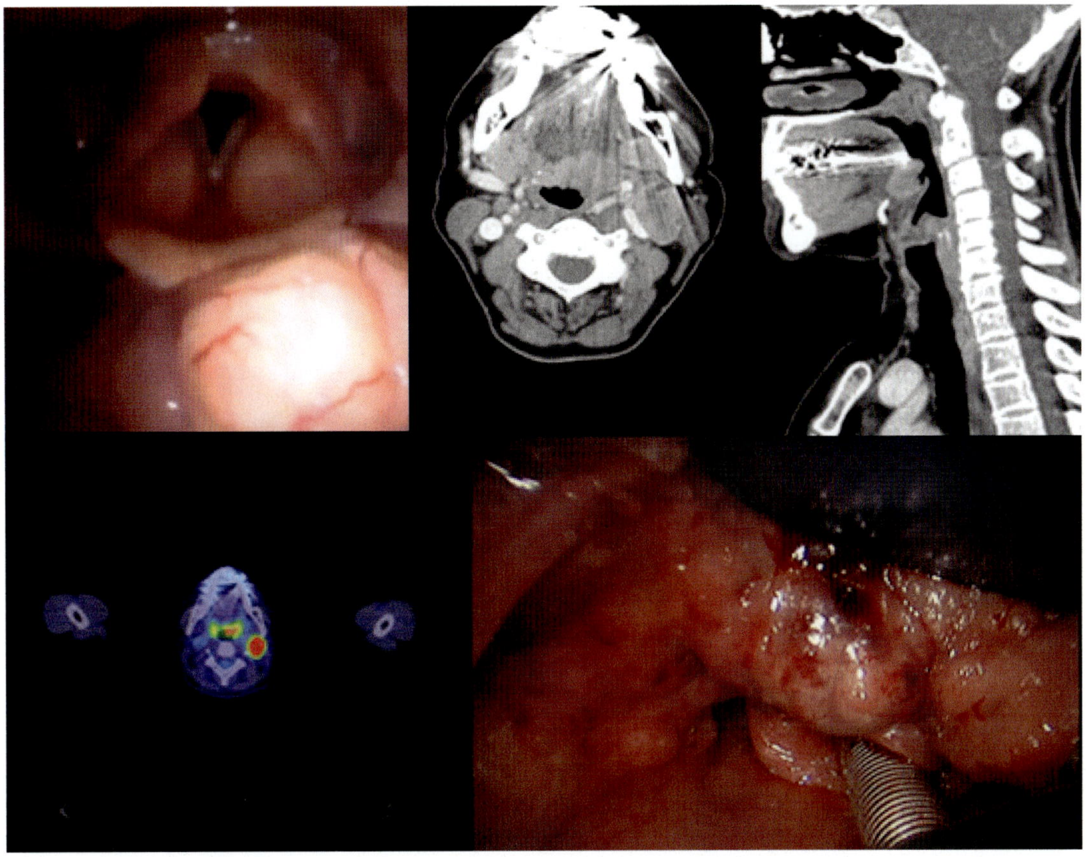
a, b
c
d
e

Fig. 5.6 The surgeon can use both physical exam and imaging to help create a mental image of the tumor to aid with operative planning. **(a)** Left base of tongue tumor visualized on flexible nasopharyngolaryngoscopy. **(b)** Axial CT scan with contrast showing a left well-encapsulated lingual mass abutting the facial artery. **(c)** Sagittal CT scan showing that the tumor does not extend beyond the hyoid bone, making the patient a good TORS candidate. **(d)** PET scan establishing the tumor to be a T3 N2b lesion. **(e)** Intraoperative view of the tumor.

tumor should be visualized, and adjustments may need to be performed throughout the procedure to maintain maximum exposure (**Fig. 5.7**).[4,7]

With exposure maximized, the surgeon can make a vertical cut through the tumor, exposing its greatest depth. This is useful since tangential cuts (to the tumor) across the BOT can fail to include the full tumor depth and unintentionally leave tumor within the deep intrinsic tongue musculature (**Fig. 5.7**). For the first step, the initial mucosal cuts are made anteriorly, allowing the tumor to fall posteriorly into the operative field (**Fig. 5.8**).

In order to recognize the inferior extent of the tumor throughout dissection, the first inferior cut should be made at the level of the vallecula. For countertraction along the plane of dissection, the surgeon can retract along the healthy mucosa of the anterior margin. Tumor extent helps to guide the placement of both the medial and lateral cuts. Dissection is then carried out either in an anterior to posterior or superior to inferior direction through the mucosa, lymphoid tissue, and tongue musculature, while making sure to preserve a cuff of normal tissue encircling the tumor.[7] Once the tumor is freed, it is grasped by the surgical assistant, oriented, and passed along to pathology for frozen section analysis (**Fig. 5.5**).

During the procedure, the surgeon should be aware of the dorsal lingual artery laterally along with contributions of the lingual artery. This is especially true for tumors that extend deeply and laterally beyond the hyoid bone, reaching the hyoglossus muscle, where both the lingual artery and hypoglossal nerve are in close proximity (**Fig. 5.9**). For adequate hemostasis, these vessels should be clipped with two to three clips on the patient's side, and one clip on the tumor side.[7,16] As described above for bleeding from the lingual artery during lateral oropharyngectomy, external pressure in the area of the greater cornu of the hyoid bone can be applied to slow blood flow until a clip can be applied. For tumors with this type of lateral extent, it may be safer to proceed with an external approach and allow for more confident resection of margins.

Neck Dissection

Pearl: If performing a concomitant neck dissection, one should do the neck portion first when unsure of location/path of great vessels. For example, if there is any lateral extension of tumor, one might consider neck dissection first. If equivocal, the authors prefer to do TORS first as there is less edema earlier on in the case.

Neck dissections are often part of the management for oropharyngeal malignancies, and either ipsilateral or bilateral

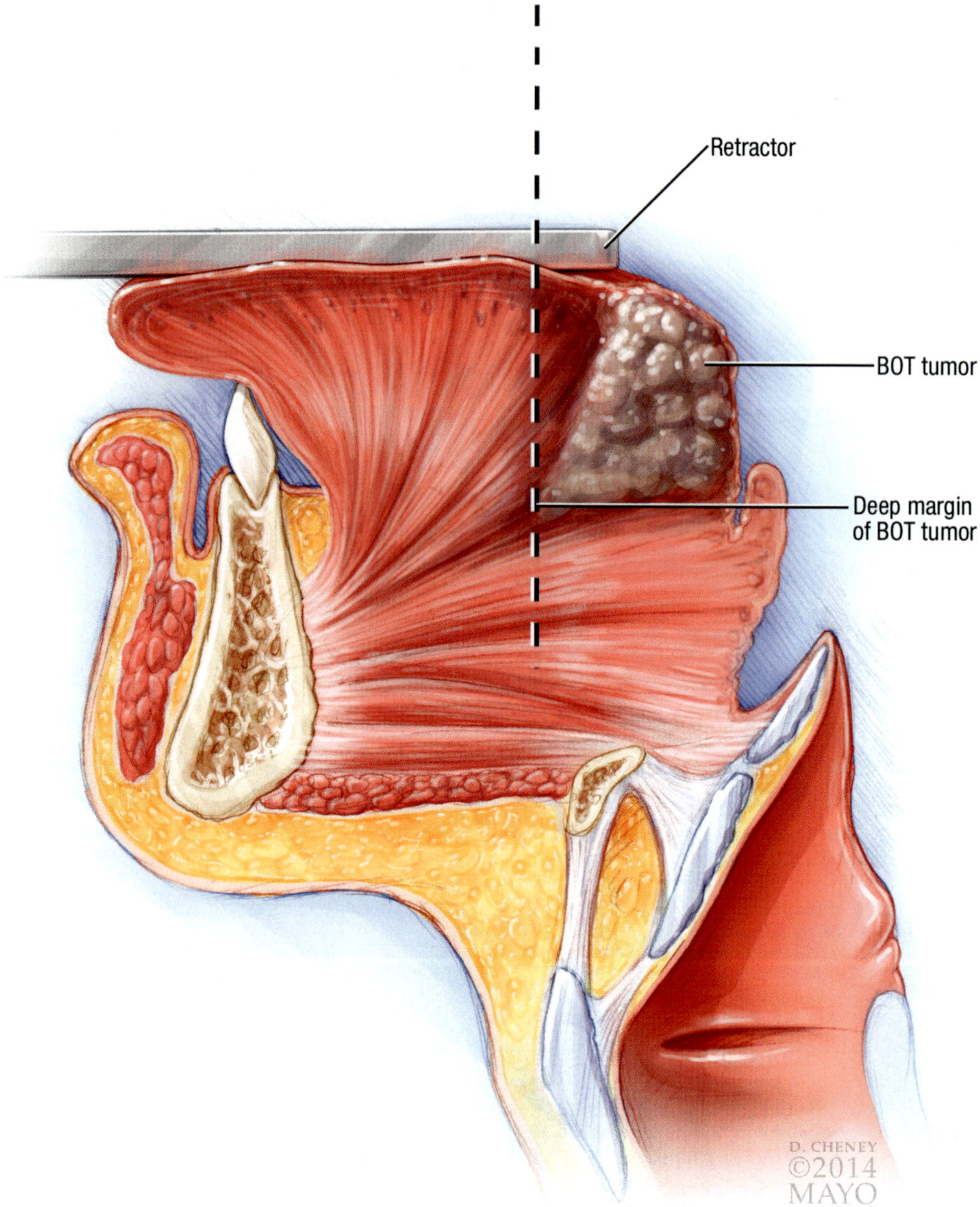

e3337946-08

Fig. 5.7 It is important to palpate the deepest extent of the base of tongue (BOT) tumor before removal. The placement of the retractor can limit tumor excision depending on the tumor's extent, and if this is the case, an open surgical technique may be required over a transoral one. (Courtesy of the Mayo Clinic, Rochester, Minnesota.)

neck dissections can be performed. If the patient has N0-N2b or N3 disease, they typically undergo an ipsilateral select neck dissection (levels II–IV). The retropharyngeal nodes are removed if there is significant invasion of the tumor into the soft palate or posterior pharyngeal wall, or if imaging shows metastasis to the area.[17] The procedure itself is not discussed in detail here, but the value of proceeding with neck dissection at the time of primary tumor removal versus waiting several weeks and performing a delayed neck dissections is discussed. The timing of the neck dissection if done concomitantly with primary transoral resection is also important, and is based on tumor involvement with vascular structures and the possible development of an orocervical communication or pharyngocutaneous fistula.[17]

Delayed neck dissection can be performed several weeks after transoral tumor removal, allowing time for healing. Advantages of waiting include the surgeon having a chance to review any delayed positive margins, possibly lowering the

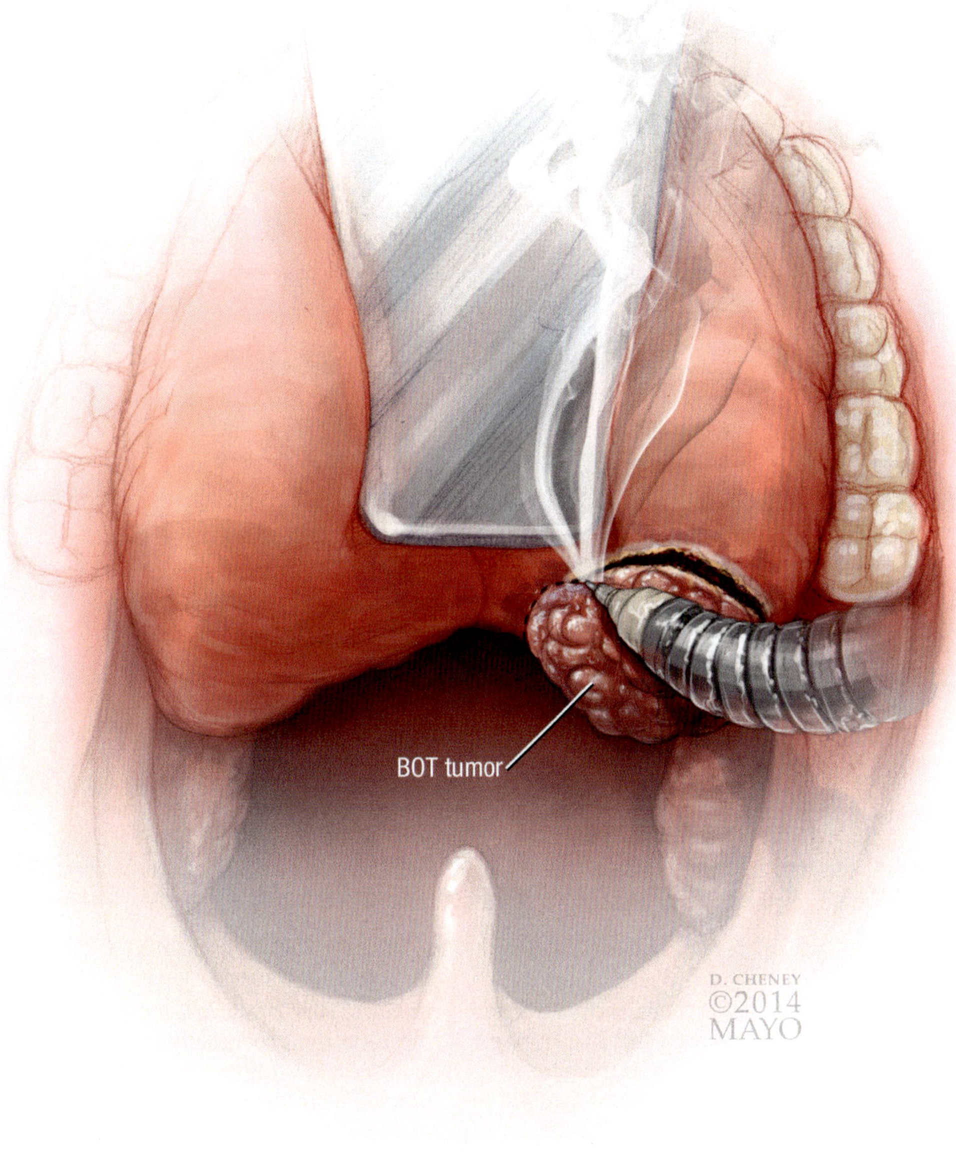

Fig. 5.8 The initial mucosal cut is made anteriorly in base of tongue (BOT) lesions, allowing the tumor to fall posteriorly. This provides proper visualization throughout the procedure. (Courtesy of the Mayo Clinic, Rochester, Minnesota.)

need for tracheostomy with less laryngopharyngeal swelling, and decreasing the risk of creating an orocutaneous communication.[12,17]

Simultaneous neck dissection is what is performed at our institution. Advantages of performing the neck dissection at the time of the transoral procedure include exposing the patient to only a single anesthetic, requiring only one hospitalization, and providing the surgeon with immediate feedback regarding staging information that can be used to initiate adjuvant therapy, which usually begins 3 to 4 weeks following surgery.[7,17] There is some concern that there is a higher risk of creating an orocutaneous fistula with simultaneous neck dissection, but even so, the rate of persistent pharyngocutaneous fistula is low.[9,15] This was emphasized in a retrospective study of

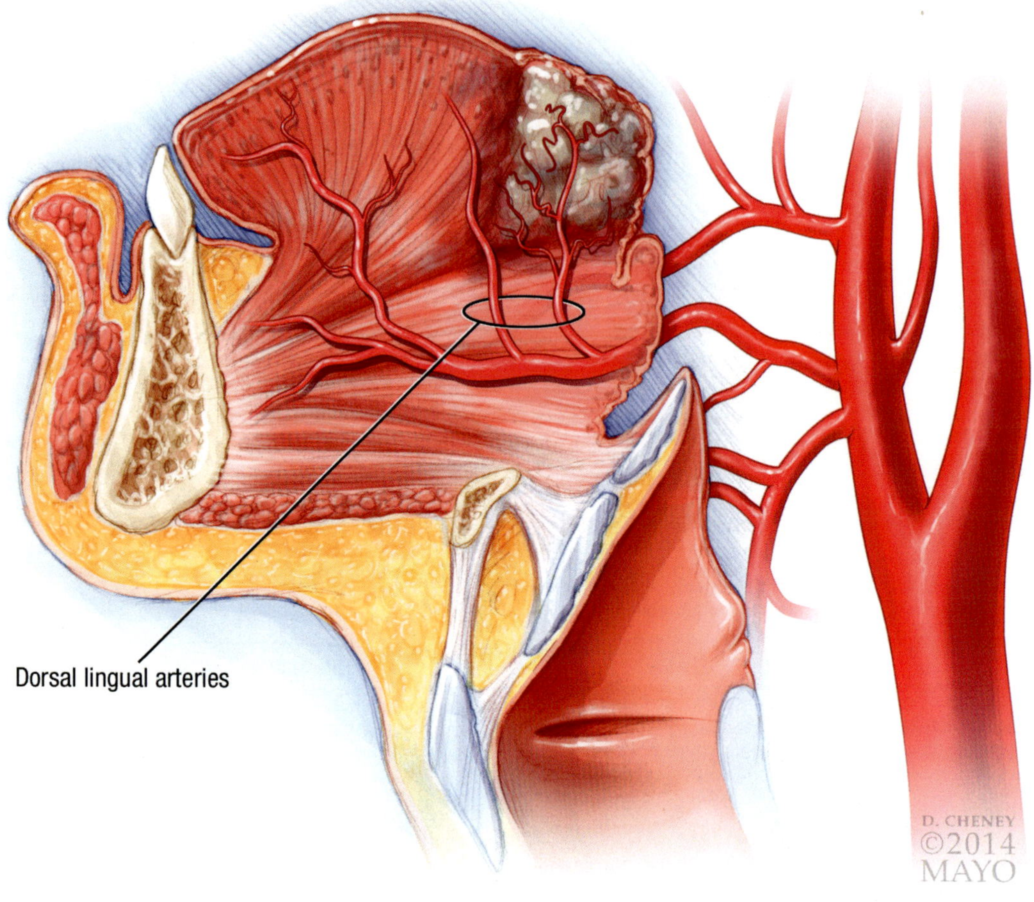

e3337946-10

Fig. 5.9 Sagittal view showing the important vasculature that the head and neck surgeon can encounter during the excision of a base of tongue lesion, with the dorsal lingual artery and its branches being the most relevant. (Courtesy of the Mayo Clinic, Rochester, Minnesota.)

patients undergoing TORS with simultaneous neck dissection that showed that although 29% of patients (42 of 148) were found to have an orocervical communication intraoperatively, only 4% (6 of 148) resulted in a pharyngocutaneous fistula.[17] To identify any orocervical communication, the nares are plugged and then sterile saline is used to irrigate the oropharynx vigorously. One should be able to see the pharynx swell into the neck without a fluid leak. Any leak that is identified should be repaired intraoperatively. If the communication is less than 1 cm, primary closure followed by Tisseel (Baxter Healthcare Corp.) application on the cervical side can be performed. A suction drain needs to be placed in the neck. This can be removed once output is less than 10 mL over 24 hours, and a clear liquid diet can be started on postoperative day 1.

In the case that the communication is greater than 1 cm, Moore et al recommend suturing the constrictor muscle, closing part of the digastric muscle to the sternocleidomastoid muscle lateral to the defect, and then applying Tisseel over the repair.[17] In these patients a suction drain with the same removal protocol is placed, as well as prohibiting oral intake for the initial 24 to 48 hours with a nasogastric feeding tube in place. This is followed by slowly advancing to a clear liquid diet, and then eventually to a regular diet as long as no leak is observed. With this method of vigilant observation for any orocutaneous fistula intraoperatively and its immediate repair, along with aggressive management of any developing orocutaneous fistulas postoperatively, simultaneous neck dissections can be safe and effective.

The timing of the neck dissection, before or after transoral resection, can be decided based on any concern of extension of disease around the great vessels. If this is the case, an ipsilateral neck dissection should be performed first with a cotton patty placed over the carotid for isolation and protection during transoral dissection.[11] Even though complications associated with transoral surgery are reduced compared to open approaches, bleeding postoperatively can be life threatening if serious. With this in mind, Salassa et al recommend tying off the entire external carotid system when pharyngeal defects are large enough to expose named arteries.[16] If the pharyngeal defects are only moderate, ligation of the lingual, facial, and superior laryngeal arteries can be considered depending on their involvement.

Reconstruction Options

Pearl: Local flaps can sometimes be useful if the buccopharyngeal fascia (BPF) is violated laterally. This possible violation emphasizes why it is important to assess mobility of a tonsil lesion. If it invades the BPF, it will not be mobile, making the patient a poor TORS candidate.

Pearl: If the defect you make with TORS requires extensive reconstruction, this defeats the purpose of the minimally invasive philosophy. This is why doing proper candidacy evaluation prior to surgery is so important.

A detailed discussion of oropharyngeal defect reconstruction is beyond the bounds of this chapter, but it is important to have a basic understanding of what options are available when performing transoral reconstruction of defects left behind by oropharyngeal malignancies. Most often, transoral wounds are left to heal by secondary intention. The advantages of this are multiple, but the resulting healed wound is mucosalized, sensate, contracted, and mimics the surrounding oral environment better than most reconstructions. Reconstruction can be necessary in large defects, and options include skin grafts or local mucosal flaps, local/regional pedicle flaps, or ultimately large regional pedicle or free flaps. We focus our attention on local/regional pedicle flaps as this is the most advanced option that is feasible when transoral resection is performed via TORS, as the robot can be used to sew in these flaps. Once a patient requires a larger pedicled flap or a free flap, the surgeon should reconsider if TORS is a suitable option, or if instead the resection should be done in an open fashion. Factors that can affect the choice of reconstruction include fistulization risk, bleeding, wound breakdown, and functional outcomes such as speech, deglutition, and phonation.[18]

Any defects of the soft palate or tonsillar fossa that are small enough can be allowed to heal by secondary intention or even closed primarily. Any defects that involve more than 50% of the soft palate or communicate with the neck require more extensive reconstruction, otherwise the patient risks developing rhinolalia and nasal regurgitation. Three local pedicled flaps that have the ability to be sewn in using the robot include the buccal fat pad flap, the inferiorly based facial artery musculomucosal (FAMM) flap, and the reverse submental artery island flap (**Figs. 5.10–5.12**). All three of these flaps offer excellent reconstructive options for patients with intermediate oropharyngeal defects, while at the same time avoiding the complexity of having a separate donor site with its own morbidities in a more distant part of the body.[18]

Things to keep in mind in order to successfully use a local pedicled flap include using a Doppler intraoperatively, especially when the patient has a history of a prior neck dissection or a neck dissection is being performed concomitantly. Both of these scenarios can interrupt the facial artery blood supply proximally and distally in the case of the submental flap, and only proximally in the FAMM flap (**Figs. 5.11** and **5.12**).[18] When performing a neck dissection with plans to use the submental flap, it is important to preserve the blood supply of the submental artery as well as its venous run off. For this reason, if there appears to be metastatic disease in the submental and submandibular triangle, it may be prudent to seek another reconstruction option, as dissection and preservation of the vessels is more tedious.

Tumor Margins and Pathology

Pearl: If your hospital does not have access to frozen sections, then be highly cautious of using the robot for treatment of oropharyngeal malignancies. Successful removal of the entire tumor with negative margins hinges upon proper communication with a pathologist and the ability to determine if clear margins were achieved with near immediate feedback.[20]

Pearl: Proper orientation and labeling of the specimen when it is removed and how it relates to the deficit is imperative in being able to use feedback from the pathologist about possible residual disease and being able to obtain negative margins. It is often useful to walk the specimen down to the pathologist and discuss the orientation of the specimen in person (**Fig. 5.5**).

The most common cause of patient mortality is the failure to completely eradicate a tumor at its primary source.[20] It has been a point of contention as to how much normal tissue should be excised along with the primary tumor, with suggested margins ranging from 1 mm to up to 10 mm of normal tissue.[20] Although in theory these values may ring true, practically they are less plausible. Oropharyngeal tissue contracts as much as 50% after being removed, and thus a 5-mm margin can become only a 2-mm margin once it reaches the pathologist. Most importantly, as Hinni explains, if one were to take a deep margin any greater than 2.4 mm in the tonsillar fossa, one would sacrifice the major vessels within the parapharyngeal space.[19] Hinni analyzed 128 tonsillar carcinomas that were treated transorally where the average deep margin was only 1.98 mm, but he still found the 5-year local control rate to be 99%. This helps support the notion that the success of transoral oropharyngeal cancer surgery hinges upon painstakingly accurate margin analysis. Thus it is crucial for the surgeon to be in excellent communication with the pathologist performing the frozen section analysis so that at the end of the case the surgeon can be confident the tumor has been completely removed with clear microscopic margins.[19]

Along with the importance of obtaining clear microscopic margins, the idea of tumor mapping is a crucial portion of the operation. Tumor mapping occurs via serial sectioning of the oropharyngeal cancer, thus allowing the surgeon to determine the deepest extent of the tumor. With the tumor sliced in this manner, it allows the surgeon to communicate with the pathologist and determine the true edge of the tumor, and also have the ability to take more tissue if any microscopic involvement is seen. One can proceed with this type of resection until all margins are clear of microscopic disease, or the surgeon can no longer remove tissue safely. In this fashion, one no longer describes the margins in terms of millimeters of normal tissue, but simply as margins free of microscopic involvement.

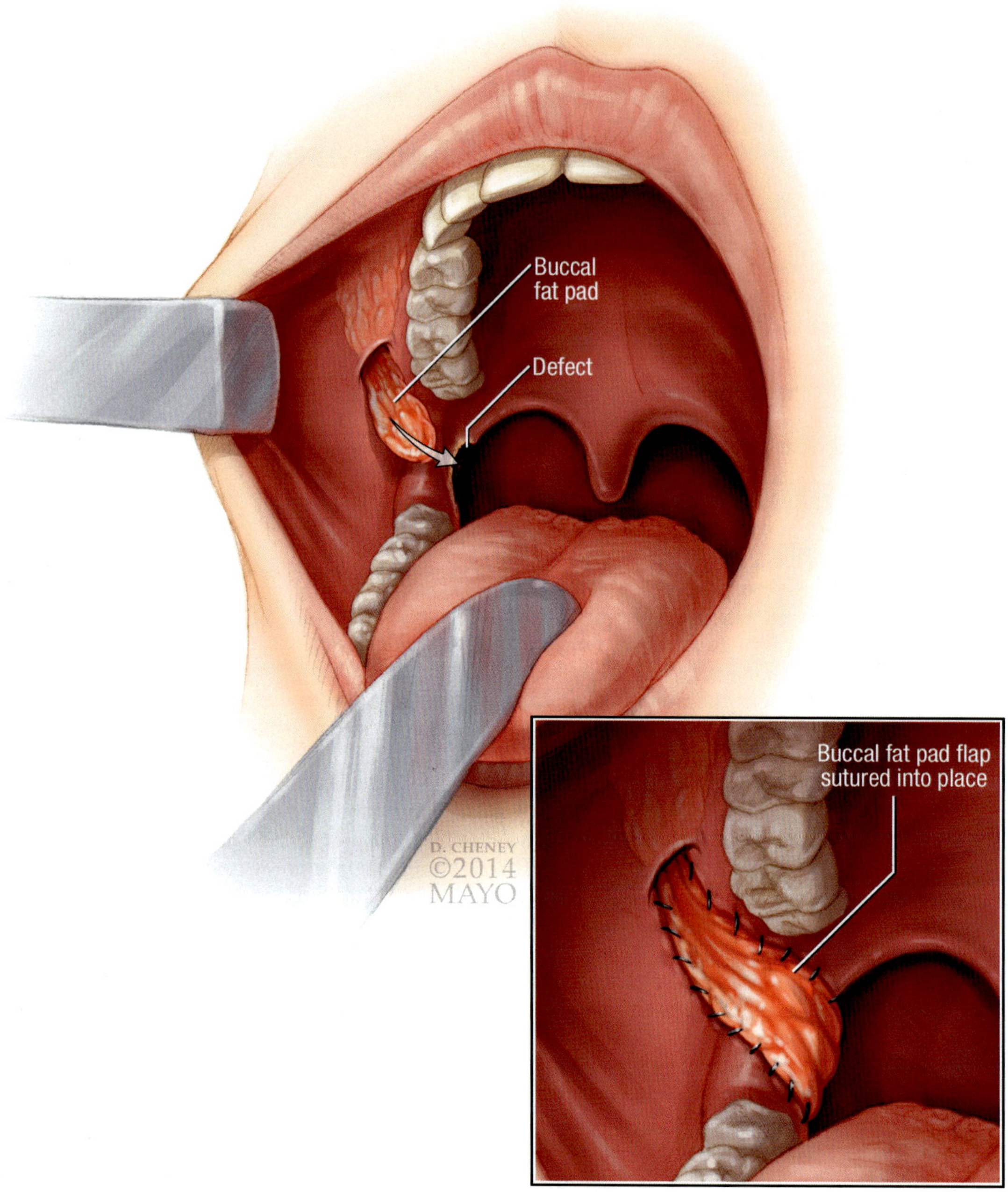

Fig. 5.10 Use of the buccal fat pad flap for oral defects following transoral removal of an oropharyngeal malignancy. (Courtesy of the Mayo Clinic, Rochester, Minnesota.)

Transoral Robotic Surgery as a Salvage Treatment Option

The decision to use TORS as a treatment option goes back to the initial description of patient candidacy. In the authors' experience, the issue with TORS as salvage therapy is twofold:

1. One needs to be able to obtain margins for adequate resection. One can imagine the primary previously untreated tumor as being contained in a box. Thus, during resection, when negative margins are obtained, one can be fairly certain the tumor in its entirety has been removed. Once a patient has had chemoradiation, the tumor is no longer confined to a box; instead, there are now islands of tumor leading to the possibility of obtaining negative margins around one island, but leaving residual tumor behind. A similar issue is seen when tumors begin to invade lymphatics or neurovascular structures and begin to spread outside of their box.

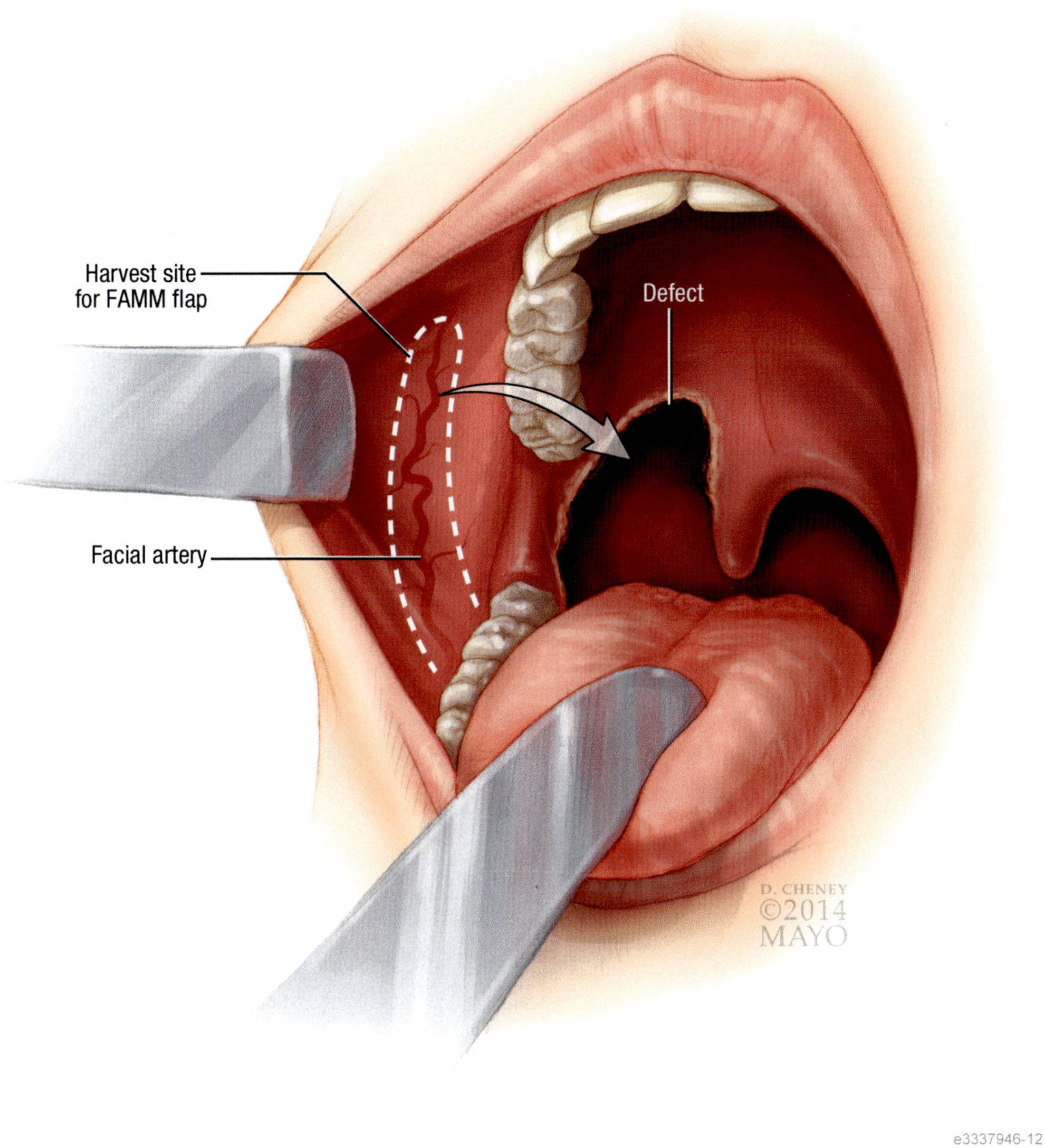

Fig. 5.11 Location of the facial artery musculomucosal (FAMM) flap used for oral defects after transoral excision of an oropharyngeal malignancy. Emphasis is on the facial artery pedicle, which can be identified with Doppler intraoperatively. (Courtesy of the Mayo Clinic, Rochester, Minnesota.)

2. The majority of TORS defects are left to heal by secondary intention. Some authorities advocate vascularized flaps in patients who have been chemoradiated, but again this somewhat defeats the purpose of the minimally invasive approach. Patients with a history of prior chemoradiation have an increased risk of developing nonhealing wounds and wound infections. In patients with TORS as the primary treatment, the chance of a cure approaches 90%,[14] whereas in patients where TORS is a salvage treatment, the chance of a cure without significant morbidities drops to 70%.[21]

Postoperative Management

Pearl: It is very important in the perioperative period to control pain, optimize nutrition and hydration, avoid bleeding, protect the airway, and monitor for any aspiration. All patients will have some extent of microaspiration and dysphagia following BOT or tonsillar resection. The extent is patient dependent. It is for the above reasons that the authors usually place a temporary nasogastric tube during the first 2 postoperative weeks.

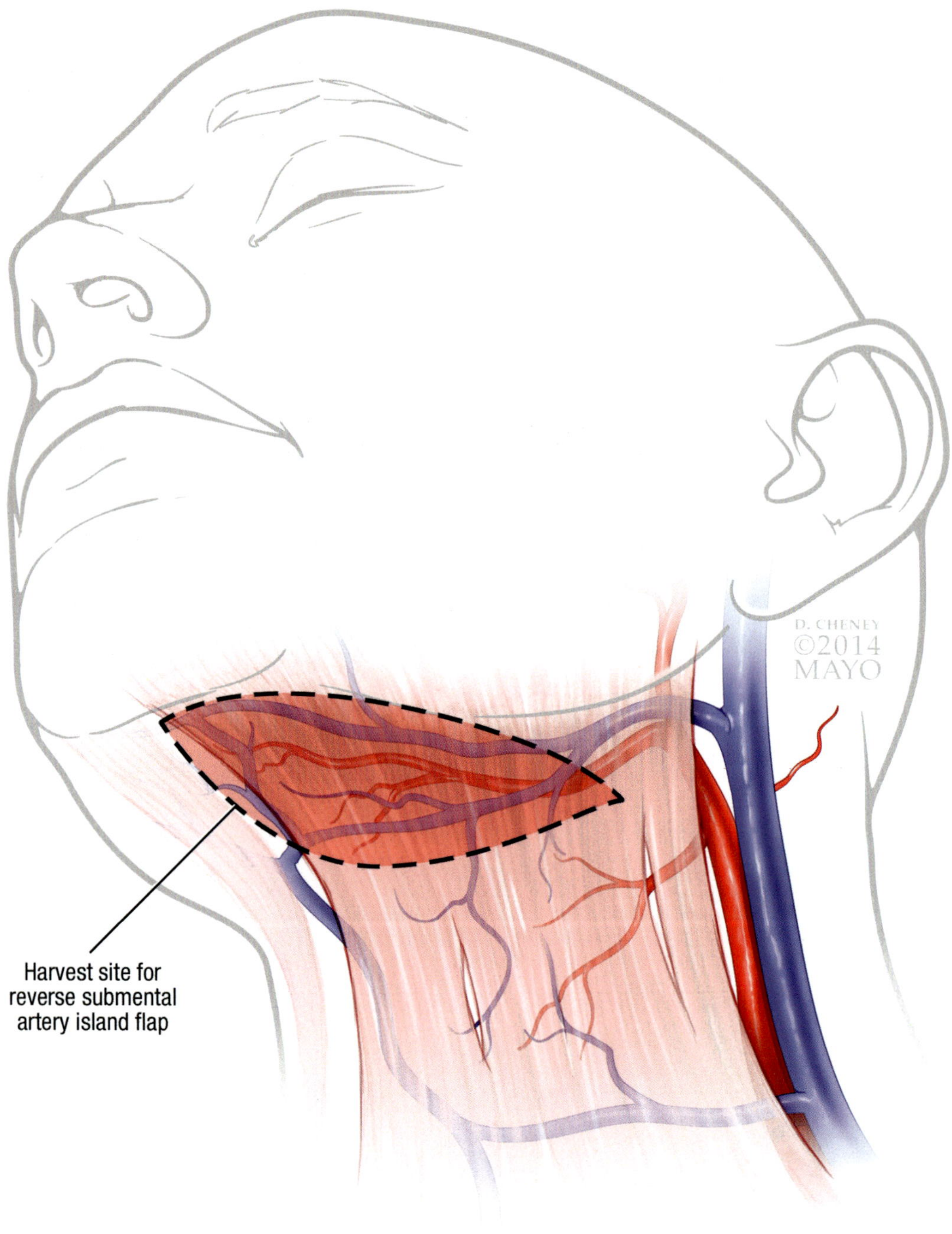

Fig. 5.12 Illustration of the location of a reverse submental artery island flap. Knowledge of both the artery's path and the venous drainage pattern is important. (Courtesy of the Mayo Clinic, Rochester, Minnesota.)

During the immediate postoperative period, things that need to be optimized include the airway, wound management, oral hygiene, diet, and nutrition. Adequate pain control is important as well, as it encourages earlier ambulation.

In regard to the airway, in any patient where a planned tracheostomy was not performed at the beginning of the procedure, a proper airway evaluation should be performed at the end prior to extubation.[12,22] Extubation can proceed as long as no epiglottic or significant laryngeal edema is noted. If edema is seen, however, then the patient should remain intubated and placed on a course of steroids for 1 to 3 days, after which the patient can be extubated or a tracheostomy placed. Unless the patient is intubated or has comorbidities that require more intensive monitoring, the patient can be admitted to a general care floor postoperatively. Most crucial during the first 24 to 48 hours, proper pulmonary toilet can help reduce the risk of considerable silent aspiration, as this is common during this period. This applies whether or not the patient has a tracheostomy placed.

Proper wound care, including adequate drain care, is important to help monitor for any signs of fistula development. If the development of a fistula is a concern, the drain should be kept in place until there are less than 10 mL of output over 24 hours; otherwise, the drain can be removed when there are less than 30 mL of output over 24 hours.[17] In any patient where an orocervical communication was observed intraoperatively, a 5-day minimum course of antibiotics should be prescribed. Oral hygiene, such as sponge brushes dipped in saline, chlorhexidine gluconate 0.12% (Peridex), or 1.5% sodium bicarbonate, helps keep the mouth moist and makes it easier for the patient to swallow and begin oral intake.

In many cases following transoral surgery, patients are able to resume swallowing immediately postoperatively and can be started on a clear diet with the goal eventually being a mechanical soft diet. A nasogastric tube (NGT) is placed in patients who are predicted to have pain, dysphagia, or an increased risk of aspiration postoperatively, as well as in patients where an orocervical communication occurred during the procedure. If pain is the only concern, the patient can be started on a clear diet immediately, but if dysphagia or aspiration is a concern, it may be prudent to obtain a speech therapy consultation while in the hospital along with a bedside swallow evaluation. For most patients with an NGT, the feeding tube can be removed once sufficient caloric intake is achieved. If the NGT was placed because of concerns for a pharyngocutaneous fistula developing, the feeding tube is left in place for 10 to 14 days until the patient is evaluated as an outpatient for speech and swallow abilities as well as their risk of aspiration.

Another key aspect to postoperative care is adequate pain control. Transoral surgery is almost always a very painful operation. At the authors' institution, the patient is started on intravenous narcotics until oral or enteral access is available, after which the patient can be changed over to oral narcotics along with scheduled acetaminophen if necessary. Due to a large majority of transoral defects being left to granulate in, the use of nonsteroidal anti-inflammatory drugs (NSAIDs) or any anticoagulation medications are not recommended.[15] By controlling a patient's pain, it encourages earlier ambulation, which in turn helps with pulmonary toilet and gastrointestinal ileus. Ambulation is encouraged to begin on postoperative day 1, along with sitting in a chair when not sleeping or resting.

■ Complications

Bleeding

Although rare, with only an incidence of 3 to 8%, postoperative hemorrhage after oropharyngeal surgery can be life threatening.[16] Prevention of postoperative bleeding can already begin at the time of surgery by carefully placing two to three clips on the patient side of any vessel greater than 2 mm in diameter, and also by identifying any vessels that may be in spasm and then retract into the soft tissue, and subsequently cauterizing them. As discussed previously, the lingual, facial, and superior thyroid arteries or even the entire external carotid artery system for large pharyngeal defects should be ligated during the neck dissection.[16] Following surgery, in the immediate postoperative period, bleeding can also be prevented by performing a cautious extubation, controlling a patient's hypertension, keeping the patient "nothing by mouth" (NPO) for 7 to 10 days (with placement of NGT), having the patient avoid Valsalva maneuvers or vigorous activities, and finally telling the patient not to take any anticoagulants for 3 weeks.[15]

Postoperative bleeding can be divided into major and minor bleeds. Minor bleeds usually occur at around 9 to 14 days after surgery, with the patient noticing blood-tinged sputum that occurs for minutes to hours. Conservative management tends to be the mainstay of treatment for minor mucosal bleeds and includes the use of ice water, stopping any anticoagulants, observation, or bedside cautery.

Major bleeding is attributed to erosion into already controlled vessels or vasodilation of vessels that were previously in vasospasm during surgery and thus not clipped. There are two reasons why major bleeding can quickly progress to catastrophic bleeding: first, large named vessels are frequently clipped during surgery and then simply left within the open wound bed as it slowly granulates in over a period of 3 to 4 weeks; and, second, most patients undergoing transoral resection have compromised swallowing ability and cannot protect their airway properly in the event of a major bleed.

It is not hypotension or exsanguination that is so dangerous with oropharyngeal bleeding, but rather the risk of asphyxiation and airway compromise.[16] With most bleeding occurring within 7 days of the surgery, it is important for both the surgical team and the patient with their family to have a plan in place in the event of a significant bleed. Foremost the patient should be instructed to place their head in the dependent position to prevent aspiration and then pressure should be applied to the affected side of the neck. Even if the patient becomes unconscious, the head of the patient should remain in the dependent position.[16] Any patient in whom the physician does not believe the bleed is superficial or can be treated with observation should go back to the operating room. The patient should then be intubated allowing the surgeon to carefully evaluate the source of bleeding and control it.

Neck Abscess

A neck abscess can result if, even with careful intraoperative evaluation, an orocervical communication occurs and is not repaired. The patient will present with swelling and erythema in the neck along with possible spontaneous rupture and drainage of the abscess. Treatment includes incision and drainage, obtaining cultures, and beginning broad-spectrum antibiotics while waiting for antibiotic susceptibilities from the culture. Wound care should include debridement and cleaning the wound with half-strength hydrogen peroxide followed by packing it with iodoform gauze. In order to allow the wound to heal by secondary intention, it should be packed twice daily, with slightly less gauze each time. If during evaluation of the cavity a pharyngocutaneous fistula is identified, an NGT should be placed so that the patient can be kept NPO for 10 to 14 days. Before oral intake can begin, the patient must show clinical improvement as well as undergo a swallow study demonstrating closure of the leak.[8]

Dental Damage and Paresthesias of the Oral Cavity

Pressure is often placed on the teeth during surgery, and dental injuries or paresthesias can result. With the use of thermoplastic splints, dental damage occurs only rarely, but if a loose tooth is recognized it should be removed to prevent aspiration. Patients with large tongues, narrow mandibular arches, or those subjected to long operative times are at a higher risk of developing paresthesias. It is important for the surgeon to keep this in mind and relax the retractor or scope when not operating. Treatment is usually conservative and resolves within a few days.[8]

Rhinolalia and Velopharyngeal Insufficiency

In patients whose tumors have superior extension and undergo lateral pharyngectomy, or those who require palatectomy for extensive soft palate lesions, palatal insufficiency is not uncommon.[15] When less than 50% of the palate has been removed, conservative management is often sufficient, as the patient's symptoms will commonly improve over the next several months. On the other hand, if more than 50% of the palate is resected without reconstruction at the time of the initial operation, then the patient can be given an obturator or return to the operating room for reconstruction. The risk of velopharyngeal insufficiency is higher in patients undergoing salvage surgery.[15]

Aspiration and Pneumonia

Aspiration can occur in patients in the immediate operative period secondary to poor pulmonary toilet and swallow function. These patients can subsequently develop pneumonia and present with a rising leukocyte count, fever, as well as thick, foul-smelling tracheal secretions. Treatment involves aggressive pulmonary toilet, aspiration precautions, and starting proper antibiotic coverage.[8]

■ Review of Available Data

Since its original introduction into the field of otolaryngology–head and neck surgery in 2005, TORS and its application for oropharyngeal malignancies, primarily OPSCC, has provided a constant stream of information in the literature. Here we review how the use of TORS in oropharyngeal malignancies has continued to expand, again emphasizing the importance of establishing which patients are proper candidates. We also address TORS' functional and oncologic outcomes, the more common complications in TORS, and lastly its use as salvage surgery.

In 2007, Weinstein and his colleagues published a prospective phase I clinical trial outlining the use of TORS for radical tonsillectomy in 27 patients.[12] This study buoyed the idea that TORS could be used for radical tonsillectomy in malignant disease. Even so, the authors had one unplanned tracheostomy, two patients with positive margins, and one case each of trismus, hypernasality, and postoperative mucosal bleeding. Since TORS offered the potential to not only decrease morbidity but also to provide better or equivalent long-term oncologic and functional outcomes when compared to open techniques, these acute morbidities were found to be acceptable.

With the expanding use of TORS in oropharyngeal pathology, as seen with Weinstein's use of TORS for radical tonsillectomy, surgeons became more comfortable with the technique and subsequently moved on to more complex resections. In 2009, Desai et al published a prospective study on TORS lateral oropharyngectomy.[23] It was in that same year that Boudreaux et al published a prospective, nonrandomized clinical trial that, in opposition to previous reports, included T1–T4 tumors of the upper aerodigestive tract that were managed via the TORS approach.[9] Even with advanced tumors, Bordeaux achieved negative margins with outstanding functional results for the majority of cases. There were two patients in this series that were unable to undergo TORS due to technical issues with the robot, and two patients where inadequate exposure was obtained including a T2 vallecula and a T4 BOT. Deeply infiltrative tumor characteristics prevented two other patients from undergoing TORS resection. Although this study did expand the range of TORS surgery, it also emphasized certain limitations for oropharyngeal lesions including the value in proper preoperative patient selection.

Moore et al have expanded on both what defines tumor candidacy, as well as reported functional outcomes of TORS. They published a prospective series of 45 patients where TORS was performed for OPSCC with all patients undergoing complete resection.[7] With their prior experience using TLM, they reported that the T stage of the tumor was less crucial for adequate exposure than which adjacent structures were invaded by tumor.[7] These findings helped to define the tumor candidacy for TORS as presented earlier in this chapter. Not only did this study show TORS to be a safe and efficacious method of surgically managing primary tumors, but it also argued against the need for staged surgical intervention by describing the feasibility of concomitant neck dissections. These were performed in 95.6% of the patients (31 unilateral, 12 bilateral). A pharyngotomy was reported in 40% of cases, all of which were repaired primarily. Only three patients (6.7%) developed orocutaneous fistulas and were treated conservatively without any further sequelae. In 2011, Moore et al published a retrospective review of 148 patients who underwent TORS for oropharyngeal malignancy along with a concomitant neck dissection.[17] In 42 patients (29%), an orocervical communication was observed intraoperatively. All cases were managed surgically followed by conservative management in the postoperative period with only six patients developing a subcutaneous fluid collection that required incision and drainage. In no patient was postoperative adjuvant treatment delayed.[17]

Another important complication to be aware of in the use of TORS for oropharyngeal malignancies is bleeding. This risk in minimally invasive surgical techniques is always important to assess as visibility and access are often limited when compared to the standard open technique. Pollei et al presented a group of 906 patients whose OPSCC was treated transorally and reported postoropharyngectomy hemorrhage rates as well as associated risk factors. They reported an incidence of 5.4% of postoperative bleeding, where 67.3% required operative intervention. There was no significant difference in bleeding rate or severity when the transcervical external carotid system was ligated or not. In addition, no difference in bleeding rates was observed when comparing patients treated with laser versus the robot. It is important to note that patients with significantly higher T-stage tumors were treated with laser instead of robotic technique.[24]

Although there is an abundance of data supporting the safety and efficacy of TORS for oropharyngeal malignancy, data of long-term oncologic outcomes for this technique are relatively recent. Weinstein et al presented the first study with long-term data showing that even with advanced tumors, TORS offers disease control comparable to standard treatment protocols as well as similar survival. His study group was comprised of 47 patients who underwent TORS for advanced OPSCC (stages III and IV) with an average follow-up of 26.6 months.[22] These outcomes only pertain to primarily treated oropharyngeal malignancies, which has been the focus of most authors when evaluating TORS.

Dean et al did evaluate the use of TORS as a salvage option when they compared TORS for primary versus recurrent OPSCC with the use of open surgical approaches for recurrent disease.[10] A significant difference was seen between TORS and the open surgical groups with regard to length of hospital stay, postoperative diet, gastrostomy tube dependence, and tracheostomy tube dependence. They also reported that patients with primary OPSCC overall fared better functionally compared to those with recurrent OPSCC. Of note, no patient in either of the TORS treatment groups developed any immediate postoperative complications, but two postoperative wound infections and two hematomas were seen in the open resection group.[10]

■ Future Directions and Conclusion

From the initial debut of TORS for oropharyngeal malignancies almost 20 years ago to today, we have made huge advances now allowing for access to difficult to reach tumors coupled with minimal morbidity and the possibility for reduced or no adjuvant therapy, but there is still more to be done. The future direction for TORS will most likely move toward advancements in instrumentation, real-time intraoperative imaging, and improved margin analysis.

Initial robotic arms and instrumentation were designed for use in the abdomen; thus the future for robotic instrumentation in the head and neck will move toward miniaturization of robotic arms as well as the creation of innovative robotic platforms tailored to the otolaryngologist's needs. There has even been a start in establishing the use of a highly flexible robotic for exploration of the oropharynx by Rivera-Serrano et al.[25] This tele-operated robot was adapted from the CardioARM (Medrobotics Corp.) and allows for 102 degrees of freedom while being steered on a nonlinear path that is self-supported. The benefit of this new technology is that it may eliminate the need for laryngeal suspension. The other possible benefit of a more flexible robotic arm is the potential to have patients positioned in the seated position during the procedure, as they are in the clinic for nasopharyngeal laryngoscopy. The seated position avoids the effects that gravity can have on anatomical structures and soft tissue while in the supine position. Looking to other specialties, the urology literature describes in vivo robots providing both video and illumination that have been trialed in both porcine and canine models performing intraperitoneal surgeries.[26] Even with these moves toward perfecting instrumentation intraoperatively, surgeons still struggle to be able to identify important landmarks during surgery that have shifted from preoperative scans.

Preoperative imaging is an extremely useful tool to help the surgeon decide on the best surgical approach. However, many of the bony landmarks such as the mandible, which are seen on initial imaging, are mobile and become unreliable points of reference intraoperatively with the placement of retractors. There has been some research focusing on overcoming this limitation. King and his colleagues evaluated the use of intraoperative cone-beam computed tomography (CT) with a mobile C-arm. Although it would be useful in situations with complex 3D anatomy seen in oropharyngeal surgeries, its primary focus is bony anatomy and less detail is seen of the soft tissues, which is also important during transoral surgery. Another approach to intraoperative real-time imaging in TORS of oropharyngeal malignancies is the adaptation of image guidance systems such as BrainLAB, which was explored by Desai, Sung, and Genden in 2008.[27] Image guidance potentially provides the surgeon with orientation in regard to pertinent vasculature. Desai and his colleagues concluded that it is a reliable method to assess tumor extent, but did warn that soft tissues shift throughout the procedure due to repositioning compared to preoperative scans, as does the mandible. The idea of using an intraoperative 3D navigation system can also be used in combination with positron emission tomography/CT image fusion since it has the ability to show the surgeon areas of hypermetabolic activity. This method was used in patients undergoing major head and neck resection and successfully identified four patients with residual positive margins.[28]

Leaving behind positive margins leads to a very poor prognosis; thus much emphasis has been placed on developing a method of identifying microscopically positive margins, which is both efficient and improves patient outcomes. Photothermal imaging was used in an in vivo study by Jakobsohn et al for the detection of head and neck neoplasms, where cancer cells were targeted by gold nanoparticle therapy with the goal of improving real-time margin analysis.[29] With a similar goal in mind, Keereweer and his associates studied the ability to target epidermal growth factor receptors or glucose receptors in a murine model using tumor-specific near-infrared fluorescent agents.[30] Both of these studies address the hope to eventually be able to directly visualize positive margins while in the operating room.

The use of TORS for oropharyngeal malignancies has provided surgeons improved access to difficult to reach tumors as well as reduced patient morbidities. All of the advantages of TORS only hold true if the surgeon adheres to using this new technology for the proper patient candidates. The surgeon must remain comfortable with all methods of surgical management including open techniques. The ultimate goal continues to be to leave the patient free of disease while preserving as much functionality as possible. Otolaryngologists now have access to a myriad of approaches to oropharyngeal malignancies, allowing treatment to be tailored to each individual patient.

References

1. Harreus U. Cummings Otolaryngology: Head & Neck Surgery. 5th ed. Maryland Heights, MO: Mosby, Inc.
2. Chaturvedi AK, Engels EA, Pfeiffer RM, et al. Human papillomavirus and rising oropharyngeal cancer incidence in the United States. J Clin Oncol 2011;29:4294–4230
3. Van Abel KM, Moore EJ. The rise of transoral robotic surgery in the head and neck: emerging applications. Expert Rev Anticancer Ther 2012;12(3):373–380
4. Steiner W, Fierek O, Ambrosch P, Hommerich CP, Kron M. Transoral laser microsurgery for squamous cell carcinoma of the base of the tongue. Arch Otolaryngol Head Neck Surg 2003;129(1):36–43
5. Pearson BW, Salassa JR. Transoral laser microresection for cancer of the larynx involving the anterior commissure. Laryngoscope 2003;113(7):1104–1112
6. Hockstein NG, Nolan JP, O Malley BW Jr, Woo YJ. Robot-assisted pharyngeal and laryngeal microsurgery: results of robotic cadaver dissections. Laryngoscope 2005;115(6):1003–1008
7. Moore EJ, Olsen KD, Kasperbauer JL. Transoral robotic surgery for oropharyngeal squamous cell carcinoma: a prospective study of feasibility and functional outcomes. Laryngoscope 2009;119:2156–2164
8. Van Abel KM, Moore EJ. Surgical management of oropharyngeal squamous cell carcinoma. Curr Otorhinolaryngol Rep 2013;1: 137–144
9. Boudreaux BA, Rosenthal EL, Magnuson JS, Newman JR, Desmond RA, Clemens L, et al. Robot assisted surgery for upper aerodigestive tract neoplasms. Arch Otolaryngol Head Neck Surg 2009;135(4):397–401
10. Dean NR, Rosenthal EL, Carroll WR, Kostrzewa JP, Jones VL, Desmond RA, et al. Robotic assisted surgery for primary or recurrent oropharyngeal carcinoma. Arch Otolaryngol Head Neck Surg 2010;136(4):380–384
11. Moore EJ, Janus J, Kasperbauer J. Transoral robotic surgery of the oropharynx: clinical and anatomic considerations. Clin Anat 2011;25(1):135–141
12. Weinstein GS, O'malley BW, Snyder W, Sherman E, Quon H. Transoral robotic surgery: radical tonsillectomy. Arch Otolaryngol Head Neck Surg 2007;133(12):1220–1226
13. White HN, Moore EJ, Rosenthal EL, et al. Transoral robotic-assisted surgery for head and neck squamous cell carcinoma: one- and 2-year survival analysis. Arch Otolaryngol Head Neck Surg 2010;136(12):1248–1252
14. Holsinger FC, McWhorter AJ, Menard M, Garcia D, Laccourreye O. Transoral lateral oropharyngectomy for squamous cell carcinoma of the tonsillar region: I. Technique, complications, and functional results. Arch Otolaryngol Head Neck Surg 2005;131(7):583–591
15. Park YM, Lee JG, Lee WS, Choi EC, Chung SM, Kim S-H. Feasibility of transoral lateral oropharyngectomy using a robotic surgical system for tonsillar cancer. Oral Oncol 2009;45(8):e62–e66
16. Salassa JR, Hinni ML, Grant DG, Hayden RE. Postoperative bleeding in transoral laser microsurgery for upper aerodigestive tract tumors. Otolaryngol Head Neck Surg 2008;139(3):453–459
17. Moore EJ, Olsen KD, Martin EJ. Concurrent neck dissection and transoral robotic surgery. Laryngoscope 2011;121(3):541–544
18. Moore EJ. Masters Techniques in Otolaryngology-Head and Neck Surgery. Volume: Reconstruction of the Head and Neck, 1st ed. Philadelphia: Lippincott Williams & Wilkins; in press.
19. Hinni ML, Zarka MA, Hoxworth JM. Margin mapping in transoral surgery for head and neck cancer. Laryngoscope 2013;123(5):1190–1198
20. Looser KG, Shah JP, Strong EW. The significance of "positive" margins in surgically resected epidermoid carcinomas. Head Neck Surg 1978;1(2):107–111
21. White H, Ford S, Bush B, et al. Salvage Surgery for recurrent cancers of the oropharynx: comparing TORS with standard open surgical approaches. JAMA Otolaryngol Head Neck Surg 2013;139(8):773–778
22. Weinstein GS, O'Malley BW, Cohen MA, Quon H. Transoral robotic surgery for advanced oropharyngeal carcinoma. Arch Otolaryngol Head Neck Surg 2010;136(11):1079–1085
23. Desai SC, Sung CK, Jang DW, Genden EM. Transoral robotic surgery using a carbon dioxide flexible laser for tumors of the upper aerodigestive tract. Laryngoscope 2008;118:2187–2189
24. Pollei TR, Hinni ML, Moore EJ, et al Analysis of postoperative bleeding and risk factors in transoral surgery of the oropharynx. JAMA Otolaryngol Head Neck Surg 2013;139(11):1212–1218
25. Rivera-Serrano CM, Johnson P, Zubiate B, et al. A transoral highly flexible robot. Laryngoscope 2012;122(5):1067–1071
26. Shah BC, Buettner SL, Lehman AC, Farritor SM, Oleynikov D. Miniature in vivo robotics and novel robotic surgical platforms. Urol Clin North Am 2009;36(2):251–263
27. Desai SC, Sung C-K, Genden EM. Transoral robotic surgery using an image guidance system. Laryngoscope 2008;118(11): 2003–2005
28. Feichtinger M, Pau M, Zemann W, Aigner RM, Kärcher H. Intraoperative control of resection margins in advanced head and neck cancer using a 3D-navigation system based on PET/CT image fusion. J Craniomaxillofac Surg 2010;38(8):589–594
29. Jakobsohn K, Motiei M, Sinvani M, Popovtzer R. Towards realtime detection of tumor margins using photothermal imaging of immune-targeted gold nanoparticles. Int J Nanomedicine 2012;7:4707–4713
30. Keereweer S, Kerrebijn JDF, Mol IM, et al. Optical imaging of oral squamous cell carcinoma and cervical lymph node metastasis. Head Neck 2011;34(7):1002–1008

6 Robotic Reconstruction of the Oropharynx

Eric M. Genden

■ Description of the Clinical Problem

In the 1970s and 1980s, surgery was a common therapeutic approach for the management of oropharyngeal carcinoma. The lip-splitting incision combined with a mandibular osteotomy and pharyngotomy was necessary to gain access to the oropharynx. Although this approach provided excellent visualization, the morbidity of the approach is not insignificant.[1,2,3,4,5,6,7] The post-operative recovery was often extensive and, in some series, this approach was associated with major morbidity rates ranging from 20 to 48%.[8,9] Following a transmandibular approach, the ablative defect often required a regional or free flap reconstruction, extending the surgical time and further increasing the rate of morbidity. The extensive surgery associated with the transmandibular approach prompted the introduction of several clinical trials using primary radiotherapy (RT) and chemoradiotherapy (CRT). The goals of these trials were to achieve similar oncologic control but with less morbidity. In spite of the different treatment combinations, alcohol- and tobacco-related disease was associated with an aggressive biology and poor survival. The genetic changes and field cancerization associated with tobacco and alcohol are associated with disease-free survival rates seldom better than 50% for all sites and all stages. In the final analysis, nonsurgical trials did not demonstrate an improved overall survival nor did they minimize morbidity.

The last decade has been met with a new form of oropharyngeal disease: human papillomavirus (HPV)-associated squamous cell carcinoma. Distinct from tobacco- and alcohol-associated disease, HPV-associated carcinoma is a nonkeratinizing form of the disease that is characteristically basaloid, with poorly differentiated histology. In contrast to the tobacco-associated disease in which a zone of epithelial dysplasia can be found peripheral to the invasive carcinoma, HPV-associated disease is a focal disease with minimal peripheral epithelial dysplasia (**Fig. 6.1**). These findings may account, at least in part, for the excellent local control rates achieved with surgical resection.

The popularization of transoral approaches for the management of oropharyngeal carcinoma coincident with the epidemic of HPV-induced disease prompted resurgence in primary surgical treatment. Unlike open approaches, transoral approaches do not require a midline mandibulotomy or lip-splitting incision. Therefore, the operative time and surgical morbidity are reduced. Transoral approaches are also associated with a reduced rate of tracheostomy, gastrostomy tube dependence, and hospital length of stay. In spite of these advantages, there are shortcomings associated with this approach. Whether working under direct vision with a headlight or through a laryngoscope and a microscope, these techniques restrict both wide-field visual access and the ability to adequately and safely manipulate surgical instruments. Germaine to this discussion, defects that require reconstruction represent a specific challenge because of the restricted access. Through a transoral approach, it is difficult to both place sutures and perform a reconstruction because it is difficult to manipulate the tissue bimanually. Therefore, it is a challenge to suture the flap into place and ensure a water-tight closure. These limitations represent several of the shortcomings associated with transoral approaches, and arguably, these shortcomings have precluded the widespread adoption of non-robotic transoral laser microsurgery.

■ Current Standard Treatment

Until recently, the standard of care for the treatment of oropharyngeal carcinoma has been concurrent chemoradiotherapy. The 1991 Veterans Administration Laryngeal Cancer Study Group trial randomized patients with locally advanced larynx cancer to standard treatment with a laryngectomy followed by radiation or to the induction chemotherapy using cisplatin and 5-fluorouracil followed by radiation in chemotherapy responders. Survival proved equivalent in both arms, and 64% of patients randomized to the induction chemotherapy arm did not require laryngectomy. This study and several others inspired an era of nonsurgical management protocols throughout the 1990s and early 2000s. The data derived from these early laryngeal trials were applied to other head and neck sites like the oropharynx, a move that has been the subject of controversy. Many argue that oropharyngeal tumors are biologically distinct from the laryngeal malignancy and the data in the laryngeal trials cannot be reliably applied to other sites. We now know that although the oral cavity, oropharynx, and larynx may be close in anatomical proximity, the biology of these tumors is very different. Similarly, each site responds differently to therapy.

In spite of these controversies, concurrent chemoradiation was introduced as an organ preservation strategy for treatment of oropharynx carcinoma. It was proposed that this technique might provide superior functional outcomes with survival outcomes that were comparable to the combination of open surgery and adjuvant chemoradiation.[10] Since this concept was proposed, data have shown that concurrent chemoradiotherapy

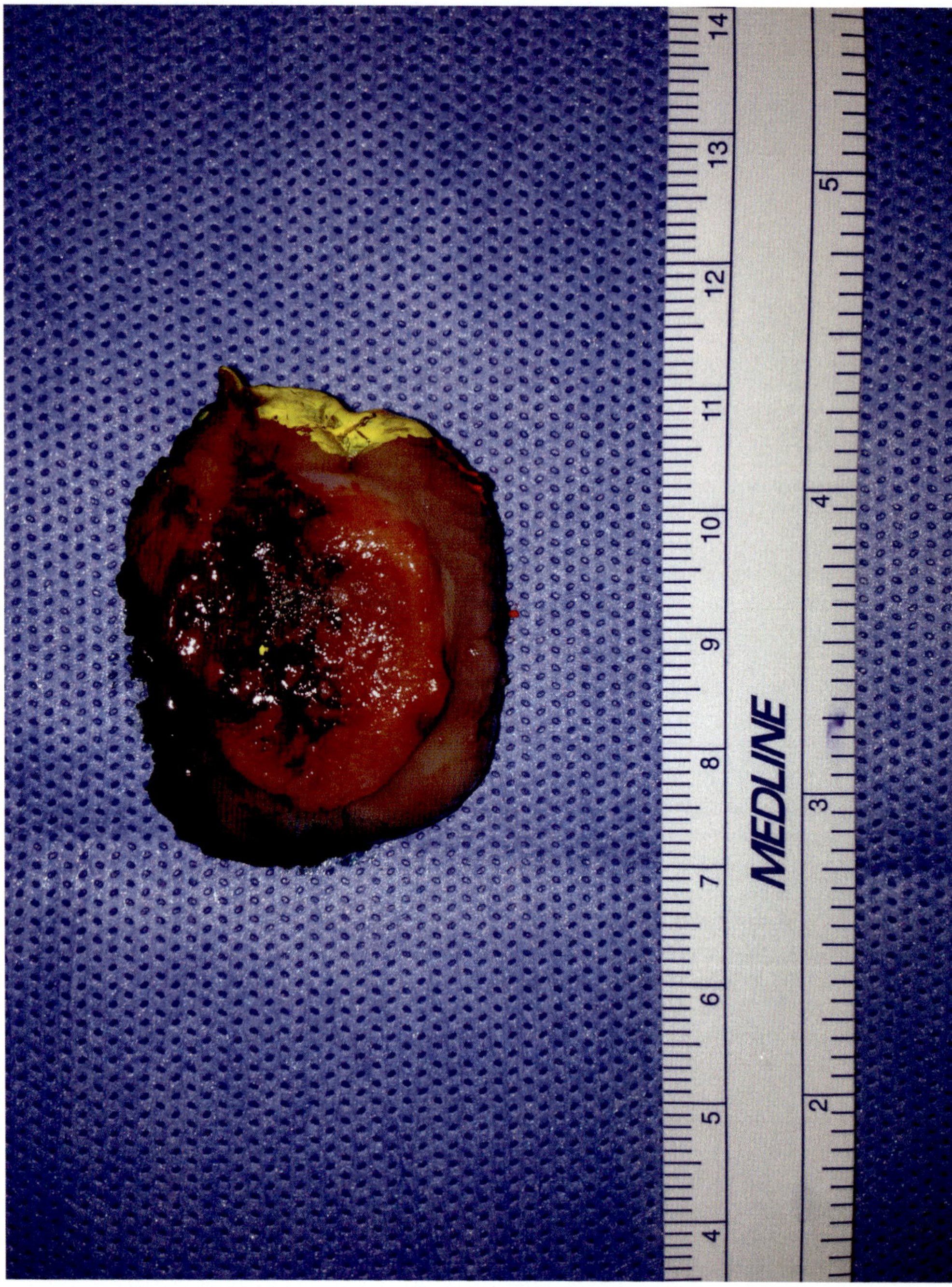

Fig. 6.1 While tobacco-related malignancy is typically associated with epithelial dysplasia that is peripheral to the carcinoma, human papillomavirus-associated disease is a focal disease with minimal peripheral epithelial dysplasia.

is associated with an unexpectedly high risk of late permanent toxicities including dysphagia and functional disturbances related to the therapy.[2,3,11] The growing numbers of patients with significant chronic treatment-related morbidity has prompted many to reconsider the use of primary chemoradiotherapy. This is particularly true given the rise in young patients presenting with HPV-positive disease. Treatment protocols that provide an opportunity to mitigate or reduce the dose of adjuvant radiotherapy would provide an advantage to this patient population by minimizing or mitigating the need for radiotherapy.

■ Benefits and Drawbacks of the Transoral Robotic Approach

If new surgical techniques are going to be adopted for the treatment of oropharyngeal carcinoma, at the very least, these approaches should achieve oncologic and or functional equipoise.

Transoral robotic surgery (TORS) has benefits and drawbacks. In several studies, TORS demonstrates superb functional outcomes and in many cases allows for deescalation or mitigation of adjuvant therapy.[12,13,14,15,16,17] Several reports demonstrate that TORS achieves functional outcomes that are equivalent or superior to those achieved following CRT.[12,14,17,18,19] Similarly, the oncologic outcomes are excellent.[14,15,17] While the U.S. Food and Drug Administration (FDA) approved TORS for the management of early stage oropharyngeal carcinoma, there has been an evolution to apply this technology to more advanced disease and in the salvage setting. Treating patients with advanced disease results in more extensive defects of the oropharynx that often involve multiple anatomical regions including the soft palate, tonsil, base of tongue, and pharynx. While TORS provides an excellent ablative approach for early oropharyngeal disease, larger tumors and larger defects represent a reconstructive dilemma. While smaller defects may heal by secondary intention, management of more extensive defects often requires reconstructive approaches that heretofore have not been applicable through the transoral approach. Until recently, the reconstruction of large oropharyngeal defects using regional or free tissue transfer required an open approach to gain access to the area. The mandibulotomy approach provides access required to achieve the defect reconstruction; however, the functional impairment associated with this approach is significant. Transoral reconstruction of extensive defects provides an excellent solution to the dilemma if a functional water-tight reconstruction can be reliably achieved. There is a paucity of data related to the benefits and drawbacks related to robotic-assisted reconstruction; however, the concept is gaining popularity. The potential to reconstruct extensive TORS-related defects using TORS techniques has the potential to advance the field of head and neck reconstruction.

■ Review of Available Data

There are four reconstructive techniques commonly applied to oropharyngeal defects following TORS. These include healing by secondary intention, local flap reconstruction, regional flap reconstruction, and free tissue transfer. Based on the current literature, most TORS defects are managed by secondary intention or local flap reconstruction. The options for local flap reconstruction include pharyngeal flaps, buccal fat pad flap, and the facial artery musculomucosal (FAMM) flap. The options for regional flap reconstruction include the submental island flap and the sternocleidomastoid (SCM) flap. Finally, the options for free tissue transfer include the radial forearm, anterolateral thigh, or tensor fascia lata flap (**Table 6.1**). Each option has an indication, and the best options are often determined by the expertise and biases of the operating surgeon. There are, however, some guidelines that may help achieve optimal outcomes.

Postablative defects associated with smaller tumors are generally managed with secondary intention; they can be left to remucosalize. This approach is used in the majority of small defects of the tonsillar fossa, tongue base, and pharynx. The primary advantage of healing by secondary intention is that the resulting remucosalized surface is sensate and therefore reduces the aspiration risk. It also preserves the functional dynamic

Table 6.1 Reconstructive options

Local flap	Regional flap	Free flap
Pharyngeal flap	Submental island flap	Radial forearm flap
Buccal fat pad flap	Sternocleidomastoid flap	Anterolateral thigh flap
Facial artery flap	Digastric flap	Tensor fascia flap

of the pharynx. In contrast, when the great vessels are exposed through an extensive neck-penetrating defect or the patient has been previously radiated, a more substantial reconstructive technique may be required. The goals of the reconstruction include closure of pharyngocervical communication, protection of great vessels, and reconstitution of the velopharyngeal complex (**Table 6.2**). Closure of the pharyngocervical communication and protection of the great vessels are critical to prevent a salivary fistula that can lead to a neck abscess or carotid rupture. Reconstitution of the velopharyngeal complex is important to preserve swallowing and speech.

The complex neuromuscular anatomy of the oropharynx is critical to speech and swallowing. Following TORS, alteration of the anatomy often disturbs both the oral and pharyngeal phases of swallowing. During the oral phase of swallowing, the tongue drives the food bolus back into the oropharynx. Concomitantly, the velopharyngeal sphincter provides the closure necessary to propel food downward toward the lower oropharynx. The oropharyngeal phase of swallowing relies on both the muscular drive of the tongue, the coordinated peristalsis of the upper pharynx, and the pressure gradients produced by adequate velopharyngeal closure and complex muscular coordination.[20] Any disruption in either the bulk or muscular contraction of the tongue will lead to dysphagia and/or dysarthria. Similarly, any disturbance in velopharyngeal competence or pharyngeal contraction will result in dysphagia. When possible, local tissue is always the best option for reconstruction. Reattachment of the muscular complex preserves a functional sphincter critical to velopharyngeal closure. In cases where the defect encroaches on the palate, velopharyngeal closure may be disturbed leading to velopharyngeal incompetence. Reconstruction of this defect can be achieved by reconstituting the velopharyngeal sphincter by reapproximating the posterior pharyngeal muscular–mucosal complex with the cut edge of the uvulopalatal complex (**Fig. 6.2**). The long-term results should provide a diminished velopharyngeal port that provides dynamic closure (**Fig. 6.3**).

Table 6.2 The goals of robot-assisted reconstruction

Goals	The rationale
Closure of pharyngocervical communication	Prevent salivary fistula and neck infection
Protection of great vessels	Prevent great vessel rupture
Reconstitution of the velopharynx	Prevent velopharyngeal insufficiency

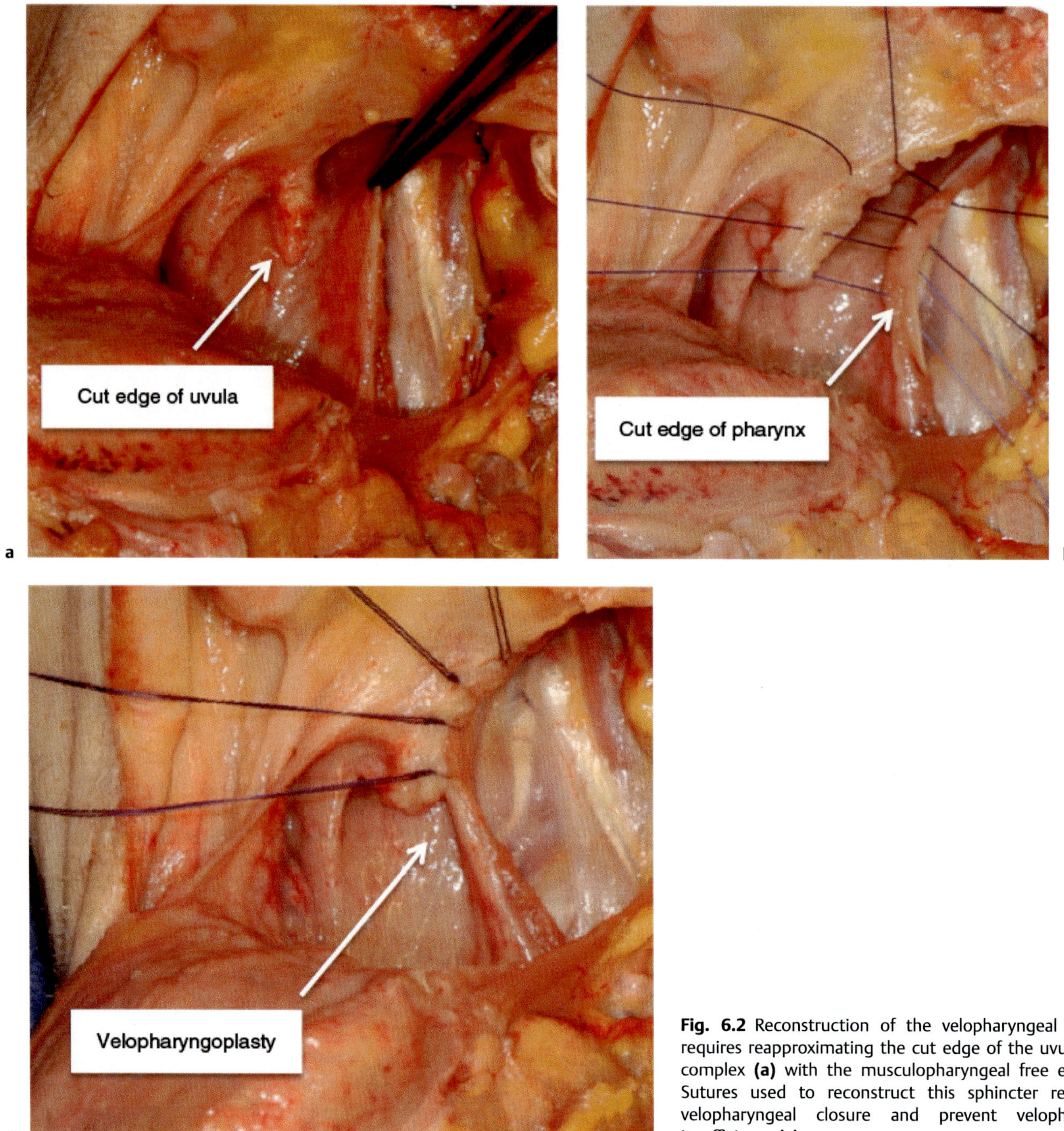

Fig. 6.2 Reconstruction of the velopharyngeal complex requires reapproximating the cut edge of the uvulopalatal complex **(a)** with the musculopharyngeal free edge **(b)**. Sutures used to reconstruct this sphincter reestablish velopharyngeal closure and prevent velopharyngeal insufficiency **(c)**.

Prior to the popularization of TORS, reconstruction of the oropharynx was necessary after open approaches to achieve separation of the visceral compartment from the neck, protect the great vessels, and restore function. The literature is replete with studies celebrating the impact of free tissue transfer on function, and the literature strongly suggests that free and pedicle flap reconstruction provides superior functional results when compared with primary closure, skin grafts, and adjacent tissue transfer for extensive defects.[1,21,22,23] However, less appreciated is the negative impact that nonsensate and adynamic free flaps have on function. Free tissue transfer is often necessary to partition the oropharynx from the neck, but paradoxically, the interposition of this tissue may hinder function because of the nonsensate adynamic nature of the flap. This highlights the importance of choosing the appropriate modality of reconstruction to ultimately achieve optimal functional outcomes.

The four questions to consider when evaluating the TORS defect for reconstruction include: (1) is the velopharynx intact; (2) are the great vessels exposed; (3) is there communication with the neck; and (4) has the patient previously been treated with radiotherapy? Considering these questions, we advocate a defect classification to guide our decisions on reconstruction.

The Classification for Oropharyngeal Robotic Defects (CORD) serves as a reconstructive algorithm[24] to guide and optimize

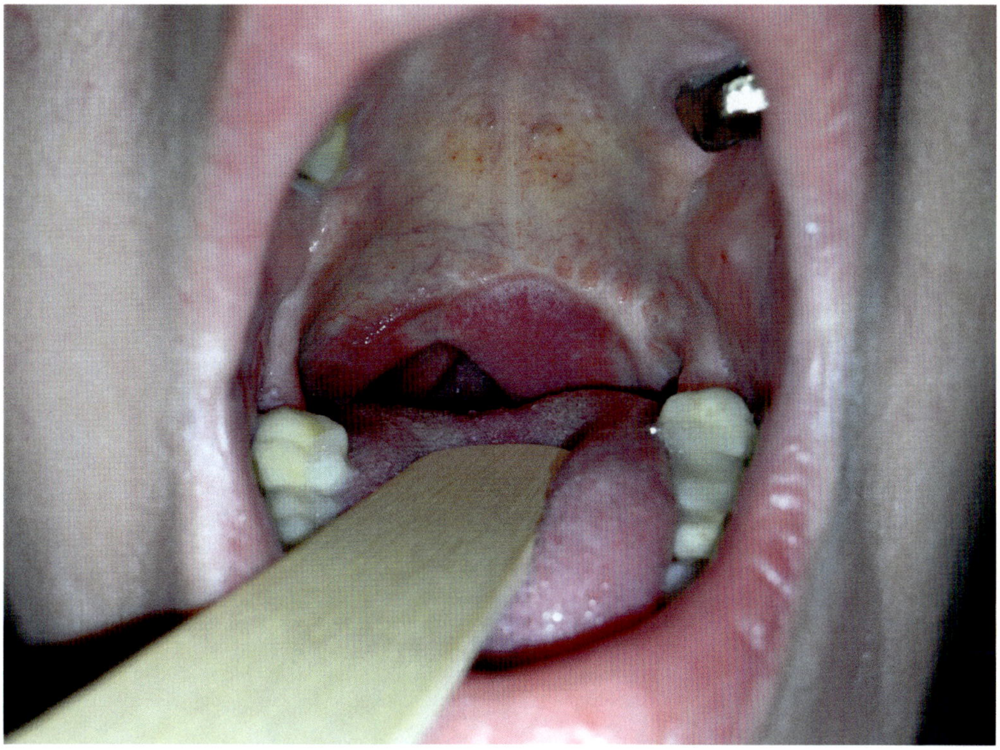

Fig. 6.3 Three months after velopharyngeal reconstruction, the nasopharyngeal port is well mucosalized and dynamic function has returned. The patient has no nasal escape or velopharyngeal insufficiency.

TORS reconstruction. This classification system is based on the site of the defect, number of subsites involved, exposure of the internal carotid artery, communication of the neck with the oropharynx, and the extent of the palatal resection. Defects are categorized into one of four classes in order of increasing complexity with higher classifications requiring more advanced reconstructive techniques. As with any reconstructive effort, reconstructive goals should include structural and functional considerations when reconstructing oropharyngeal defects following TORS. Structural considerations include preventing cervicopharyngeal fistulas by creating an adequate barrier separating the neck and pharynx and ensuring adequate coverage of the vascular structures of the neck. Functional considerations include restoration of swallowing function, preservation of speech and articulation, and maintaining velopharyngeal competence. The CORD system accounts for both functional and structural considerations by dividing defects into four classes.

Class I defects include any single subsite of the oropharynx without any complicating features such as carotid artery exposure, pharyngocervical communication, or extensive palatal defect (**Table 6.3**, **Fig. 6.4**). The majority of these defects are typically left to remucosalize secondarily and often do so with minimal functional morbidity. For tongue base defects, exposed deep intrinsic tongue muscles serve as the vascularized bed for remucosalization (**Fig. 6.5**, **Video 6.1**).

In posterior pharyngeal defects wherein the prevertebral fascia is exposed, mucosa will reline the area within several weeks. After pharyngectomy, fat from the parapharyngeal space provides vessel coverage and a surface for epithelialization. Small defects of the palate, however, may require a series of sutures to close the free edge of the remaining palate to the posterior pharyngeal wall, thus closing the enlarged nasopharyngeal aperture. The goal of this technique is to minimize velopharyngeal insufficiency to improve speech and swallowing. Our work on reconstituting the functional nasopharyngeal unit was based on the initial work published by Seikaly et al, who described reconstruction of the palate using a size-based classification system with defects classified into one of three categories.[25] For defects of less than one-fourth of the palate, they suggest primary closure of the palate to the posterior pharyngeal wall. In their series of 22 patients with small defects closed primarily, only one patient complained of nasopharyngeal

Table 6.3 Classification of oropharyngeal robotic defects

Classification	Defect characteristics
Class I	A defect involving one subsite of the oropharynx with no adverse features.[a]
Class II	A defect involving more than one subsite with no adverse features.
Class III	A defect involving only one subsite with adverse features.
Class IV	A defect involving more than one subsite with adverse features.

[a]Adverse features include carotid artery exposure, pharyngocervical communication, and/or a palatal defect that is greater than 50% of the palate.

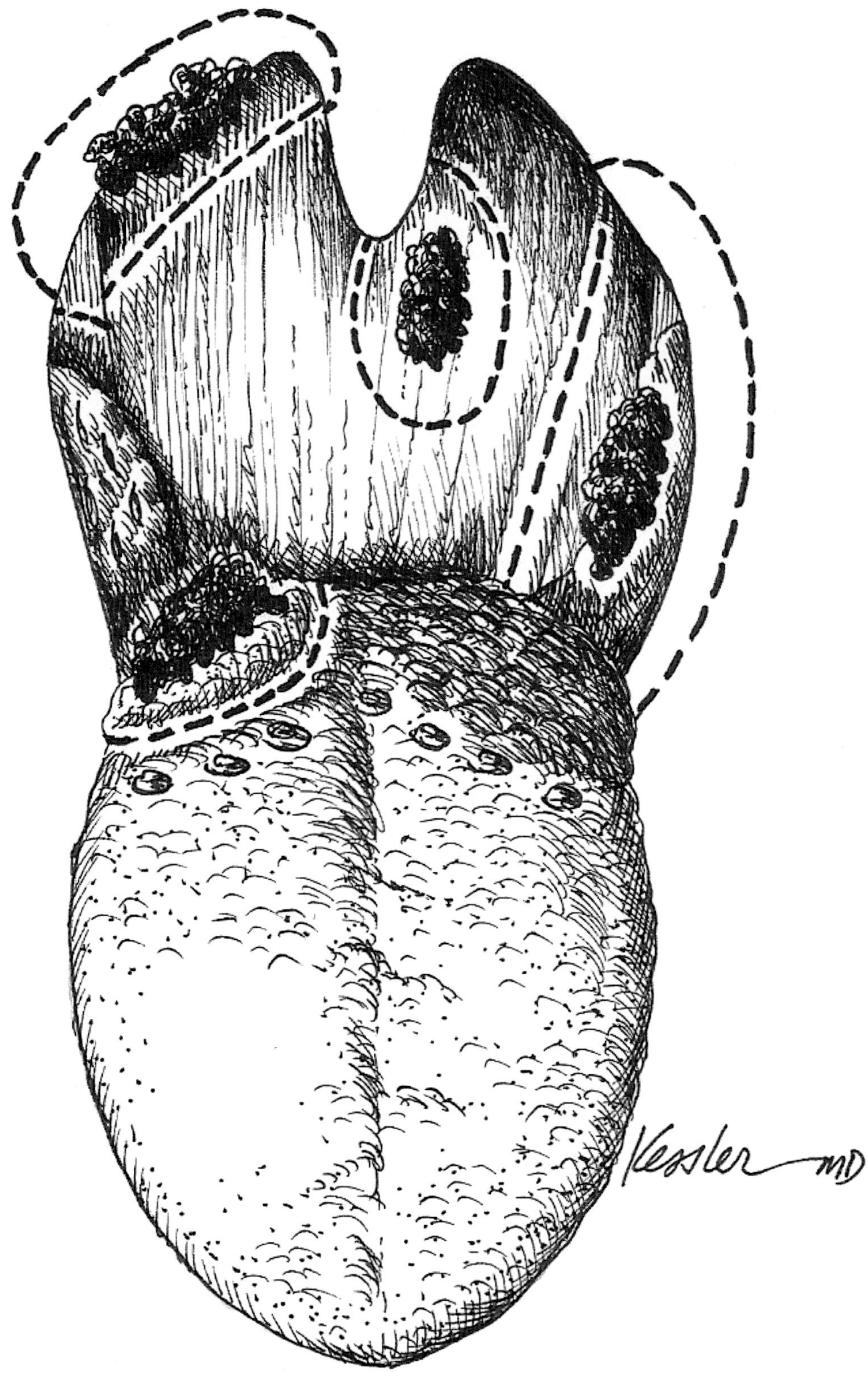

Fig. 6.4 Class I defects include any single subsite of the oropharynx without any complicating features such as carotid artery exposure, pharyngocervical communication, or extensive palatal defect. (Used with permission from de Almeida JR, Park RCW, Villanueva NL, Miles BA, Teng MS, Genden EM. Reconstructive algorithm and classification system for transoral oropharyngeal defects. Head Neck 2014;36(7):934–941.)

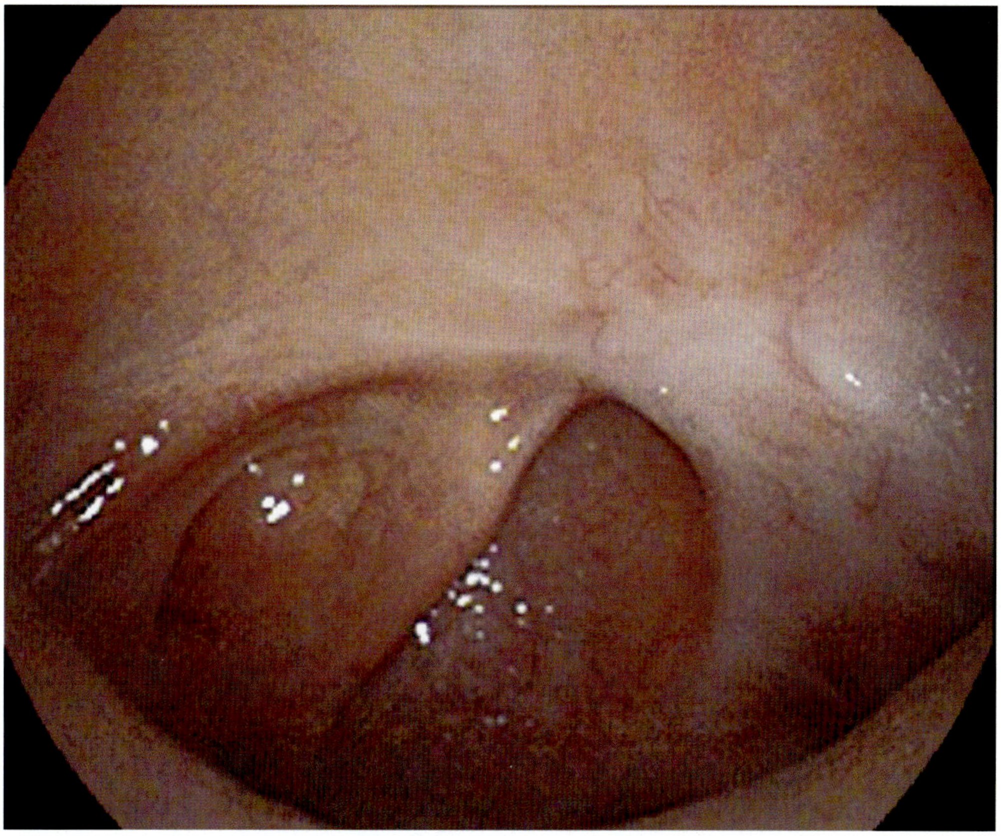

Fig. 6.5 The base of tongue and lateral pharynx will remucosalize after several weeks. This figure demonstrates defect of the pharynx and base of tongue 12 weeks following therapy. The surgical site has remucosalized.

regurgitation at 1 year after operation. In the same cohort, one patient remained gastric tube–dependent and three required nutritional supplementation. Our technique for velopharyngeal reconstruction as described in **Fig. 6.2** has proven effective and durable in our patient population. In over 300 patients treated with TORS for oropharyngeal carcinoma, the incidence of velopharyngeal incompetence is < 2% as measured by barium swallow and patient history.

Class II defects are similar to class I defects in that they have no complicating features; however, they are more advanced in that more than one subsite is involved (**Fig. 6.6**). Rarely do class II defects require a regional or free flap for reconstruction. Defects involving the tongue base extending into the tonsil are often left to heal secondarily.

For defects of the tonsillar–palatal complex, a local musculomucosal flap may be used to seal the nasopharyngeal port. This flap is typically based on the mucosa and the superior constrictor muscle of the posterior pharyngeal wall. A monopolar cautery or contact laser is typically mounted in one of the robotic arms and used to raise this flap in the submuscular plane carefully to avoid potential injury to the internal carotid artery. This flap can then be rotated toward the posterior edge of the palate and sutured in order to reduce the size of the nasopharyngeal port. This technique has been previously described by Gehanno[26] and has also been referred to as a superior constrictor advancement rotation flap. The advantage of this local flap is that it is theoretically a neurotized flap and can preserve the dynamic function of the constrictor muscles during swallowing.

Class III defects involve one subsite of the oropharynx but have adverse features such as internal carotid artery exposure, communication with the neck, or > 50% soft palate defect (**Fig. 6.7**). The author advocates regional or free flap reconstruction for class III defects. The rationale for this approach is based on the potential for a salivary fistula, contamination of the neck and great vessels, and great vessel rupture.

Class IV defects involve multiple subsites of the oropharynx and one or more of the adverse features including internal carotid artery exposure via the pharynx, communication with the neck, or > 50% soft palate defect (**Fig. 6.8**). We advocate regional or free flap reconstruction for class IV defects or smaller defects in patients who have received prior radiotherapy.

In a review of 92 TORS patients at Mount Sinai Medical Center in New York, the majority of the patients fell in the class II category (n = 45, 49%), while class I, III, and IV defects were seen in 34% (n = 31), 3% (n = 3), and 14% (n = 13), respectively.[27] The goals of TORS-assisted microvascular reconstruction are to patch the pharyngocervical communication, protect the great vessels, and manage extensive defects of the palate that would otherwise result in significant functional deficit.

■ Surgical Procedure

TORS-assisted microvascular reconstruction requires planning and a coordinated effort. Preoperative assessment is important

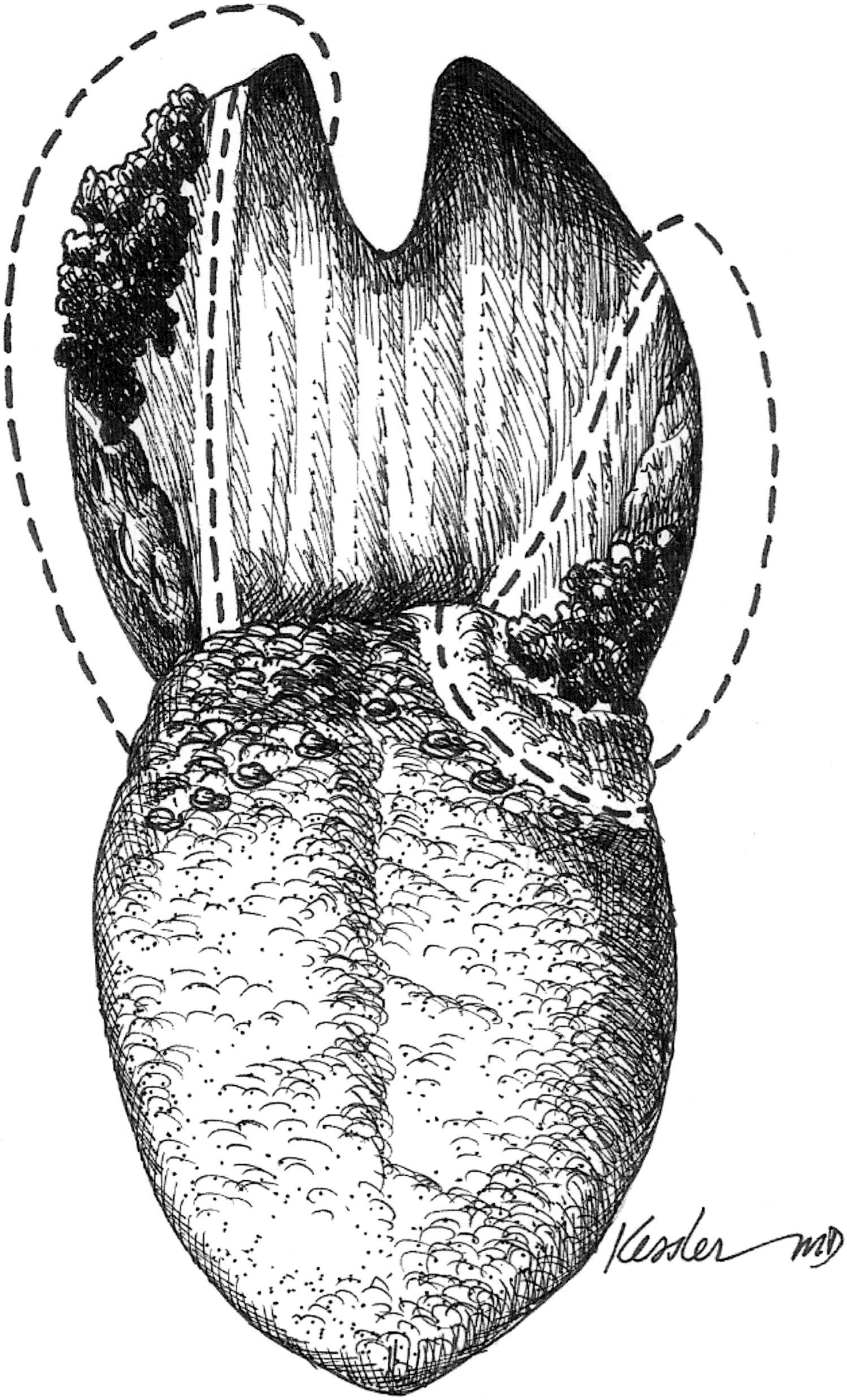

Fig. 6.6 Class II defects are similar to class I defects in that they have no complicating features; however, they are more advanced in that more than one subsite is involved. (Used with permission from de Almeida JR, Park RCW, Villanueva NL, Miles BA, Teng MS, Genden EM. Reconstructive algorithm and classification system for transoral oropharyngeal defects. Head Neck 2014;36(7):934–941.)

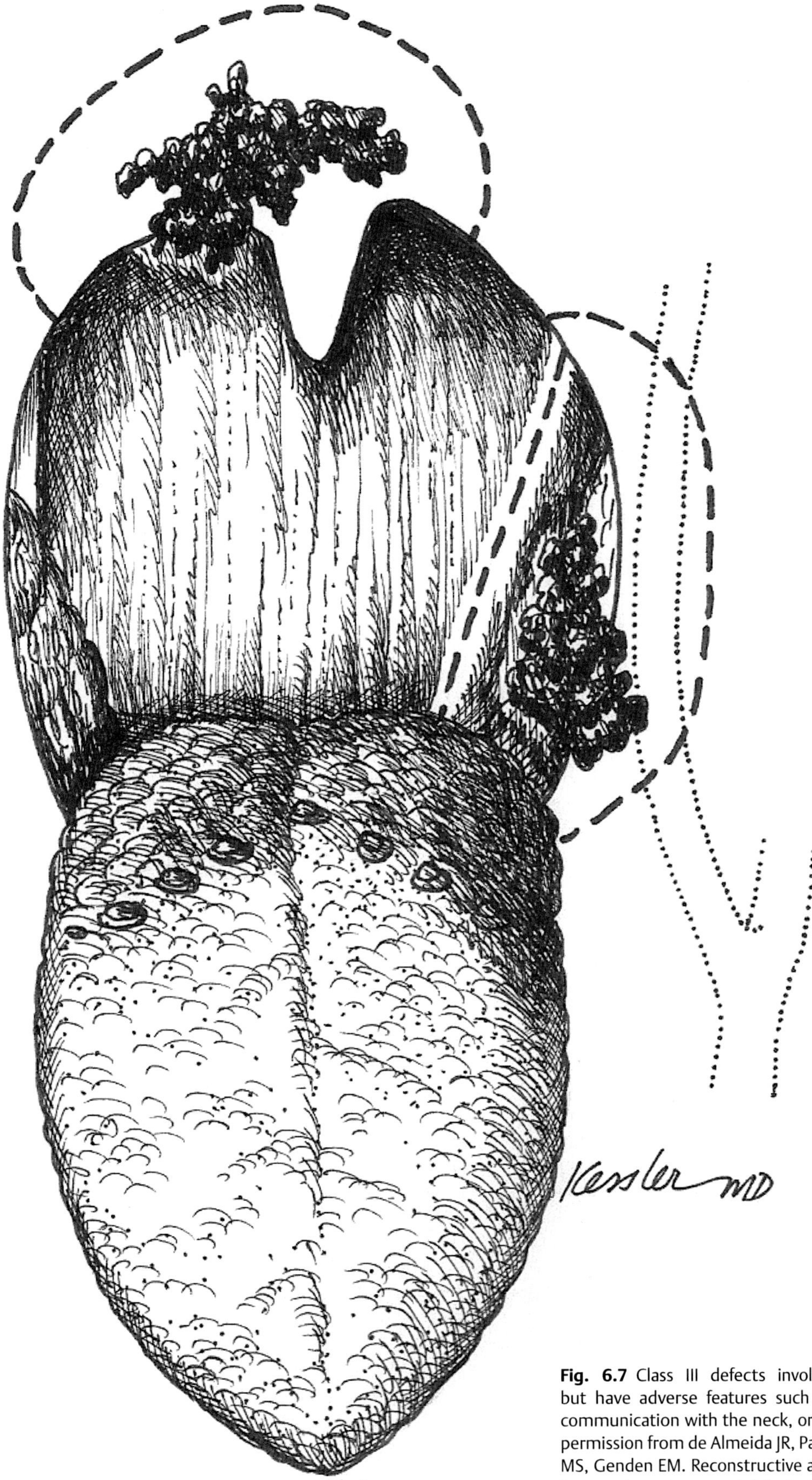

Fig. 6.7 Class III defects involve one subsite of the oropharynx but have adverse features such as internal carotid artery exposure, communication with the neck, or > 50% soft palate defect. (Used with permission from de Almeida JR, Park RCW, Villanueva NL, Miles BA, Teng MS, Genden EM. Reconstructive algorithm and classification system for transoral oropharyngeal defects. Head Neck 2014;36(7):934–941.)

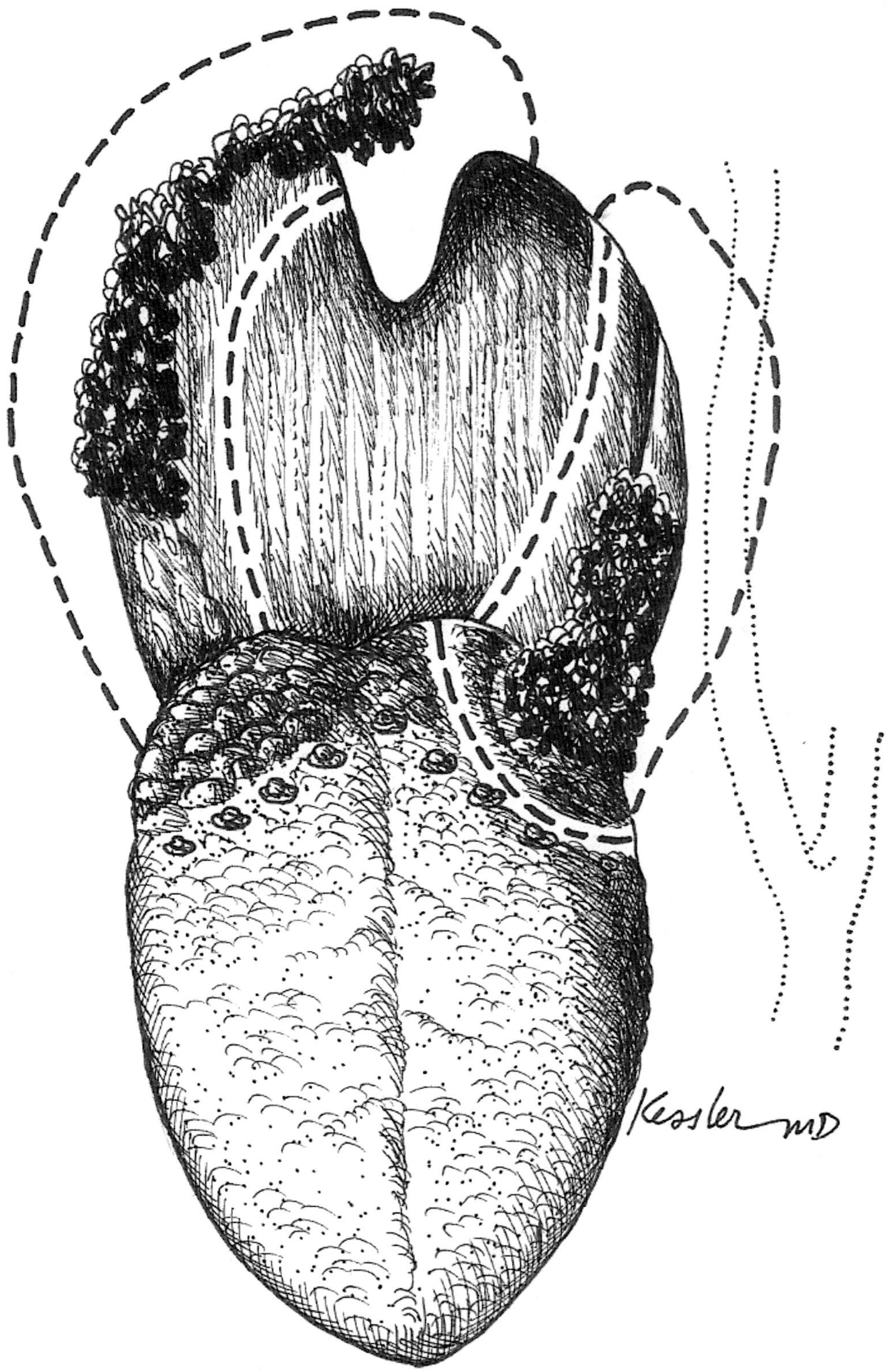

Fig. 6.8 Class IV defects involve multiple subsites of the oropharynx and one or more of the adverse features including internal carotid artery exposure via the pharynx, communication with the neck, or > 50% soft palate defect. (Used with permission from de Almeida JR, Park RCW, Villanueva NL, Miles BA, Teng MS, Genden EM. Reconstructive algorithm and classification system for transoral oropharyngeal defects. Head Neck 2014;36(7):934–941.)

in anticipating the defect. The use of gadolinium-enhanced magnetic resonance imaging as well as contrast-enhanced computed tomography may be necessary to assess the extent of tumor involvement of the oropharynx in those patients with suspected deep pharyngeal invasion. In those patients who are undergoing salvage surgery after radiotherapy who may sustain extensive defects of the oropharynx and require free tissue transfer, we start by selecting the optimal donor site. In most cases, the radial forearm donor site provides a source of thin and pliable tissue that can be manipulated to achieve the native contouring of the oropharynx. In select cases the anterolateral thigh or lateral arm or submental donor sites may be appropriate. Most importantly, preoperative coordination, the instrument setup, and room setup are critical. Ideally a large operating room (OR) should be utilized to provide space for robotic and microscopic instrumentation. We find that bringing the microscope into the room after resection of the primary tumor and neck dissection provides better logistical use of the OR space and prevents congestion.

For large tumors, we may perform the mucosal and pharyngeal muscle incisions around the tumor with the robot and then convert to a transcervical pharyngotomy to complete the inferior incisions and final resection. This provides a careful assessment of the deep margin by palpating the tumor through the neck in order to achieve safe inferior mucosal and deep margins. If a combined transcervical approach is warranted we then remove the patient from suspension and proceed with neck dissection, mobilization of the hypoglossal nerve and great vessels, and transcervical pharyngotomy with completion of the inferior resection. Alternatively, the complete tumor resection may be achieved transorally without conversion to a transcervical approach. Determining which of these two approaches is best suited is predicated on the anatomy of the patient, the exposure, and the ability to safely control the great vessels and the carotid branches during the course of the operation. If at any time we are unsure of our surgical position relative to the great vessels, we convert to a transcervical approach and ensure control of the great vessels.

Before completing the transoral resection, we robotically place a series of sutures along the inferior, lateral, and medial surgical margins. These sutures are left with the needles in place and will be used during the reconstruction to guide placement of the flap and ensure that there is a water-tight closure of the defect. Defects that are confined to the soft palate and the tonsil can be closed transorally with traditional transoral or robotic techniques often without the use of anchoring sutures. However, defects that extend inferiorly into the base of tongue, the glossotonsillar sulcus, or hypopharynx are more complex and require anchoring sutures. Occasionally, these sutures are placed transcervical to achieve a reliable distal mucosal closure. If the defect is very inferior we recommend placing the initial two or three sutures transcervical and then pushing the flap into the defect. This will allow for positioning of the vascular pedicle as it is tunneled into the neck as well.

The robot is then brought into place and the patient is suspended. If we decide that the defect can be closed with the robot completely then—using a 30-degree camera—the caudal aspect of the flap can be sutured to the adjacent native tissue of the hypopharynx (**Video 6.2**). Then complete inset of the flap is performed before microvascular anastomosis. Even in large defects that require prolonged suturing times with the use of the robot we establish flap inset in less than 90 minutes. When robotically tying knots, sutures should be trimmed to an approximate length of 10 cm to avoid tangling with instrumentation, which complicates robotic knot throwing. In tight spaces, urologic needles may be used, which have a smaller radius and aid dramatically in robotic suturing. We do recommend practice with robotic suturing prior to embarking on this technique. Experience with smaller defects can provide valuable practice time in preparation for robotic-assisted microvascular flap inset.

It is our experience the robot provides the access, visualization, and dexterity necessary to achieve complex microvascular reconstruction without the need for mandibulotomy. In more than half of the cases, a portion of the closure was achieved transcervically. This is often done to assure a reliable caudal closure. This is often accomplished by placing a series of sutures peripherally around the defect. The flap can then be placed into position and reliably sutured into the defect. Once the flap is inset, the microvascular anastomosis is performed.

Complication Avoidance and Management

When TORS is performed with a concomitant neck dissection, a pharyngocutaneous fistula may develop inadvertently or as part of the planned resection. A study by Moore and colleagues showed that 29% of patients had experienced a pharyngocervical communication intraoperatively while only 4% of these developed a permanent communication.[28] While some have advocated for a staged neck dissection to reduce the risk of fistula formation, tumors invading through the pharyngeal constrictor muscles may require a resection resulting in a surgically created fistula. Several techniques have been advocated for management of a fistula in the acute setting; however, in large defects or in patients who have received previous external beam radiotherapy, regional or free tissue transfer may represent the only reliable method of reconstruction. Flap reconstruction may be accomplished with the use of local muscle flaps such as the digastric muscle flap (**Figs. 6.9** and **6.10**) or the sternocleidomastoid muscle flap (SCM). The SCM flap can be harvested as a superior based flap (**Fig. 6.11**) and draped across the neck to achieve closure of the defect (**Fig. 6.12**).

These can be applied to the external neck component of the defect leaving the lumen to remucosalize. This technique is indicated for defects that do not expose the great vessels. When the great vessels are exposed, an epithelial-lined barrier between the pharyngeal lumen and the great vessels is ideal. Local flaps such as the submental island flap or free tissue transfer can provide the necessary reconstruction (**Figs. 6.13–6.16**).[29,30] Irrespective of the technique used to reconstruct the defect, it is important to separate the upper aerodigestive tract from the neck to prevent postoperative fistula and vascular complications associated with the great vessels of the neck.

(text continued on page 66)

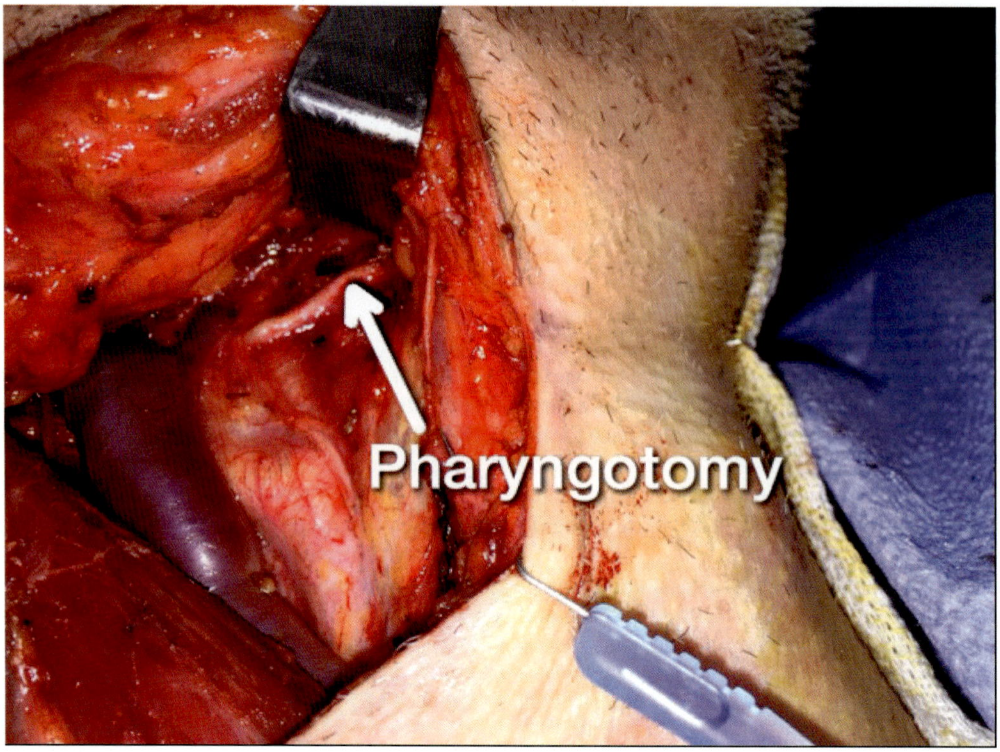

Fig. 6.9 Small pharyngotomy defects can be managed with a digastric flap.

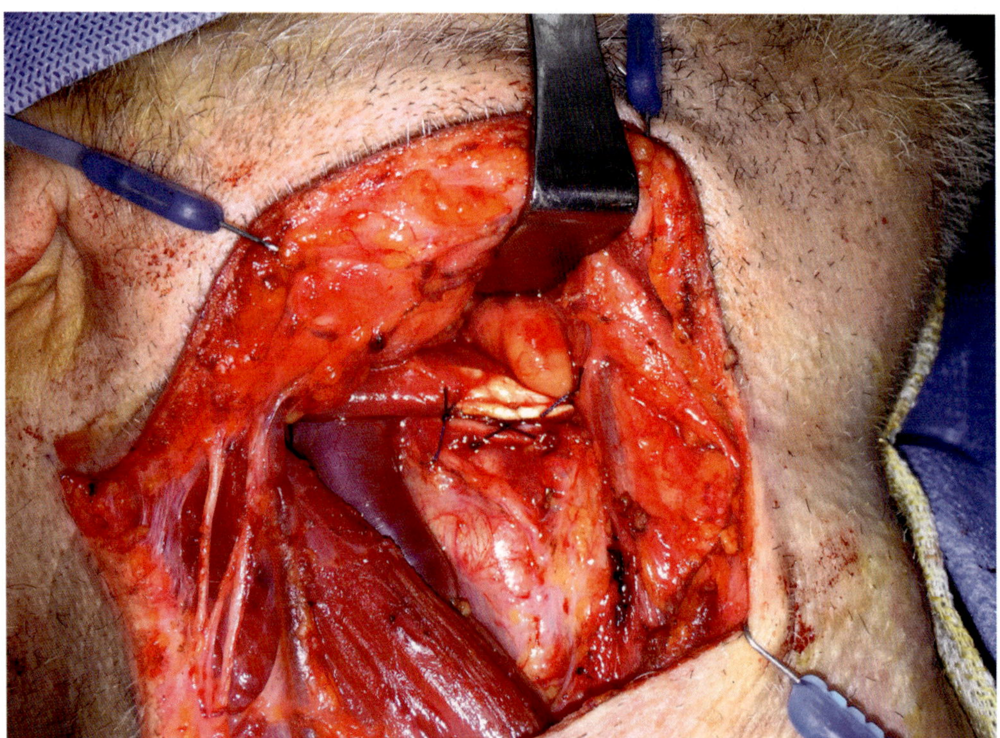

Fig. 6.10 The muscle is transposed over the defect to achieve closure of the fistula.

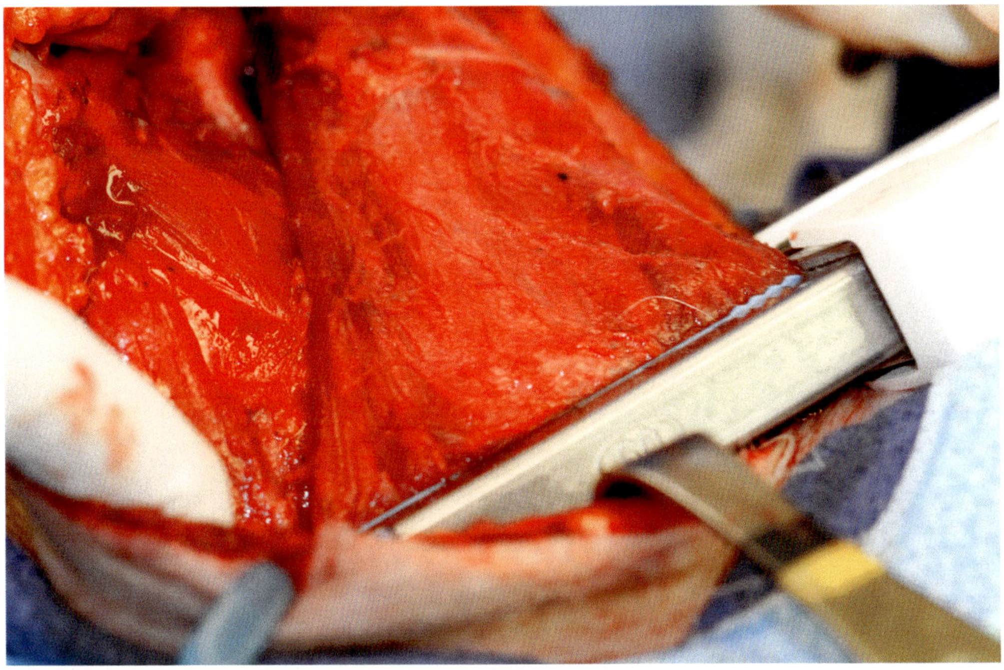

Fig. 6.11 Larger defects may require the sternocleidomastoid flap. The muscle flap is harvested using a stapling device to achieve a uniform muscle edge.

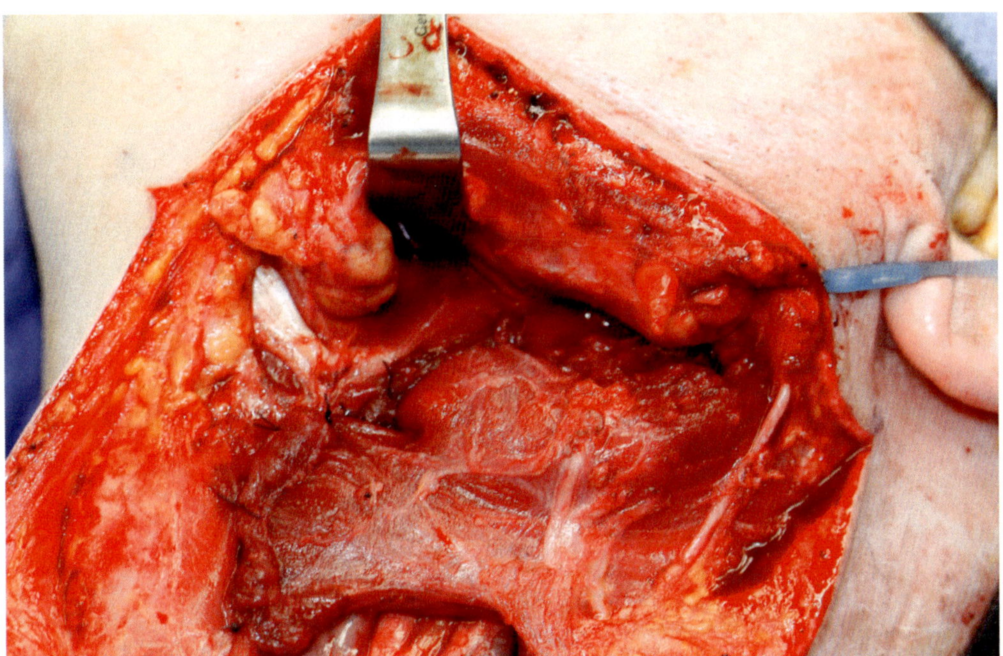

Fig. 6.12 The sternocleidomastoid flap. The superior vascular supply is kept intact to maintain blood supply to the flap. The flap can be transposed across the defect to manage the pharyngeal defect.

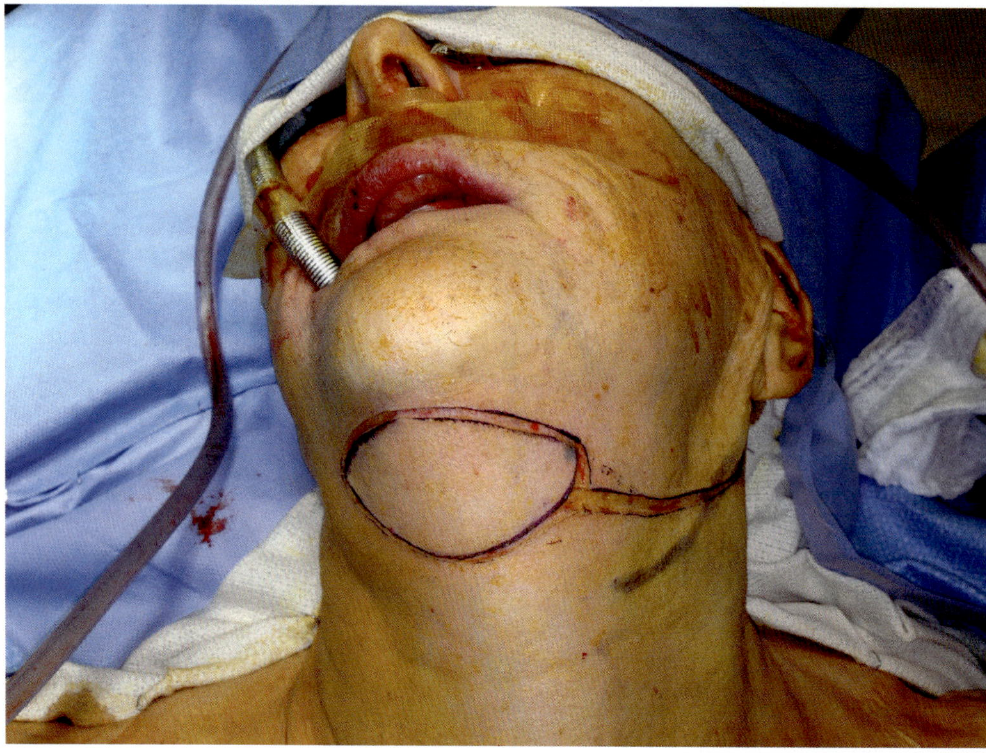

Fig. 6.13 More extensive defects can be managed with local flaps like the submental island flap.

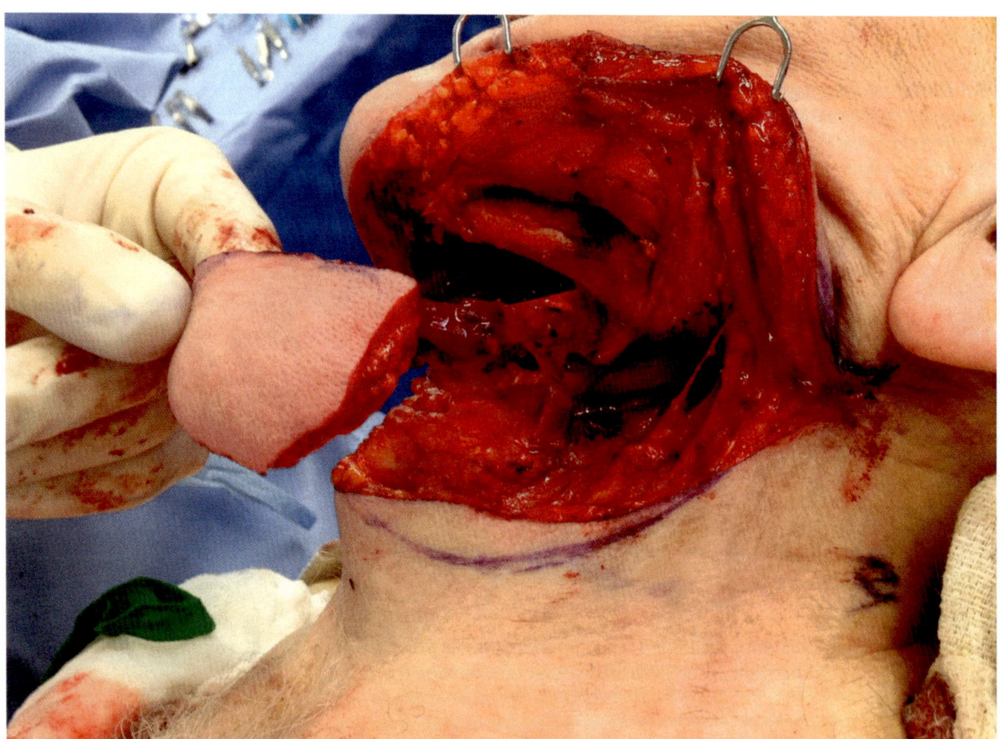

Fig. 6.14 The flap can be harvested according to the size of the defect.

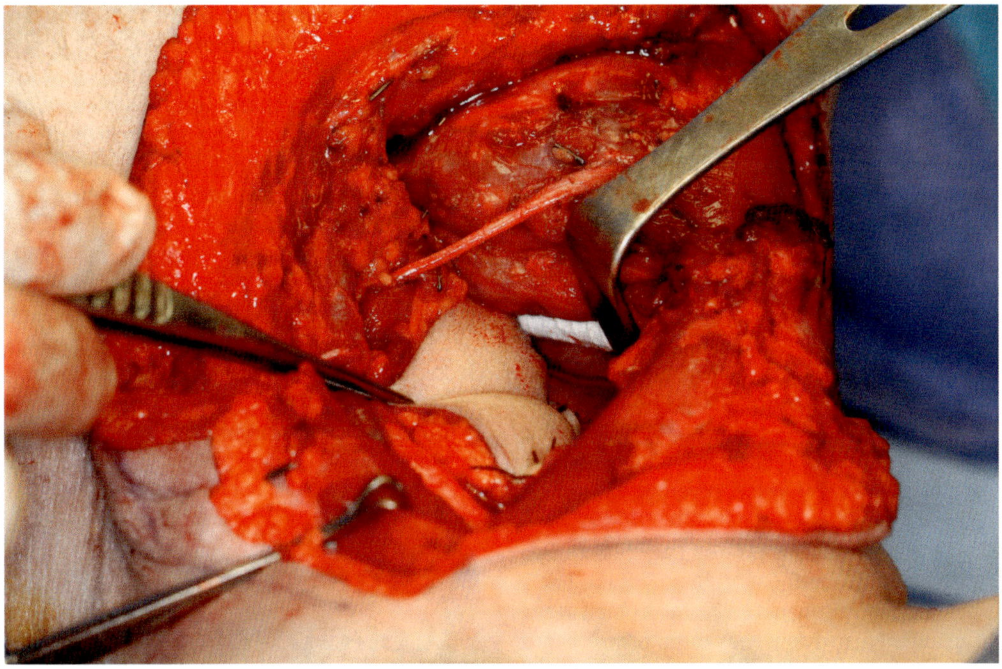

Fig. 6.15 The flap is then transposed into the defect and sutured into place using transcervical and transoral robotic–assisted sutures.

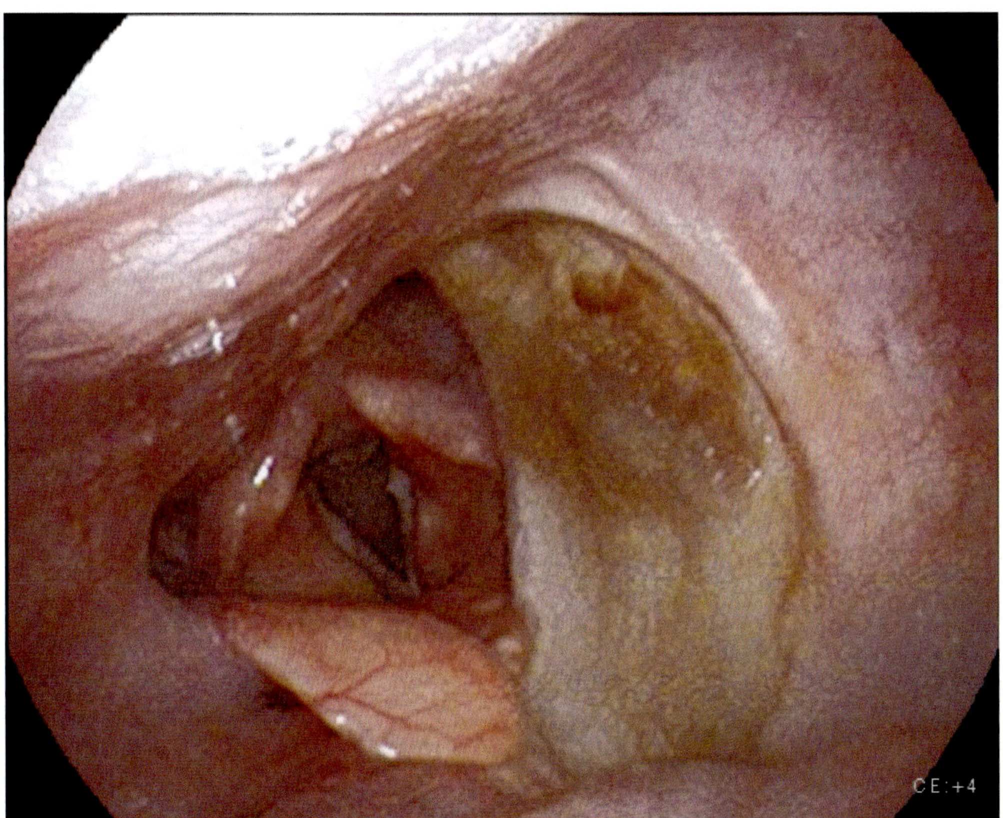

Fig. 6.16 Eight weeks following surgery, the flap is well healed and integrated into the pharynx.

Rupture of the carotid artery is a well-known complication following surgery when the great vessels are exposed to salivary contaminants and in the setting of prior external beam radiotherapy. It can occur in 3 to 14%[31,32] of patients after oropharyngeal surgery. In most cases of tonsil cancer resection, the parapharyngeal fat is left in place to protect the carotid artery and provide a vascularized surface or remucosalization. In advanced cancers of the pharynx, the fat pad may require resection resulting in exposure of the carotid artery. In such cases, it is important to provide coverage and protection of the great vessels. A recent electronic survey of TORS surgeons across the United States revealed the rate of postoperative hemorrhage to fluctuate between 2.5 and 4.5% in a total of 2,015 reported procedures. They also reported 6 deaths within 30 days after TORS—all from hemorrhage related to the surgery.[33] While the majority of these events are likely related to branches of the external carotid, the importance of vessel coverage cannot be underestimated.

Defects of the soft palate that involve more than 50% of the soft palate represent a unique functional problem.[21] It has been shown that such defects of the soft palate result in high rates of velopharyngeal insufficiency, dysphagia, and a compromise in quality of life.[34] These defects often require a velopharyngoplasty in addition to soft tissue reconstruction. The soft tissue coverage of the palatal defect is best achieved with a regional or free tissue transfer. This approach has proven effective in reestablishing speech and swallowing.[25]

The impact of external beam radiotherapy on wound healing has been well documented. In patients who have undergone prior external beam radiotherapy, transoral robotic salvage surgery can be fraught with complications if the surgical defect is not managed appropriately.[35] Because the tissue has been compromised and the wound healing is suboptimal, free tissue transfer provides an opportunity to interpose well-vascularized tissue into the defect. This approach has been shown to be safe and effective for the management of these complex wounds.[36] In contrast to the extensive defects described previously, we advocate the use of free tissue transfer for modest defects of the pharynx because of the high risk of fistula, great vessel exposure, and catastrophic complications. In our experience, failure to reconstruct these patients with free tissue transfer leads to adverse and uncontrollable scarring, high risk of fistula, and significant compromise and decreased functional performance.

Much of the data related to TORS-assisted free flap reconstruction is in the process of analysis, and initial data seem to indicate that the technique provides an excellent tool to manage complex and extensive defects of the oropharynx. Importantly, this technique mitigates the need for a mandibulotomy. However, data demonstrate that with the exception of the extensive soft palate defect, the functional performance following free tissue transfer is rarely equivalent to local musculomucosal flap reconstruction. Patients healing by secondary intention or reconstructed with local musculomucosal flaps perform significantly better than patients requiring a free flap reconstruction.[2,37] Older studies suggest the same finding when comparing speech and swallowing outcomes of oropharyngeal reconstruction with primary closure or secondary intention healing versus flap reconstruction.[38] Although the size of the defect and tumor stage have been well documented to impact functional outcome in open surgery, in the TORS group, age (> 50 years) and preoperative functional performance status had a significant impact on early (< 30 days) and long-term (> 30 days) function as assessed by the need for a gastrostomy.[39] As such, patients with potential indications for TORS-assisted free flap reconstruction should be counseled regarding the risk of gastrostomy dependence.

Our experience suggests that the risk of flap failure, fistula formation, or wound infection in the TORS-assisted free flap reconstruction group is not statistically different from age-matched, stage-matched, and performance-matched patients treated with open surgery. The length of hospital stay is less in the former group, and although not quantified, patients value an opportunity to forgo a mandibulotomy and lip-splitting incision.

■ Future Directions and Conclusion

TORS provides an outstanding opportunity to treat disease of the oropharynx, particularly in an era dominated by HPV-associated disease. Unlike tobacco-related carcinoma, the surrounding tissue rarely demonstrates field effect dysplasia and HPV-associated oropharyngeal carcinoma is commonly a focal entity. For this reason, HPV-associated disease is more amenable to surgical resection. Locoregional recurrence rates are significantly lower than documented in tobacco-related disease. Transoral surgical resection can be achieved through transoral laser microsurgery (TLM), TORS, or direct transoral approaches. While there are merits of each approach, TORS provides the unique ability to manipulate and suture tissue using a two-handed approach: the design of the robotic instrumentation provides the operator the advantage of the ability to manipulate the tissue with one instrument while driving the suture with the second instrument. Because of this unique advantage, TORS is the only transoral technique that allows for complex reconstruction of the deep oropharynx, supraglottic larynx, and base of tongue. TORS-assisted free flap reconstruction provides a reliable method to achieve a safe reconstruction without the functional and aesthetic disturbance associated with traditional transmandibular approaches. As discussed, the rate of short- and long-term gastrostomy dependence rises when free tissue reconstruction is required, and patients should be aware of this risk.

In its current form, the da Vinci robotic system (Intuitive Surgical, Inc.) has many limitations for head and neck reconstruction. Until the instrumentation is specifically designed for transoral application, the acute angles of approach necessary to access the deep recess of the hypopharynx limit what can be achieved. For this reason, we often place the caudal sutures using a combination of transcervical and transoral approaches. In spite of these limitations, TORS-assisted reconstruction holds great promise by obviating the need for a mandibulotomy. Future goals will be directed toward improved instrumentation and modifications in technique that provide improved access to the hypopharynx.

References

1. Rieger JM, Zalmanowitz JG, Li SY, Sytsanko A, Harris J, Williams D, Seikaly H. Functional outcomes after surgical reconstruction of the base of tongue using the radial forearm free flap in patients with oropharyngeal carcinoma. Head Neck 2007;29: 1024–1032
2. Logemann JA, Pauloski BR, Rademaker AW, McConnel FM, Heiser MA, Cardinale S, et al. Speech and swallow function after tonsil/ base of tongue resection with primary closure. J Speech Hear Res 1993;36:918–926
3. Jantharapattana K. Oncologic and functional outcomes in advanced laryngeal and hypopharyngeal cancer treated with concurrent chemoradiation versus primary surgery followed by adjuvant treatment. J Med Assoc Thai 2013;96:1164–1168
4. Suntornpong N, Sukkasem M, Uwattanasombat C, Samasanti N, Thephamongkol K. The effectiveness of clinical practice guideline for nasopharyngeal and oropharyngeal cancer to reduce acute treatment toxicity from concurrent chemoradiation. J Med Assoc Thai 2011;94:585–591
5. Barkati M, Fortin B, Soulieres D, Clavel S, Despres P, Charpentier D, et al. Concurrent chemoradiation with carboplatin-5-fluorouracil versus cisplatin in locally advanced oropharyngeal cancers: is more always better? Int J Radiat Oncol Biol Phys 2010;76: 410–416
6. Boscolo-Rizzo P, Stellin M, Fuson R, Marchiori C, Gava A, Da Mosto MC. Long-term quality of life after treatment for locally advanced oropharyngeal carcinoma: surgery and postoperative radiotherapy versus concurrent chemoradiation. Oral Oncol 2009;45:953–957
7. Machtay M, Rosenthal DI, Hershock D, Jones H, Williamson S, Greenberg MJ, et al. Organ preservation therapy using induction plus concurrent chemoradiation for advanced resectable oropharyngeal carcinoma: a University of Pennsylvania Phase II Trial. J Clin Oncol 2002;20:3964–3971
8. Dubner S, Spiro RH. Median mandibulotomy: a critical assessment. Head Neck 1991;13:389–393
9. Shah JP, Kumaraswamy SV, Kulkarni V. Comparative evaluation of fixation methods after mandibulotomy for oropharyngeal tumors. Am J Surg 1993;166:431–434
10. Gillespie MB, Brodsky MB, Day TA, Lee FS, Martin-Harris B. Swallowing-related quality of life after head and neck cancer treatment. Laryngoscope 2004;114:1362–1367
11. Bhayani MK, Hutcheson KA, Barringer DA, Lisec A, Alvarez CP, Roberts DB, et al. Gastrostomy tube placement in patients with oropharyngeal carcinoma treated with radiotherapy or chemoradiotherapy: factors affecting placement and dependence. Head Neck 2013;35:1634–1640
12. Hutcheson KA, Holsinger FC, Kupferman ME, Lewin JS. Functional outcomes after TORS for oropharyngeal cancer: a systematic review. Eur Arch Otorhinolaryngol 2015;272(2):463–471
13. Sinclair CF, McColloch NL, Carroll WR, Rosenthal EL, Desmond RA, Magnuson JS. Patient-perceived and objective functional outcomes following transoral robotic surgery for early oropharyngeal carcinoma. Arch Otolaryngol Head Neck Surg 2011; 137:1112–1116
14. Moore EJ, Olsen KD, Kasperbauer JL. Transoral robotic surgery for oropharyngeal squamous cell carcinoma: a prospective study of feasibility and functional outcomes. Laryngoscope 2009;119:2156–2164
15. Hurtuk A, Agrawal A, Old M, Teknos TN, Ozer E. Outcomes of transoral robotic surgery: a preliminary clinical experience. Otolaryngol Head Neck Surg 2011;145:248–253
16. Genden EM, Park R, Smith C, Kotz T. The role of reconstruction for transoral robotic pharyngectomy and concomitant neck dissection. Arch Otolaryngol Head Neck Surg 2011;137:151–156
17. Weinstein GS, O'Malley BW Jr., Cohen MA, Quon H. Transoral robotic surgery for advanced oropharyngeal carcinoma. Arch Otolaryngol Head Neck Surg 2010;136:1079–1085
18. Iseli TA, Kulbersh BD, Iseli CE, Carroll WR, Rosenthal EL, Magnuson JS. Functional outcomes after transoral robotic surgery for head and neck cancer. Otolaryngol Head Neck Surg 2009; 141:166–171
19. Weinstein GS, O'Malley BW Jr., Desai SC, Quon H. Transoral robotic surgery: does the ends justify the means? Curr Opin Otolaryngol Head Neck Surg 2009;17:126–131
20. Giraldez-Rodriguez LA, Johns M 3rd. Glottal insufficiency with aspiration risk in dysphagia. Otolaryngol Clin North Am 2013; 46:1113–1121
21. Seikaly H, Rieger J, Wolfaardt J, Moysa G, Harris J, Jha N. Functional outcomes after primary oropharyngeal cancer resection and reconstruction with the radial forearm free flap. Laryngoscope 2003;113:897–904
22. Bozec A, Poissonnet G, Chamorey E, Laout C, Vallicioni J, Demard F, et al. Radical ablative surgery and radial forearm free flap (RFFF) reconstruction for patients with oral or oropharyngeal cancer: postoperative outcomes and oncologic and functional results. Acta Otolaryngol 2009;129:681–687
23. Arce K, Bell RB, Potter JK, Buehler MJ, Potter BE, Dierks EJ. Vascularized free tissue transfer for reconstruction of ablative defects in oral and oropharyngeal cancer patients undergoing salvage surgery following concomitant chemoradiation. Int J Oral Maxillofac Surg 2012;41:733–738
24. de Almeida JR, Genden EM. Robotic assisted reconstruction of the oropharynx. Curr Opin Otolaryngol Head Neck Surg 2012;20:237–245
25. Seikaly H, Rieger J, Zalmanowitz J, Tang JL, Alkahtani K, Ansari K, et al. Functional soft palate reconstruction: a comprehensive surgical approach. Head Neck 2008;30:1615–1623
26. Gehanno P, Guedon C, Veber F, Perreau P, Alalouf P, Moisy N. Velopharyngeal rehabilitation after transmaxillary buccopharyngectomy extending to the soft palate. Ann Otolaryngol Chir Cervicofac 1985;102:135–137
27. de Almeida JR, Park RC, Villanueva NL, Miles BA, Teng MS, Genden EM. A reconstructive algorithm and classification system for transoral oropharyngeal defects. Head Neck 2014;36(7): 934–941
28. Moore EJ, Olsen KD, Martin EJ. Concurrent neck dissection and transoral robotic surgery. Laryngoscope 2011;121:541–554
29. Selber JC, Robb G, Serletti JM, Weinstein G, Weber R, Holsinger FC. Transoral robotic free flap reconstruction of oropharyngeal defects: a preclinical investigation. Plast Reconstr Surg 2010;125:896–900
30. Perrenot C, Berengere P, Mastronicola R, Gangloff P, Dolivet G. Infrahyoid myocutaneous flap for reconstruction after robotic transoral surgery for oropharyngeal tumors. Plast Reconstr Surg 2014;133:236e–237e
31. Marks JE, Freeman RB, Lee F, Ogura JH. Pharyngeal wall cancer: an analysis of treatment results complications and patterns of failure. Int J Radiat Oncol Biol Phys 1978;4:587–593
32. Righini CA, Nadour K, Faure C, Rtail R, Morel N, Beneyton V, et al. Salvage surgery after radiotherapy for oropharyngeal cancer. Treatment complications and oncological results. Eur Ann Otorhinolaryngol Head Neck Dis 2012;129:11–16
33. Chia SH, Gross ND, Richmon JD. Surgeon experience and complications with Transoral Robotic Surgery (TORS). Otolaryngol Head Neck Surg 2013;149:885-892

34. Rieger J, Dickson N, Lemire R, Bloom K, Wolfaardt J, Wolfaardt U, et al. Social perception of speech in individuals with oropharyngeal reconstruction. J Psychosoc Oncol 2006;24:33–51
35. Teknos TN, Myers LL, Bradford CR, Chepeha DB. Free tissue reconstruction of the hypopharynx after organ preservation therapy: analysis of wound complications. Laryngoscope 2001;111:1192–1196
36. Fung K, Teknos TN, Vandenberg CD, Lyden TH, Bradford CR, Hogikyan ND, et al. Prevention of wound complications following salvage laryngectomy using free vascularized tissue. Head Neck 2007;29:425–430
37. Pauloski BR, Logemann JA, Rademaker AW, McConnel FM, Stein D, Beery Q, et al. Speech and swallowing function after oral and oropharyngeal resections: one-year follow-up. Head Neck 1994;16:313–322
38. McConnel FM, Pauloski BR, Logemann JA, Rademaker AW, Colangelo L, Shedd D, et al. Functional results of primary closure vs flaps in oropharyngeal reconstruction: a prospective study of speech and swallowing. Arch Otolaryngol Head Neck Surg 1998;124:625–630
39. Dziegielewski PT, Teknos TN, Durmus K, Old M, Agrawal A, Kakarala K, et al. Transoral robotic surgery for oropharyngeal cancer: long-term quality of life and functional outcomes. JAMA Otolaryngol Head Neck Surg 2013;139:1099–1108

7 The Prevention and Management of Complications in Robotic Surgery for Malignancy

Julia A. Crawford, Hilliary N. White, and J. Scott Magnuson

■ Introduction

Transoral robotic surgery (TORS) is an emerging treatment option in the management of head and neck malignancy, particularly for oropharyngeal squamous cell carcinoma (OPSCC). The publication of the Department of Veterans Affairs report in 1991 shifted the paradigm of treatment for head and neck tumors from surgical intervention to primary chemoradiotherapy. This report showed that the morbidity associated with chemoradiotherapy was considerably less than with surgical intervention.[1] This was reinforced by a meta-analysis by Parsons et al that found similar oncologic outcomes for patients treated with either primary surgery or chemoradiotherapy but a much higher morbidity in those treated with primary surgery.[2]

Over the past decade, however, the epidemiology of OPSCC has changed to p16- or human papillomavirus (HPV)- positive tumors. The affected patients present at a predominantly younger age and have a better long-term survival compared to those patients who have HPV-negative tumors.[3,4,5] There is significant long-term morbidity associated with primary chemoradiotherapy, and the aim of minimally invasive surgery for head and neck carcinomas has been the desire to offer a less morbid alternative to chemoradiation without compromising local and regional tumor control rates.[6,7]

These minimally invasive surgical approaches have included transoral laser microsurgery (TLM) and, in more recent years, TORS.[8,9,10,11,12,13,14] In contrast to traditional open surgical resection, these endoscopic procedures provide excellent oncologic outcomes while preserving speech and swallowing function.[15,16,17] With appropriate adjuvant therapy, early studies have shown that TORS can achieve equivalent oncologic results when compared to other surgical and nonsurgical treatments while also achieving excellent functional outcomes. The key to preserving function of the oropharynx is to minimize damage to the surrounding musculature and motor and sensory nerves of the pharynx. One of the main advantages of TORS is that it produces minimal disruption to these structures.[16,17]

With any new technique, however, it is important to understand both the prevention and management of any potential complications. This chapter aims to identify the preoperative, intraoperative, and postoperative complications that may occur during the application of TORS for malignancy.

■ Applied Anatomy

One of the keys to avoiding complications is to have a thorough understanding of the anatomy that may be encountered during surgery. The transoral approach to the oropharynx needs a significantly different conceptual understanding to the open approach. This "inside-out" approach is different than the traditional open approach, and an understanding, particularly of the vascular and neurologic anatomy, will help prevent both intraoperative and postoperative complications.

Limited Pharyngectomy

For TORS of the oropharynx, the first muscular landmark of importance is the superior pharyngeal constrictor muscle with the underlying buccopharyngeal fascia. Deep to this buccopharyngeal fascia lies the medial pterygoid superiorly and parapharyngeal space more inferiorly. The internal carotid artery is protected in the region of the parapharyngeal space only by a layer of parapharyngeal fat and pulsations can often be appreciated in this region. The surgeon should avoid dissecting lateral to the pharyngeal fat pad so as not to encounter the internal carotid artery. Additionally, it is important to spare the fat pad in order to provide protection to the carotid arterial system postoperatively.[18]

The next important landmarks are the stylopharyngeus and styloglossus that form the styloid diaphragm. Most vascular structures lie lateral to these muscles. The stylopharyngeus muscle spans from the base of the styloid process lateral to the superior constrictor before passing between the superior and middle constrictor muscles to attach onto the posterior border of the thyroid cartilage and the palatopharyngeus muscle. The styloglossus muscle is positioned more superficially and laterally to the stylopharyngeus and arises from the inferior and lateral edge of the styloid process, broadening out as it descends to insert into the lateral aspect of the tongue. Following identification of these muscles, the surgeon will typically encounter the tonsillar branch of the glossopharyngeal nerve; this often courses between the two muscles. The vascular supply of this area arises from the external carotid artery and its branches, including the facial, lingual, ascending pharyngeal, and internal maxillary arteries.

The lingual nerve may also be encountered during lateral dissection so it is important to have a conceptual understanding of its inside-out location. The lingual nerve is one of the branches of the posterior division of the mandibular nerve and while initially deep to the lateral pterygoid, as it descends inferiorly it lies on the medial pterygoid anterior to the inferior alveolar nerve passing under the free lower border of the superior constrictor muscle. From here it runs anteriorly on the mylohyoid muscle, grooving the lingual plate of the mandible just below the last molar tooth. It is this location, as it lies directly on the mandible heading anteriorly on mylohyoid, that is most at risk during TORS.

Base of Tongue Resection

The pharyngeal part of the tongue is covered by lymphoid tonsillar tissue and this is contiguous with the palatine tonsil at the glossotonsillar sulcus. Immediately deep to this tissue lies the intrinsic tongue musculature. The main issue when considering the vasculature of the base of tongue is to understand the course of the lingual artery and its branches. It arises from the external carotid artery at the level of the hyoid bone and continues lateral to the middle constrictor muscle until the hypoglossal nerve crosses it. From here it passes deep to the hyoglossus muscle and runs along the superior surface of the hyoid bone. It is in this location that it will most likely be encountered during TORS. At this juncture it divides into four branches. The most important branch for consideration in TORS is the dorsal lingual artery that predominantly supplies the base of tongue.

Supraglottic Laryngectomy

The dissection in supraglottic laryngectomy (SGL) typically begins at the lateral pharyngoepiglottic fold and immediately deep to this lies the fibers of the middle constrictor muscles. The dissection continues medial to the hyoid bone and the superior laryngeal vascular bundle is predictably encountered early in the dissection. This bundle lies inferior and anterior to the greater cornu of the hyoid bone and anterior to the superior horn of the thyroid cartilage. The branches of the superior laryngeal artery (SLA) that are clinically important to a supraglottic laryngectomy are the superior branch that runs along the aryepiglottic fold to the epiglottis and the anterior branch that runs through the superior portion of the paraglottic space toward the superior border of the thyroid cartilage. It is important to manage these with endoscopic clips as secondary hemorrhage can be severe.[19]

■ Preoperative Assessment

For TORS, there are specific considerations that affect the feasibility of robotic surgical intervention. A detailed preoperative assessment can limit the number of complications encountered during surgery. Access to the tumor can be an issue for TORS and physical examination to assess limitations to access and tumor resectability is an important first step to avoiding intraoperative complications. Any degree of trismus and limitation to neck extension should be assessed prior to intervention. Even a mild degree of trismus could indicate extension beyond the superior constrictor muscles into the pterygoid musculature. Additionally, on palpation, the tumor should not be fixed to the lateral tissues as this may also indicate extension of the tumor beyond surgical resectability. Radiographic imaging, such as computed tomography or magnetic resonance, may aid in determining the degree of infiltration of the tumor into adjacent structures.

■ Indications and Contraindications for Transoral Robotic Surgery

Oropharyngeal Malignancy

The primary indication for TORS is any biopsy-proven squamous cell carcinoma of the oropharynx where there is adequate intraoral access. Currently, the U.S. Food and Drug Administration (FDA) has approved TORS for T1 and T2 stage benign and malignant tumors only. The contraindications for TORS can be relative and absolute and then further broken down into tumor- and nontumor-related reasons.

The relative contraindications to TORS relate to access issues and whether the resultant TORS defect will leave the patient with significant morbidity. If the patient has poor mouth opening or significant macroglossia, micrognathia, or retrognathia this may make intraoral access difficult. If the tumor has a large soft palate component and resection could result in significant long-standing velopharyngeal insufficiency then other treatment options should be considered. If preoperative imaging is highly suspicious for extracapsular lymph node spread and the patient is likely to require postoperative chemoradiotherapy regardless of the surgical pathology, then primary nonsurgical therapy should be considered. Absolute contraindications include locally advanced tumors involving bone, extrinsic muscles of the tongue, prevertebral muscles, or the carotid, and unresectable neck disease. Nontumor-related absolute contraindications include significant medical comorbidities that increase anesthesia risk or increase post surgical risk. The need for anticoagulation may relatively impact on the decision to pursue a surgical route.

Indications for oropharyngeal malignancy TORS are:

- Biopsy-proven squamous cell carcinoma of the oropharynx
- T1, T2 stage tumors (FDA)

Relative contraindications for oropharyngeal malignancy TORS are:

- Anatomical limitations to intraoral access
- Anatomical limitations to neck extension
- Aberrant carotid artery anatomy
- Medical contraindications to transoral surgery in which an open wound heals by secondary intention
- Resultant defect after resection that limits patient's speech and/or swallowing
- Likely treatment requiring chemoradiotherapy

Absolute contraindications for tumor-related oropharyngeal malignancy TORS are:

- Stage IVC disease
- Pharyngeal involvement requiring resection of > 50% of the posterior pharyngeal wall
- T4a disease with mandibular or hard palate invasion, medial pterygoid involvement with resultant trismus, or deep involvement of the tongue base to the level of the genioglossus
- Radiological evidence of carotid artery involvement

- Fixation on palpation with radiological evidence of invasion lateral to the constrictors or posterior into the prevertebral fascia
- Unresectable neck disease

Absolute contraindications for nontumor-related oropharyngeal malignancy TORS are:

- Medical contraindications for either general anesthesia or surgery

Supraglottic Laryngectomy

Similarly to tumors of the oropharynx, the indication for an SGL is any patient with a biopsy-proven T1 or T2 stage tumor of the supraglottis. Relative contraindications relate to the accessibility of the tumor secondary to patient anatomy. A limited subset of T3 tumors, those without vocal cord fixation, or invasion of the thyroid cartilage may be considered for robotic surgical treatment. The absolute contraindications for SGL are patients who have an FEV_1/FVC ratio of < 50% and patients with locally advanced tumors or unresectable neck disease.

Indications are:

- Biopsy-proven squamous cell carcinoma of the oropharynx
- T1, T2 stage tumors (FDA approval)

Relative contraindications are:

- T3 tumors
- Tumors with minimal pyriform sinus involvement
- Limited transoral exposure

Absolute contraindications are:

- Poor pulmonary reserve
- Involvement of the thyroid cartilage or anterior commissure
- Vocal cord fixation or paraglottic space invasion
- Bilateral arytenoid cartilage involvement
- Tumor extension into pyriform apex or postcricoid mucosa
- Unresectable neck disease

Intraoperative Complications

Bleeding

The high-definition, three-dimensional (3D) optics available with the robotic system allow for clear identification of the different tissue. The enhanced visualization aids in the identification and dissection of vessels from surrounding muscles and fascia. As the best principle to overcoming bleeding is avoidance, an understanding of the vascular anatomy is vitally important.

Management of vessels as they are encountered intraoperatively will depend on the caliber of the vessel involved. For smaller vessels, it is possible to apply cautery in order to control bleeding. Additionally, the bedside assistant may use a flexible suction cautery device to stop low-flow vascular bleeding.

For larger caliber vessels, vascular clips may be employed. The options available for the application of the hemoclips are the EndoWrist clip-applying instrument used with the da Vinci system (**Fig. 7.1**), or a laryngeal endoscopic clip applier

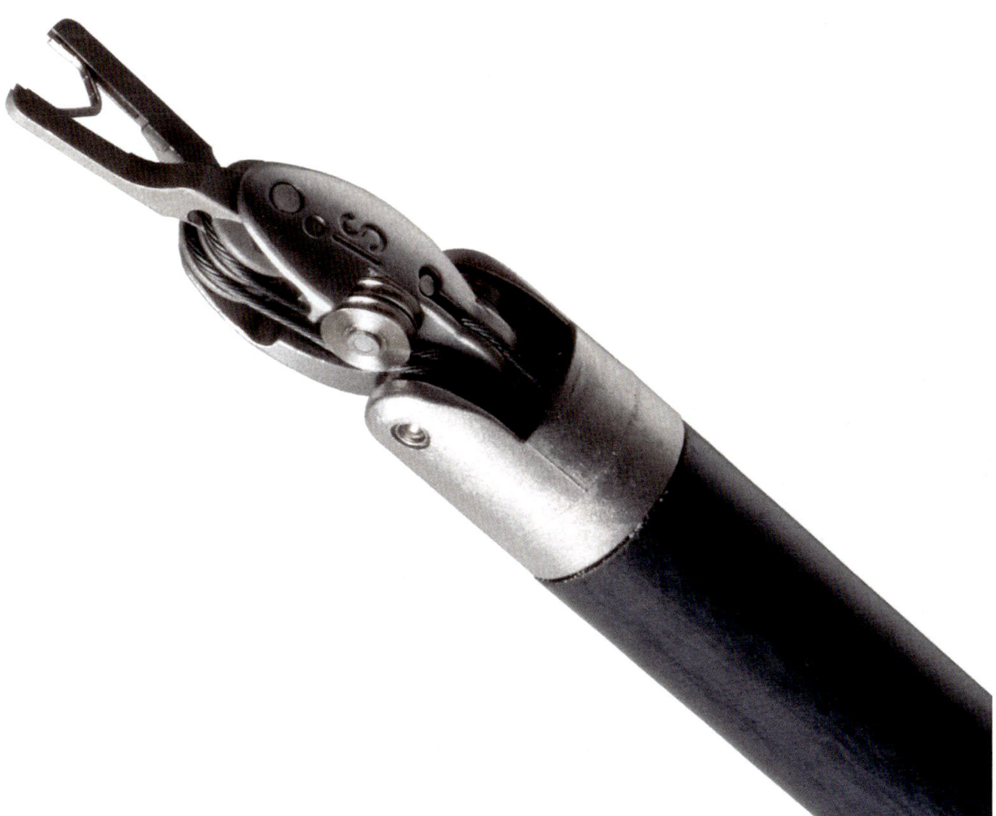

Fig. 7.1 An 8-mm EndoWrist small clip applier. (Courtesy of Intuitive Surgical, Inc.)

(see Chapter 4, Fig. 4.8) that is used by the bedside assistant. The difficulty with the EndoWrist clip appliers is that they are only available as 8-mm instruments. Exchanging between 5- and 8-mm robotic instruments requires the exchange of the 5- and 8-mm robotic cannulas at the end of the robotic arm. In the event of significant hemorrhage, this may be too time consuming and will take control of the robotic arms away from the console surgeon. The laryngeal endoscopic clip appliers allow for application of endoscopic clips by the bedside assistant. There is a right and left angled clip and the console surgeon can use the robotic arms to display the vessel so that multiple clips can be applied to the distal end and one to the proximal end prior to transecting the vessel.

Several strategies exist for the prevention and management of intraoperative bleeding. Preoperative planning is crucial in the avoidance of catastrophic bleeding. For larger tumors of the tonsil and for most tumors of the tongue base, it is beneficial to perform the neck dissection prior to the TORS procedure. This allows for ligation of the lingual and facial arteries, so that when they are encountered during TORS, the chance of significant bleeding is less.

During TORS, the Maryland dissector can be used to grasp the bleeding vessel in order to tamponade the bleeding. The spatula tip monopolar cautery instrument can then be used to bluntly dissect the tissue around the vessel in order to prepare the vessel for application of a hemoclip. If needed, the cautery instrument may be replaced easily with another grasping instrument to aid in controlling the bleeding. It is critical to state that removing the robot from the field in order to control bleeding at the bedside, with the intention to control the bleeding in a transoral manner, places the surgeon at a disadvantage. The best way to control bleeding in this fashion is by using all advantages the robot affords: magnification, overcoming line of sight limitations, multiple instruments in the field, etc. If it is not possible to stop bleeding in a transoral way, then the surgeon must consider control via a transcervical approach.

One useful technique that may be utilized during significant bleeding at the tongue base is to have the assistant apply external neck pressure just above the ipsilateral greater cornu of the hyoid bone. This will apply pressure to the external carotid and lingual artery, resulting in decreased blood flow, and better visualization of the surgical field. The surgeon may then stop the bleeding in an appropriate manner. Finally, at the end of the case, the surgeon may utilize hemostatic agents such as Tisseel or FloSeal hemostatic matrix (Baxter Healthcare Corp) to cover the mucosal defect.

Mucosal and Dental Injury

Risk of dental injury is low during TORS.[20] The majority of risk comes from the mouth gag device. The upper central incisors may be injured by the steel edge of the mouth gag. The risk of trauma may be minimized by the use of a device for dental protection, such as a thermoplastic splint or surgical gauze over the teeth. The posterior mandibular molars may be injured from both the mouth gag device or by the robotic instruments. Depending on the width of the mandibular arch, the blades from the mouth gag may overlap the molars and cause injury. In this case, it is important to choose the width of the blade carefully. Less commonly, the robotic instruments may rub against the molars and cause injury. Avoidance can be done by proper placement of the robotic arms and checking the range of motion of the arms prior to beginning the TORS procedure.

Intraoral mucosal trauma is uncommon during placement of the mouth gag. Areas at risk are the mucosa on the ventral surface of the tongue and the lips. Injury to the ventral mucosa of the tongue results from the pressure of the blade on the tongue pressing against the lower teeth. This can be minimized by covering the lower teeth, as done with the upper teeth, so they do not sharply press against the tongue. Also, the robotic instruments may rub against the lips and cause harm. As previously stated, this can be avoided by assessing the range of motion of the arms prior to beginning the procedure.

While not reported, hypothetically the lips and oral mucosa can suffer thermal injury from the shaft of the cautery instrument. The shaft of each instrument is covered with a protective layer. Any damage to this layer may place the patient at risk of thermal injury. Therefore it is necessary to inspect each instrument prior to use.

Nerve Injury

Both hypoglossal and lingual nerve palsy are possible complications during TORS. Lingual nerve paresis is usually secondary to compression from the mouth gag, and decreasing the duration of the surgery will decrease the severity of this complication. Paresis will typically resolve without intervention. Similarly, hypoglossal nerve injury, resulting from either transmission from the energy device or from traction, will likely resolve given sufficient time. Surgeons must be aware of the inside-out anatomy to decrease the risk of nerve transection. The lingual nerve is most at risk during lateral dissection close to the mandible while the hypoglossal nerve may be damaged with dissection lateral to the hyoid bone.

Salivary Fistula

When a neck dissection is performed concurrently with the intraoral resection there is a potential risk of orocervical fistula formation and subsequent pharyngocutaneous fistula. However, several studies have shown that, should a communication occur intraoperatively, the rate of persistent pharyngocutaneous fistula formation is low.[21,22] Moore at al found in a retrospective review of patients undergoing simultaneous neck dissection and TORS that although 29% of patients were found to have an orocervical communication intraoperatively, only 4% of these developed a pharyngocutaneous fistula.[23]

When an intraoral fistula is identified at the time of surgery, it can be repaired primarily. For defects of 1 cm or less, Moore et al recommend primary closure followed by application of Tisseel to the cervical side of the wound. For defects over 1 cm, the constrictor muscles should be closed and the digastric muscle sutured to the sternocleidomastoid muscle lateral to the defect. This can be reinforced with Tisseel.[24] Initiation and progression of diet is dependent on clinical signs of fistula formation. If fistula formation occurs, most will resolve with daily packing changes and antibiotic therapy.[16]

Early Postoperative Complications

Airway Compromise

During the early experience with TORS for malignancy, patients were either left intubated overnight for airway protection or had placement of a tracheostomy prophylactically.[25] As experience with TORS as a new surgical modality increased, it became apparent that most patients could be extubated immediately postoperatively and monitored on a general ward. Strategies to decrease the risk of airway edema include the use of perioperative intravenous steroids and periodically removing the pressure of the mouth gag on the tongue, allowing for recirculation.

For surgery closer to the larynx, heat generated by the cautery instrument may cause edema of the mucosa around the glottis. Lower settings on the instrument may help avoid this result. It is the opinion of the authors that TORS around the larynx for salvage surgery in patients who have failed chemoradiation do best with a planned tracheotomy.

At the completion of the operation, if there is concern with edema of the tongue or larynx, it is possible to keep the patient intubated for planned extubation the next day. This delay allows for the swelling to decrease and allows for safe extubation. Also, if the swelling is not enough to warrant delayed extubation but there is still some concern, a nasal trumpet may be used to bypass the edema of the tongue.

Postoperative Hemorrhage

Postoperative hemorrhage may occur in the first 24 to 48 hours. This is typically due to inadequate hemostasis at the time of the initial surgery. Compression from the tongue blade on the mouth gag can cause vasospasm. After relaxation, oropharyngeal hemorrhage may occur. In this case, return to the operating room for hemostasis is commonly required.

Late Postoperative Complications

Delayed Postoperative Hemorrhage

The published rates of bleeding for transoral surgery range from 3 to 14%.[13,26,27,28,29,30] Asher et al published on 145 patients undergoing transoral robotic-assisted surgery for any indication. Of these patients, 11 (7.5%) developed some degree of postoperative hemorrhage with 9 (6%) requiring reoperation for examination and/or control of bleeding. The most consistent risk factor in those patients who bled was that they were on antithrombotic medication, either anticoagulants or antiplatelet agents, for other medical comorbidities. This study also found that there was a high bleeding rate in salvage surgery as opposed to primary surgery; however, this did not reach statistical significance.[28] Richmond et al found a similar bleeding rate of 7% in their series of 99 patients. As with Asher's findings, 50% of secondary hemorrhage occurred in patients who were on anticoagulant medication for medical comorbidities.[30]

Chia et al investigated surgeon preferences for the perioperative management of transoral robotic surgery in a multi-institutional retrospective survey. One of the parameters they measured was the risk of postoperative hemorrhage. A total of 2,015 procedures were included as reported by 45 TORS-trained surgeons. Postoperative hemorrhage was reported in 62 (3.1%) patients. Of note, there were seven patient deaths in the survey period and four of these were due to postoperative hemorrhage. One of the conclusions of this paper was that the rate of complications tended to decrease with surgeon experience; however, this finding was not specifically related to postoperative hemorrhage.[20]

Pollei et al conducted a multicenter retrospective review of a single institution's experience with transoral surgery from 1994 through 2012. The techniques used for the transoral surgery included both transoral laser surgery and TORS. In their analysis there was a bleed rate of 5.4% (49 of 906 patients) with 67.3% of these patients requiring operative intervention. Within this study population they did not find any statistically significant role for transcervical carotid system ligation; however, it was only performed in 15.6% of patients. Furthermore, they noticed a trend toward reduced post oropharyngectomy bleeding severity in the context of a carotid system ligation. They did determine, however, that high T-stage tumors had a higher bleeding rate.[29]

In the event of a delayed postoperative bleed, management of the bleed will depend on its severity. As with post tonsillectomy hemorrhage, conservative measures may be applied in the first instance, and if these fail then operative intervention becomes necessary. Surgical management is performed without the use of the robot. Once the airway is appropriately established, access to the point of hemorrhage can be obtained using either a typical tonsil gag such as a Boyle-Davis or Crowe-Davis for more tonsillar-based issues or with a laryngoscope for base of tongue hemorrhage. Once visualization of the bleeding has been achieved, suction monopolar cauterization will control most hemorrhage points. If the bleeding cannot be managed intraorally, then the neck can be accessed for ligation of either the external carotid artery or one of its appropriate branches.

Dysphagia

Percutaneous gastrostomy (PEG) tube dependency can be used as a surrogate indicator for the preservation of swallowing function. Iseli et al concluded that the rate of PEG dependence correlated with a high T stage, an oropharyngeal or laryngeal tumor site, and the tumor being a recurrent or second primary tumor.[31] Weinstein et al found in their early feasibility TORS study a 5% PEG dependency rate in patients treated primarily with TORS. Similarly, Moore et al found in their long-term functional analysis of TORS-treated oropharyngeal carcinomas a long-term PEG tube rate of 4.5%.[32]

Mendelsohn et al in their review of 18 patients undergoing SGL found that no patients required long-term PEG placement.[26] Similarly, Ozer and colleagues demonstrated that only 1 of 14 patients undergoing SGL required a temporary PEG placement and this was removed 40 days postoperatively.[33] Olsen and colleagues presented their experience of nine patients, seven of whom had advanced stage disease. In their cohort, seven patients (44%) required temporary PEG placement and two (22%) required long-term placement, although both of these patients had required multimodality treatment.[34]

Velopharyngeal Insufficiency

For those patients with tumors that have significant extension into the soft palate, it is not uncommon for them to experience temporary palatal insufficiency. When less than 50% of the palate has been removed, conservative management is often sufficient as it is likely that the patient's symptoms will resolve within several months. If more than 50% of the palate is involved the patient may require reconstruction with a pharyngoplasty or obturator. The risk of a patient developing velopharyngeal insufficiency is higher in patients undergoing salvage surgery. [24]

Aspiration Pneumonia

All TORS patients are potentially at risk of developing aspiration pneumonia, although those with extensive tongue base resections and supraglottic tumors are at greatest risk. In patients where oral intake is likely to be problematic secondary to the risk of aspiration, a fine-bore nasogastric tube should be placed prophylactically at the time of surgery. These patients require a bedside speech therapy assessment prior to the commencement of an oral diet. Patients who are deemed at risk following this assessment should be discharged on an enteral diet and be reassessed with an outpatient functional endoscopic assessment of swallowing or a modified barium swallow prior to advancing their diet.

■ Conclusion

The application of TORS for upper aerodigestive tract malignancy is a rapidly expanding field in otolaryngology. As with the introduction of any new technology, it is important to ensure that patients are not placed at undue or increased risk when comparing the new technology to already existing treatment modalities. Familiarity with a different surgical approach to cancer removal, an inside-out approach, is critical to ensure safety to the patient. Unique precautions for TORS must be understood for safe outcomes. While there remains a paucity of published data regarding long-term oncologic, functional, and complication outcomes of TORS, current literature supports the safety of this procedure. The reported results remain encouraging, with a similar or better risk profile to the already established treatment modalities.

References

1. Department of Veterans Affairs Laryngeal Cancer Study Group. Induction chemotherapy plus radiation compared with surgery plus radiation in patients with advanced laryngeal cancer. N Engl J Med 1991;324:1685–1690
2. Parsons JT, Mendenhall W, Stringer SP, et al. Squamous cell carcinoma of the oropharynx: surgery, radiation therapy, or both. Cancer 2002;94:2967–2980
3. Genden E. The role for surgical management of HPV-related oropharyngeal carcinoma. Head Neck Pathol 2012;6:S98–S103
4. Cohan DM, Popat S, Kaplan SE, et al. Oropharyngeal cancer: current understanding and management. Curr Opin Otolaryngol Head Neck Surg 2009;17:88–94
5. Shah KV, Westra WH. Genital HPVs in the aerodigestive tract: etiologic association with a subset of oropharyngeal/tonsillar cancers and with recurrent respiratory papillomatosis. Dis Markers 2007; 23:235–245
6. Ang KK, Surgis EM. Human papillomavirus as a marker of the natural history and response to therapy of head and neck squamous cell carcinoma. Semin Radiat Oncol 2012;22(2):128–142
7. Dowthwaite SA, Franklin JH, Plama DA, et al. The role of transoral robotic surgery in the management of oropharyngeal carcinoma: a review of the literature. ISRN Oncol 2012;2012:945162
8. Steiner W, Fierek O, Ambrosch P, et al. Transoral laser microsurgery for squamous cell carcinoma of the base of tongue. Arch Otolaryngol Head Neck Surg 2003;129:36–43
9. Grant DG, Salassa JR, Hinni ML, et al. Carcinoma of the tongue base treated by transoral laser microsurgery, part 1: a prospective analysis of oncologic and functional outcomes. Laryngoscope 2006;116:2150–2155
10. Haughey BH, Hinni ML, Salassa JR, et al. Transoral laser microsurgery as primary treatment for advanced stage oropharyngeal cancer: a United States multicenter study. Head Neck Surg 2011;33:1683–1694
11. Grant DG, Hinni ML, Salassa JR, et al. Oropharyngeal cancer: a case for single modality treatment with transoral laser microsurgery. Arch Otolaryngol Head Neck Surg 2009;135:1225–1230
12. Hockstein NG, Nolan M, O'Malley BW. Robotic microlaryngeal surgery: a technical feasibility study using the da Vinci surgical robot and an airway mannequin. Laryngoscope 2005;115: 780–785
13. O'Malley BW, Weinstein GS, Snyder W, et al. Transoral robotic surgery (TORS) for base of tongue neoplasms. Laryngoscope 2006;116:1465–1472
14. Weinstein GS, O'Malley BW, Magnuson JS, et al. Transoral robotic surgery: a multicenter study to assess feasibility, safety and surgical margins. Laryngoscope 2012;122:1701–1707
15. Sinclair CF, McColloch NL, Carroll WR, et al. Patient-perceived and objective functional outcomes following transoral robotic surgery for early oropharyngeal carcinoma. Arch Otolaryngol Head Neck Surg 2011;137(11):1112–1116
16. Moore EJ, Olsen SM, Laborde RR, et al. Long-term functional and oncologic results of transoral robotic surgery for oropharyngeal squamous cell carcinoma. Mayo Clin Proc 2012;87(3):219–225
17. Moore EJ, Olsen KD, Kasperbauer JL. Transoral robotic surgery for oropharyngeal squamous cell carcinoma: a prospective study of feasibility and functional outcomes. Laryngoscope 2009;119:2156–2164
18. Kokot N, O'Malley BW, Weinstein G. Transoral anatomy in the context of TORS. In: Weinstein GS, O'Malley BW, eds. Transoral Robotic Surgery (TORS). San Diego: Plural Publishing Inc; 2012:59–84

19. Goyal N, Yoo F, Setabutr D, et al. Surgical anatomy of the supraglottic larynx using the da vinci robot. Head Neck 2014;36(8): 1126–1131
20. Chia SH, Gross ND, Richmon JD. Surgeon experience and complications with transoral robotic surgery (TORS). Otolaryngol Head Neck Surg 2013;149(6):885–892
21. Park YM, Lee JG, Lee WS, et al. Feasibility of transoral lateral oropharyngectomy using a robotic surgical system for tonsillar cancer. Oral Oncol 2009;45(8):e62–66
22. Boudreaux BA, Rosenthal EL, Magnuson JS, et al. Robot-assisted surgery for upper aerodigestive tract neoplasms. Arch Otolaryngol Head Neck Surg 2009;135(4):397–401
23. Moore EJ, Olsen KD, Martin E. Concurrent neck dissection and transoral robotic surgery. Laryngoscope 2010;121(3):541–544
24. Moore EJ. Robotic surgery for the management of oropharyngeal malignancies. In: Grillone GA, Jalisi S, eds. Robotic Surgery of the Head and Neck; A Comprehensive Guide. New York: Springer; 2015:61–82
25. White HN, Frederich J, Zimmerman T, et al. Learning curve for transoral robotic surgery: a 4-year analysis. JAMA Otolaryngol Head Neck Surg 2013;139(6):564–567
26. Mendelsohn AH, Remacle M, Van Der Vorst S, et al. Outcomes following transoral robotic surgery; supraglottic laryngectomy. Laryngoscope 2013;123:208–214
27. Salassa JR, Hinni ML, Grant DG, et al. Postoperative bleeding in transoral laser microsurgery for upper aerodigestive tract tumors. Otolaryngol Head Neck Surg 2008;139(3):453–459
28. Asher SA, White HN, Kejner AE, et al. Hemorrhage after transoral robotic-assisted surgery. Otolaryngol Head Neck Surg 2013;149(1):112–117
29. Pollei TR, Hinni ML, Moore EJ, et al. Analysis of post-operative bleeding and risk factors in transoral surgery of the orohpharynx. JAMA Otolaryngol Head Neck Surg 2013;139(11):1212–1218
30. Richmon JD, Feng AL, Yang W, et al. Feasibility of rapid discharge after transoral robotic surgery of the oropharynx. Laryngoscope 2014;124(11):2518–2525
31. Iseli TA, Kulbersh BD, Iseli CE, et al. Functional outcomes after transoral robotic surgery for head and neck cancer. Otolaryngol Head Neck Surg 2009;141:166–171
32. Weinstein GS, O'Malley BW, Magnuson JS, et al. Transoral robotic surgery: a multicenter study to assess feasibility, safety and surgical margins. Laryngoscope 2012;122:1701–1707
33. Ozer E, Alvarez B, Kakarala K, et al. Clinical outcomes of transoral robotic supraglottic laryngectomy. Head Neck 2013; 35(8):1158–1161
34. Olsen SM, Moore EJ, Koch CA, et al. Transoral robotic surgery for supraglottic squamous cell carcinoma. Am J Otolaryngol 2012;33(4):379–384

8 Robotic Surgery for the Management of Sleep Apnea

Claudio A. Vicini, Filippo Montevecchi, Ahmed Yassin Bahgat, Mohamed Eesa, Ehsan Hendawy, Giuseppe Meccariello, and Julia A. Crawford

■ Description of the Clinical Problem

Obstructive sleep apnea hypopnea syndrome (OSAHS) is increasingly prevalent worldwide and, with a large increased risk of all-cause mortality, poses a serious social health issue.[1] The most important modifiable risk factor for OSAHS in the adult populations is obesity; over the last few decades in the United States the prevalence rate of obesity has experienced an epidemic trajectory.[2] Despite this epidemic not being as prevalent in areas such as the Gulf region and East Asia, the incidence of OSAHS remains high and this may be related to certain anatomical differences between regions, such as micrognathia. In moderate to severe disease, OSAHS is well recognized as an independent risk factor for cardiovascular, neurocognitive, and cerebrovascular diseases. Perhaps more importantly, it also has a significant impact on mood and reported quality of life.[3,4,5,6,7,8,9] The effective management of this disorder remains an important and challenging clinical dilemma.

Treatment of OSAHS can be achieved with both nonsurgical and surgical techniques. The most common nonsurgical technique is continuous positive airway pressure (CPAP) ventilation. Other nonsurgical options include oral appliances, weight loss, and positional sleep therapy. CPAP remains the most commonly utilized and effective treatment strategy for OSAHS; however, for those not able to tolerate CPAP therapy, there must be another treatment option. The effectiveness of the other nonsurgical options is variable and is largely dependent on patient selection. Even with optimal patient selection, compliance rates for nonsurgical therapies are less than 30% for a period of time greater than 1 year.

There is a wide range of potential surgical interventions for OSAHS; these include uvulopalatopharyngoplasty, mandibular-maxillary advancement, nasal surgery, and a variety of palatal advancement and hyoid advancement techniques. Like nonsurgical techniques, however, surgical approaches can have limited efficacy. Appropriate patient selection remains the mainstay of success; however, even when this is optimized, long-term success is rare. Poor treatment efficacy is a result of several issues, the most important of which seems to be that upper airway obstruction is typically a result of multilevel collapse. There is a relative paucity of surgical therapies that address the base of tongue—a common site of obstruction in those who have failed previous surgical intervention.[10] It is in the treatment of the base of tongue that robotic surgery comes to the fore due to the excellent access and visualization that is possible with the robotic camera and instrumentation.

■ Current Standard Treatment

To achieve treatment success, it is important to identify the site or sites of obstruction. This allows treatment to be tailored to the needs of the individual patient profile. The individual site or sites and the pattern of collapse must be carefully studied before planning surgery in order to perform a targeted correction of the obstructing anatomy. Following the introduction of drug-induced sleep endoscopy (DISE) as a component of the preoperative workup for OSAHS patients, tongue base and supraglottic obstruction was found to be the source of obstruction in more than 25% of patients with moderate to severe OSAHS.

Tongue base obstruction is the most common site of airway obstruction in patients with OSAHS and this remains a great challenge for both surgeon and patient. Minimally invasive techniques are rarely sufficient in satisfactorily managing these kinds of patients. Reports in the literature do not directly address the problem of tongue base hypertrophy and limit their evaluations to a generic retrolingual collapse. Furthermore, the three-dimensional (3D) anatomy of the tongue base, the complex relationship to surrounding structures, and the physiological function of the tongue make surgery on the tongue base both technically demanding and encumbered with the potential for significant complications. Traditional open tongue base approaches, regardless of the pathology, are associated with significant morbidity, making this surgery somewhat unpopular. The OSAHS literature on this topic includes a limited series of procedures (**Table 8.1**).

From an historical perspective, Chabolle was the first to propose a tongue base resection through a transcervical suprahyoid approach; however, the procedure remained confined to a very limited number of published experiences, probably because of the technical difficulties and the potential associated morbidity. At the same time, minimally invasive techniques are not sufficient when dealing with significant tongue base hypertrophy. Radiofrequency ablation surgery can be successfully used in cases of moderate tongue base hypertrophy, but it is inadequate for severe obstruction. On the other hand, surgical management of the tongue base by a microscopic laser–assisted approach is challenging from a technical point of view and requires extensive surgical training and skills. Furthermore, the manipulation of tongue base tissues causes complex distortions in the geometrical architecture of the region, thus impairing the surgeon's orientation and increasing the risk of complications. In addition, the postoperative functional and pain profiles for laser resection are problematic. For these reasons, laser resection has not gained popularity in many parts of the world.

Table 8.1 Base of the tongue surgical techniques for OSAHS treatment in adults

Technique	Reference
Laser midline glossectomy	Fujita et al, 1991[11]
Laser lingualplasty	Woodson/Fujita, 1992[12]
Palatopharyngoglossoplasty	Djupesland et al, 1992[13]
Midline glossectomy and epiglottidectomy	Mickelson/Rosenthal, 1997[14]
Radiofrequency volume reduction of the tongue	Powell et al, 1999[15]
Tongue base reduction with hyo-epiglottoplasty (TBRHE)	Chabolle et al, 1999[16]
Coblation channeling in base of tongue	Senders/Strong, 2003[17]
Radiofrequency tongue reduction through a cervical approach	Blumen et al, 2006[18]
Tongue base reduction with thyrohyodopexy (TBRTHP)	Vicini et al, 2010[19]
Submucosal minimally invasive lingual excision (SMILE)	Friedman et al, 2008[20]

Coblation is another option that has gained treatment ground; however, working with a two-dimensional scope held by one hand compels the surgeon to use just one hand for cutting and, if necessary, for hemostasis. The combination of limited view and restricted manipulation is a disadvantage that the robot can overcome.

Benefits and Drawbacks of the Transoral Robotic Approach

The first transoral robotic surgery (TORS) for OSAHS was carried out in May 2008 at the ENT Department of Forlì. It was devised as a robotically assisted transoral version of Chabolle's operation (open transcervical tongue base reduction hyoepiglottoplasty [TBRHE]) for moderate to severe obstructive sleep apnea.[21] After a few years, the technique was adopted with some personal modifications in many ENT centers all over the world the world.[22,23,24] Today, TORS is included in the surgical routine for sleep disordered breathing (SDB) treatment in a great number of ENT departments. Although few departments have series of more than 100 TORS cases, many of these have completed at least 50 consecutive TORS for OSAHS. It is one of the most published techniques in surgical management of the tongue base and has become much more popular compared to the open TBRHE that inspired TORS. The robotic setup, which permits multiplanar tissue transection at any angle, enhances the surgeon's dissecting skills in such a complex anatomical region and, as opposed to traditional open approaches, tongue base resection by means of TORS seems to be very well tolerated.[25] Apart from the postoperative pain profile that remains relatively low, the tolerability of the procedure is reflected in the minimal (if any) reduction in body mass index (BMI) during the postoperative period. Typically, in the case of impaired quality of life and problematic swallowing, the patient loses weight.

Data from the literature show that the operating time and blood loss are comparable or less than the open surgical approaches or endoscopic laser resection approaches. Additionally, the visualization is considered superior to traditional microscopic surgery because of the 3D perspective.[23,24,26,27,28,29,30,31,32] Better visualization, better manipulation, and four-handed surgery means more precision and easier management of intraoperative bleeding. Advantages and disadvantages of TORS versus competitive options are summarized here.

TORS advantages vs. open:

- Scarless procedure
- Lower pain procedure
- Lower functional impact
- Better cosmetic result
- Strong impact on quality of life

TORS advantages vs. TO (laser):

- Digitally enhanced "true" 3D view (dual endoscopic system)
- Angulated view (30 degrees) working around the corner
- Intuitive image and joysticks movement
- Bimanual
- EndoWrist (6 degrees of freedom)
- Endolaryngeal suturing made possible
- Amplitude scaling according surgical requirement
- Tremor filtering
- More rapid learning curve
- More rapid surgical procedures (vs. CO_2 laser)

TORS disadvantages:

- Cost
- Lack of reliable haptic feedback
- No dedicated robotic laser device
- Monopolar distortion of resected specimen
- Lack of evidence-based clinical data

Review of Available Data

TORS for OSAHS was devised mainly as a transoral robotic approach to the tongue base and supraglottic larynx. The high-definition and 3D view provided by the camera arm of the da Vinci robot (Intuitive Surgical, Inc.) coupled with the precision and angled manipulation of the EndoWrist 5-mm instruments has made TORS a safe and effective tool for reducing the volume of the tongue base and for reshaping a collapsing and obstructing supraglottic larynx. This area may be considered as a unique anatomical entity, defined as the subglosso-supraglottic (SGSG) region. Its obstructive role in sleep apnea may be directly observed by awake or sedated endoscopy, as well as by imaging. It should be considered as a site of potential collapse in severe OSAHS patients with minimal or no collapse in retropalatal area. A disproportionately huge tongue base may be observed behind a relatively normal oral tongue, or be a part of a whole enlarged tongue. Histology and geometry of the enlarged tongue may widely differ among patients.

If the obstructing tissue is mainly lymphoid tissue, it is a case of lingual tonsil hyperplasia, and a lingual tonsillectomy is the required procedure. In many other cases, a variably thin lymphoid mantle covers a true muscle enlargement, requiring a so-called tongue base debulking or reduction that, if necessary, includes the removal of a midline wedge of oral tongue. The anatomy of the neurovascular bundle within the tongue muscle mass is predictable and must be handled with care. As described in the Moore classification, tongue base obstruction may be mainly inferior, superior, or diffuse. In preoperative planning, the type of obstruction in each individual patient must be assessed in order to properly address the areas of obstruction. Finally, in surgical practice, the Cormack-Lehane classification for the degree of enlargement of the pharyngeal tongue as well as the Friedman staging for the oral tongue are useful guides for oral and tongue base enlargement assessment and should be incorporated into the preoperative clinical assessment.

If the epiglottis is found to contribute to airway obstruction on preoperative assessment, it may be addressed in conjunction with tongue base reduction. A primary or secondary obstructing epiglottis may be included in the main application of TORS.

According to the patient's anatomical levels of obstruction and according to the surgeon's preference, TORS in SGSG may be included in a multilevel surgical approach and addressed in the same or separate setting as nasal and palatal surgery.

The da Vinci robot may also be used in palate area reshaping (palatine tonsillectomy and palate/pharyngoplasty). This approach may be justified in the setting of TORS training when the robot is already being used for tongue base resection. However, it is our opinion that palate TORS is far less cost effective than conventional palate surgery, and in our hands TORS was not really suitable for expansion sphincter pharyngoplasty (ESP) or, more recently, for barbed reposition pharyngoplasty (BRP), which are so far our preferred palate procedures.

Most of the patients with SGSG obstruction show a moderate to severe degree of OSHAS (apnea-hypopnea index [AHI] > 20). It is the senior author's opinion that in this group of severe patients at high cardiovascular and neuropsychiatric risk, the use of this technique is justified from a cost-effectiveness viewpoint. However, in a few cases of mild to moderate OSAHS where tongue base obstruction is the primary pathology, TORS is also justifiable.

In our SDB practice, only sufficiently symptomatic patients (Epworth Sleepiness Scale [ESS] > 10) are selected for surgery as these are the patients who will have an appreciable outcome in quality of life measures. Most of our patients are overweight males, but we prefer to treat patients with a preoperative BMI less than 30. Mouth opening measured as interincisive distance of 25 mm or more is a prerequisite for a sufficient exposure. About 70% of our cases were primary surgeries after CPAP treatment failure. Nevertheless, TORS may be used as a salvage procedure in cases of failure of previous surgeries as well.

DISE is considered essential in the preoperative patient selection for our unit. From the strictly diagnostic point of view, DISE may offer additional information about the dynamic behaviors of base of tongue (BOT) and supraglottic (SG) regions. In the case of significant lateral wall collapses, shown during DISE, the surgeon should avoid TORS. Potential additional information from DISE (upper airway collapsibility, typical patterns predicting outcomes) is still under evaluation and may prove useful after further study.

■ Surgical Procedure

Nasotracheal intubation is recommended for our patients to provide unobstructed access to the base of tongue. In a select group of patients, a planned tracheostomy may be indicated. Patients with severe sleep apnea, those at high risk for postoperative bleeding, or patients who are at risk of postoperative airway obstruction should be consented for a tracheostomy. Other indications for tracheotomy include subjects with morphometric index suggesting a difficult intubation (short neck, short hyoid-mental distance, micrognathia, macroglossia) and those undergoing multilevel surgery (nasal palatal, BOT, and SG).

In preparation for surgery, the patient is positioned in supine position with the neck flexed and head extended. We place a 0-0 nonabsorbable suture through the tip of the tongue to provide traction when pulling the tongue forward. Using a Davis-Meyer or Crowe-Davis retractor system, the shortest and widest blade is placed. The Storz blades integrate a peripheral suction that is useful for removing cautery plume and blood from the surgical field. A very thin soft rubber dental protector is applied to the upper dentition to prevent dental injury from the retractor.

To provide the best surgical exposure of the tongue base both the tongue retention suture and the appropriate blade are required. In our experience, symmetrical blade positioning results in less distortion of the anatomy. Once the base of tongue is appropriately exposed, da Vinci is docked in the standard position for transoral robotic procedures. We prefer the 12-mm 30-degree videoendoscope facing upward. The instruments should be viewed during the introduction of the instrumentation onto the oral cavity to prevent any mucosal injury. We recommend using a round tip cautery and a Maryland forceps. We do not routinely use a laser (thallium or CO_2) for SGSG surgery in OSAHS patients. However, if laser is available, it may be an alternative option. Immediately before the start of surgery and after the routine operative safety checklist, we perform a TORS-specific checklist. This checklist includes the following:

1. Check proper illumination of surgeon's console.
2. Check blue endoscopic light for the head assistant.
3. Check that additional instruments are available, including a Yankauer suction, a bipolar and monopolar coagulating device, a set of clip applicators of different sizes, and an open neck tray in the event that emergent open surgery is required for vessel ligation.
4. Check video recording equipment.

The process of SGSG TORS is performed through a series of steps. These include the bilateral reduction of the BOT followed by a suprahyoid horizontal epiglottoplasty. To prepare for these procedures, the endoscope should be set on wide view to provide the best view of the anatomy. Maryland forceps provide appropriately sized jaws for working in a narrow space and are sufficient to firmly grasp the tissue. As the first step, we make a deep cut into the tongue base posterior to the circumvallate papillae to create a ledge of tissue that can be firmly gripped by the Maryland forceps. The cautery and cutting power should be enhanced by a proper tension on the tissue (see below). The round tip cautery may be used with concentrated energy set at maximal cutting power, using the flat surface (distributed energy, lower cutting power, and better coagulation), or the lateral edge (intermediate situation). A blended set (cautery + coagulation) is the best option. We use coagulation set between 20 and 30 power in order to achieve bloodless cutting.

The head assistant's role is crucial in OSAHS patients. The role encompasses using a Yankauer suction to provide a bloodless and smokeless field, retracting tissues to provide better visualization, and keeping the BOT tissues on tension for better cutting. The procedure is performed through a staged removal of three tissue layers starting from the surface mucosa (**Fig. 8.1**).

In summary, the superficial lymphoid layer is resected down to the junction between muscle and lymphoid tissue. We then resect a second muscular layer—we refer to it as the "safety trapezoid"—in order to spare the lingual artery root. Finally, we resect a third midline strip of muscular tissue. The shape of resected area is mushroomlike, with a wide superficial head and a narrow deep central root. There are several resection strategies that vary from this description including the one reported by Friedman et al.[22,25,26,32,33,34]

The BOT reduction is performed through two steps. Instrument settings include placing the forceps in the left robotic arm and the powered instrument of choice in the right arm. We first perform a midline split of the two lingual tonsils. The foramen caecum is the key point for starting the dissection. This point must be well identified because it serves to define the upper limit of the resection. This approach serves to spare circumvallate papillae and, therefore, taste. It also provides the surgeon with a reference to locate the midline. The incision point inferiorly is the center of the epiglottic tip. This can be exposed by the head assistant with a gentle lifting of the midline tongue base with a Yankauer suction. Occasionally, the epiglottis becomes evident during the midline splitting. The dissection is carried out to the depth of the lymphoid–muscle junction. Next, the surgeon locates the three limits of the tongue base dissection: superior (sulcus terminalis), lateral (amygdaloglossus sulcus), and inferior (glossoepiglottic sulcus). The borders of the right lingual tonsil are identified and, according to surgeon's preference, marked by cautery. The dissection may be performed en bloc to the lower border maintaining the dissection plane close to the lympho-muscular junction (**Figs. 8.2–8.5**).

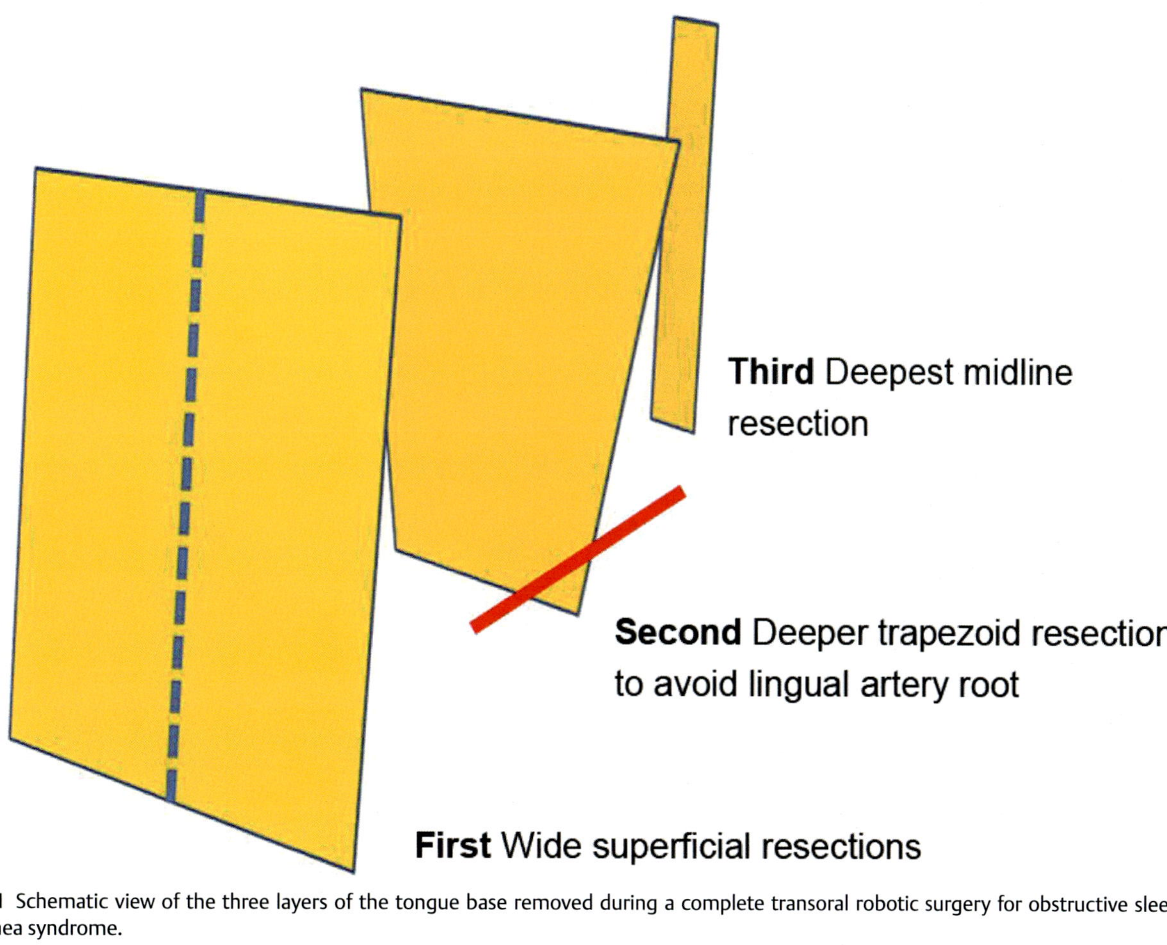

Fig. 8.1 Schematic view of the three layers of the tongue base removed during a complete transoral robotic surgery for obstructive sleep apnea hypopnea syndrome.

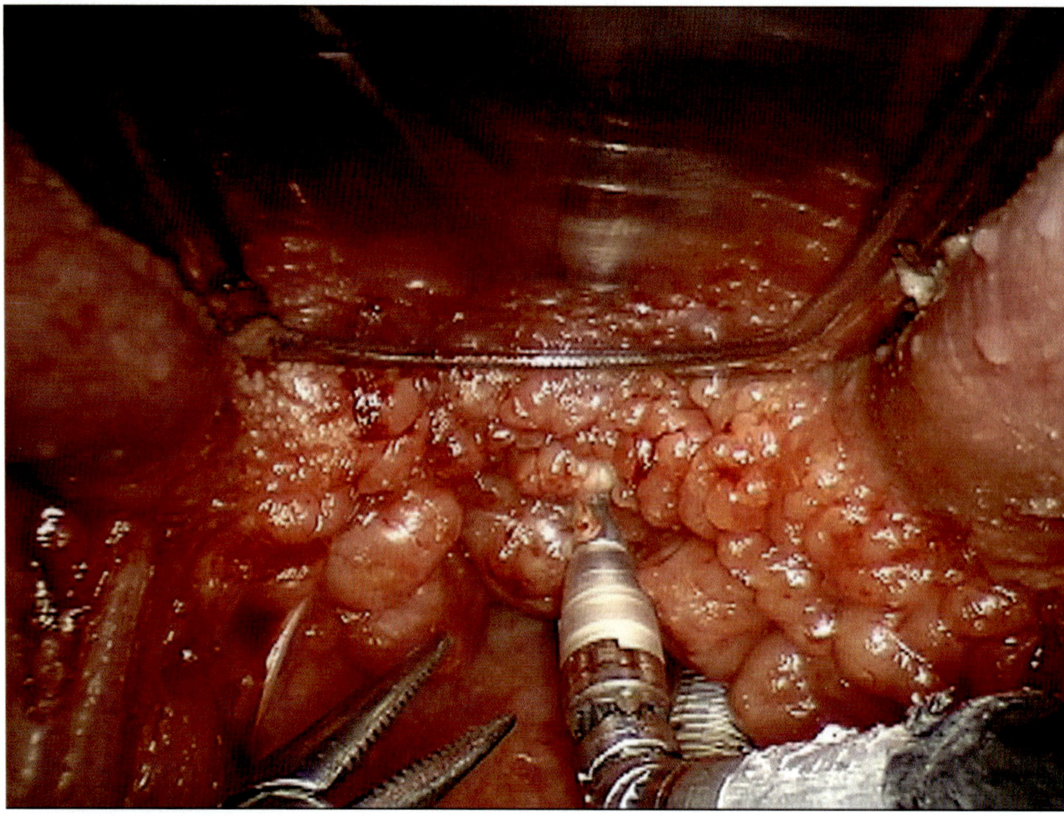

Fig. 8.2 Initial step of tongue base reduction: Maryland forceps on the left, round tip cautery on the right, and blade on the top, retracting the body of the tongue.

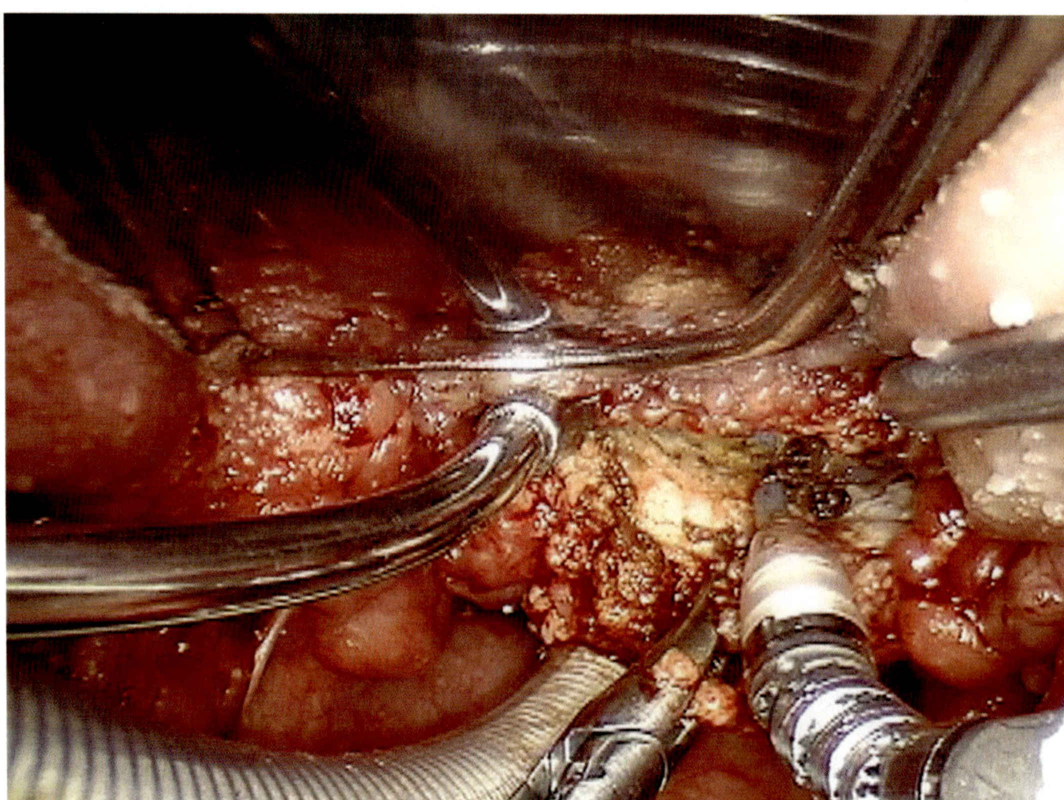

Fig. 8.3 Right side tongue base reduction, from above to below. Note, besides the robotic instruments, there is also a suction device retracting the surrounding tissue. This is being held by the bedside assistant.

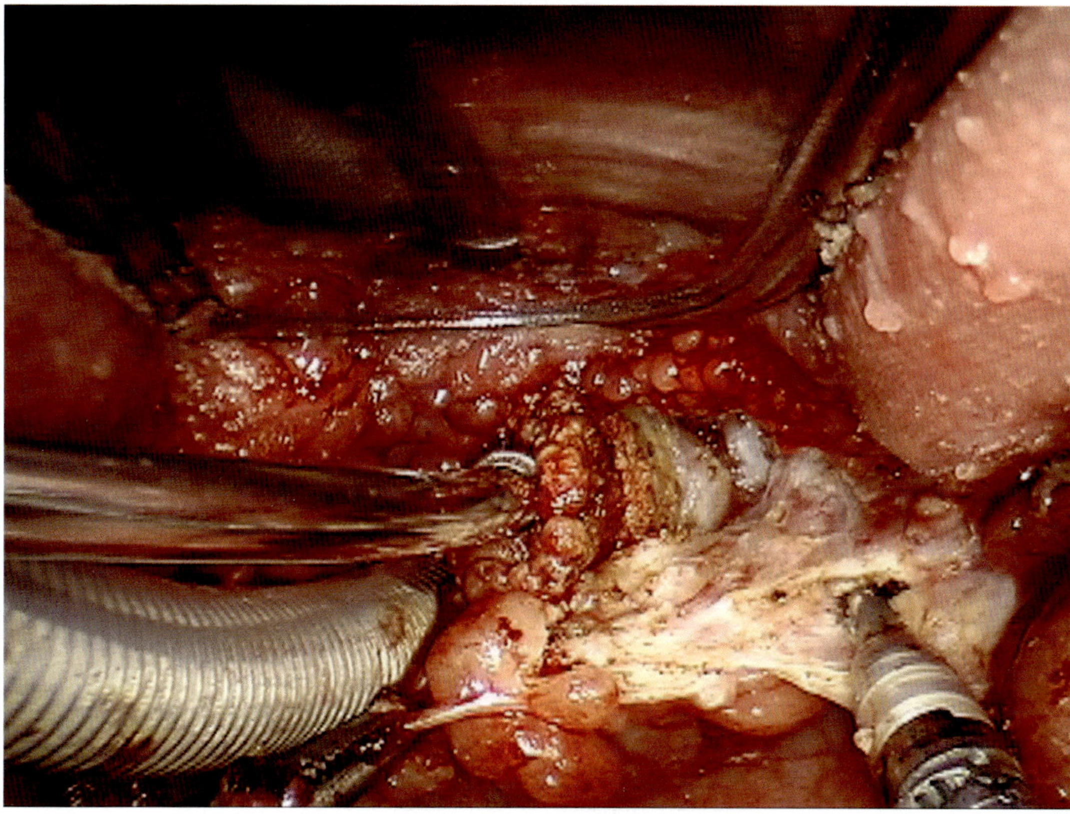

Fig. 8.4 Last step of right tongue base reduction; the dissection plane between muscle and lymphoid tissue is well demonstrated.

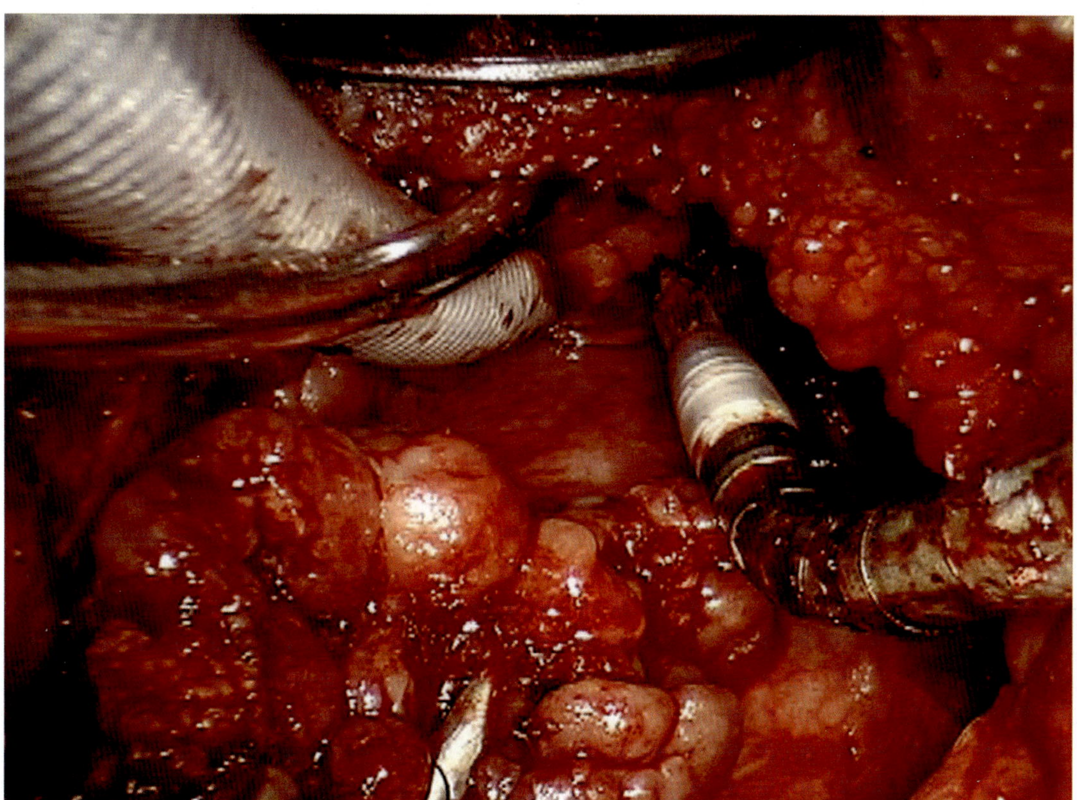

Fig. 8.5 The tongue base specimen is removed by the patient's head assistant. The epiglottis is apparent on the right side.

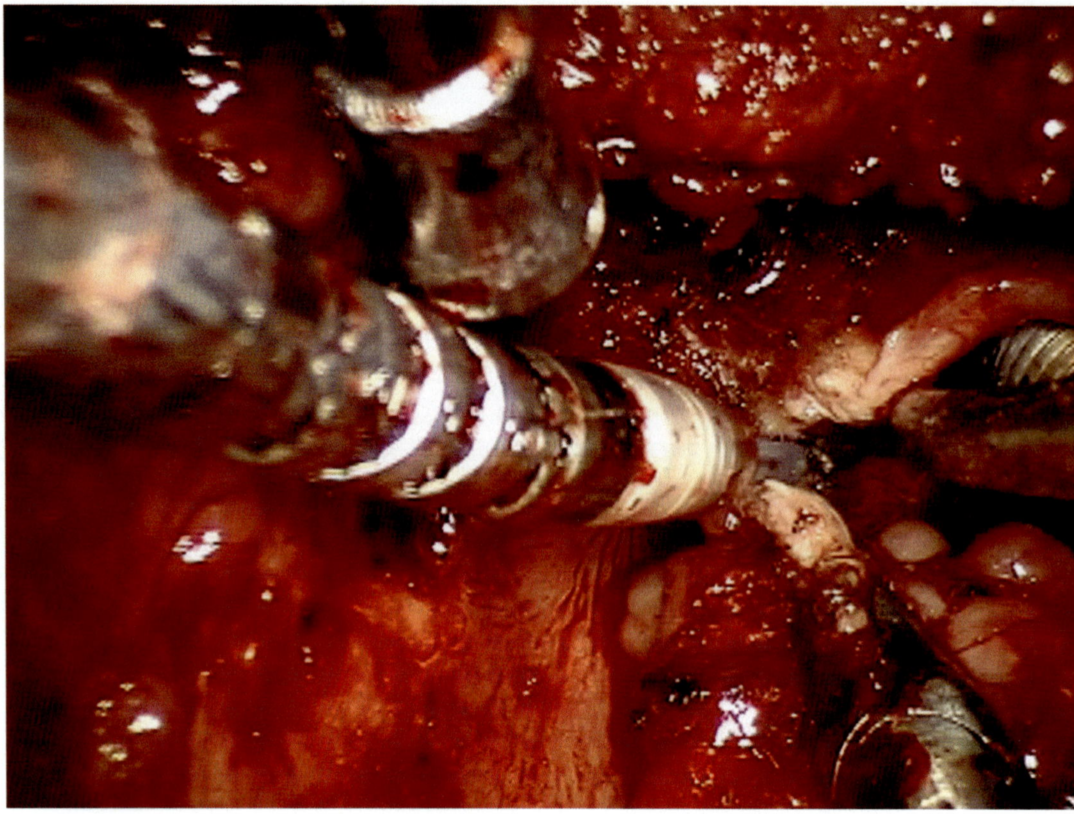

Fig. 8.6 Left side tongue base reduction almost completed.

The scope is maintained in high magnification in the surgical field for a better identification of vessels and nerves. A precise 3D resection is easily planned with the aid of the 3D view of the da Vinci optics. The proper tissue tension along the section line is maintained by applying countertraction between the surgeon's forceps and the assistant's suction tip. This ensures easy and efficient cutting. As we approach the inferior limit of the resection the vallecular mucosa becomes gradually evident. The volume of surgical specimen removed is measured. It is put into a 20-mL graduated syringe filled with saline solution: the displaced volume of the liquid is the volume of the specimen. At this point the instruments are swapped and the left lingual tonsillectomy is completed in the same way (**Fig. 8.6**).

Once lingual tonsillectomy is completed, the surgical field is inspected in order to evaluate the residual degree of obstruction (**Fig. 8.7**). The entire surgical volume of the specimen is measured. If the Cormack and Lehane grade is more than 2 and/or if the overall resected volume of tissue is less than 7 to 8 mL, an additional resection in true muscle area is required. Additional resection can be either lingual tonsil or muscle. The key is to clear the inspected airway to a reasonable level of patency at the endoscopic surgical view. The minimum of resected volume must be 7 mL, which is derived from our previous study comparing success rate to the volume of resected tissue.

The key to this next step is to remove a sufficient amount of muscle in order to open the posterior airway space as well as to avoid any possible injury to the main trunk of the lingual artery (the dorsal branches, if encountered, may be coagulated or clipped without serious problems; the hypoglossal nerve and the lingual nerve are anatomically more lateral). A muscle layer thinner than 10 mm may be removed without risk. In the midline, an additional muscle strip of 5 mm on each side and 5 mm in depth may be resected without major additional risks.[25,33,34] The high-definition, 3D, and magnified vision provided by the robotic camera is the key to identification of the crucial structures—and working carefully step by step with a mix of blunt and sharp dissection with robotic arms to avoid damage to these neurovascular structures.

A removal of the suprahyoid epiglottis is the final step (**Fig. 8.8**). The epiglottis is divided in the midline to a point at least 5 mm above the deep vallecular plane (a sufficient strip of cartilage is left for keeping in place a sort of "dam" preventing aspiration). A horizontal section on both sides is then removed leaving enough of the epiglottis to prevent aspiration and high enough to avoid any possible bleeding from the superior laryngeal vessels (**Fig. 8.9**).

If required, nasal and/or palatal procedures may be carried out at the end of the SGSG step. In most of our cases, the nasal obstruction is addressed by means of septoplasty and inferior turbinoplasty. Early in our experience the palatal area was addressed with the classic uvulopalatopharyngoplasty (UPPP). Since 2012, the so-called expansion sphincter pharyngoplasty (ESP) was adopted.[35] More recently, we introduced one different type of oropharyngeal surgery that we called barbed reposition pharyngoplasty (BRP). By means of a reabsorbable barbed suture, the pharyngoglossus muscle and the upper tongue base are suspended to the pterygomandibular raphe. This procedure is quick and has a short learning curve and its effectiveness is currently under evaluation. The preliminary results in more than 55 cases demonstrate that the technique is quick, safe, and effective as a component of multilevel surgery.

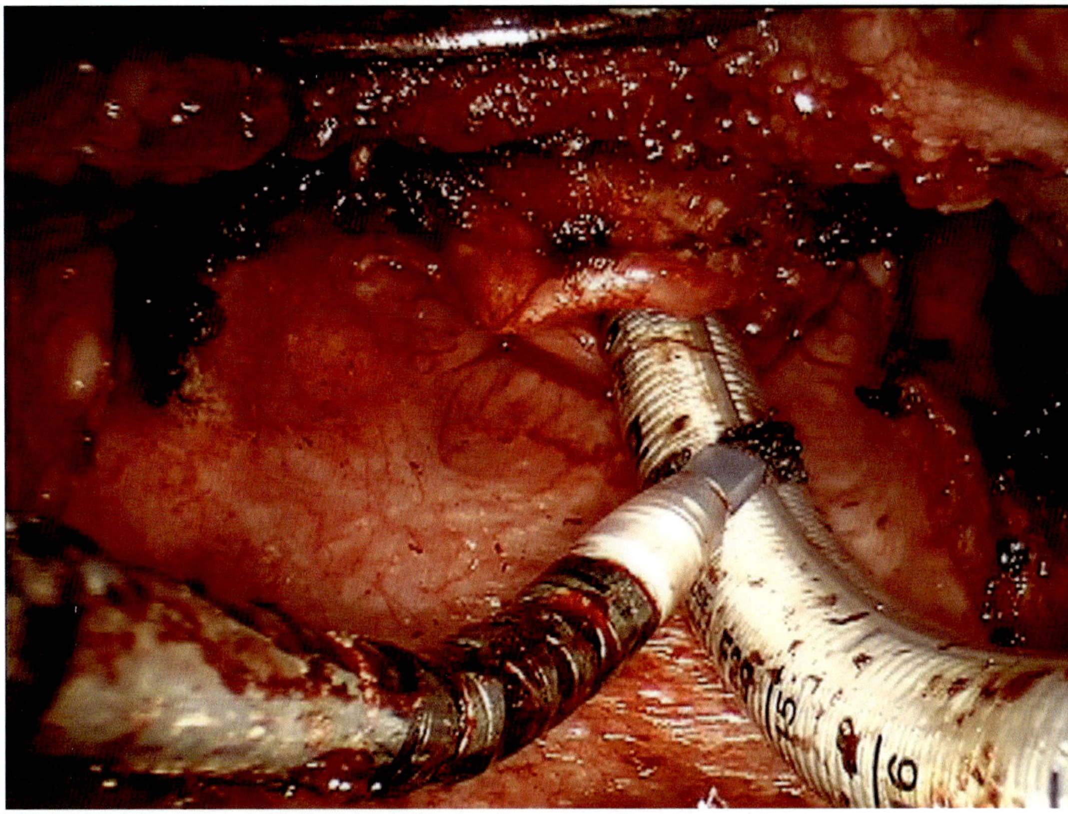

Fig. 8.7 A wide-angle view of the surgical field after tongue base reduction. Epiglottis is completely exposed. The resection of the ligaments between the anterior surface of epiglottis and tongue base may produce an iatrogenic epiglottis instability in case of a very long epiglottis.

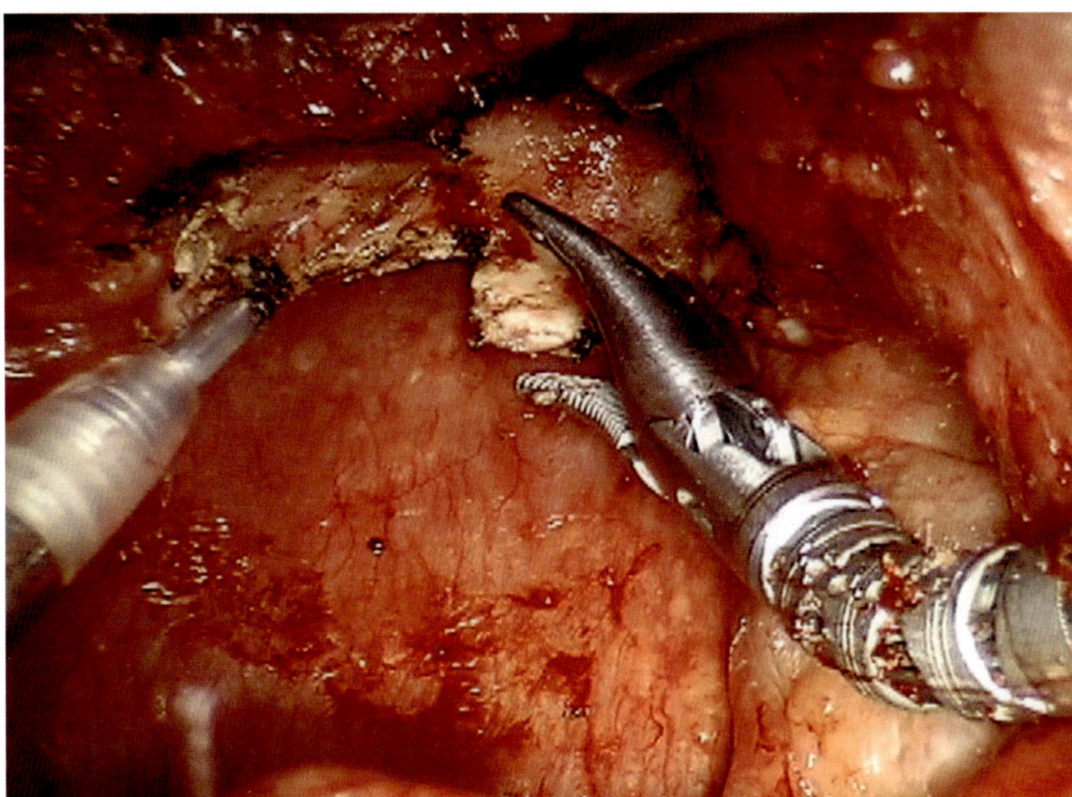

Fig. 8.8 Left side epiglottis trimming is completed. A planned resection of 3 to 5 mm of suprahyoid epiglottis is devised in order to fix the floppy epiglottis phenomenon induced by the tongue base reduction.

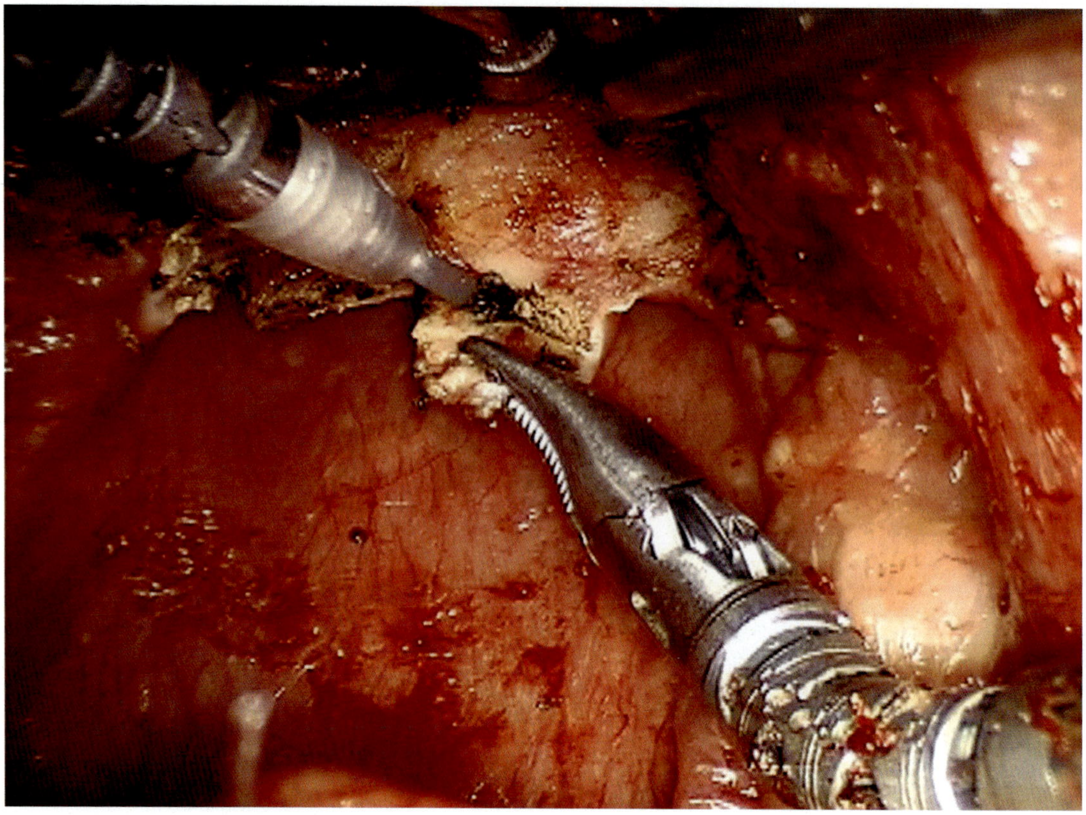

Fig. 8.9 Right side epiglottis trimming.

■ Postoperative Management

If the patient has not undergone tracheotomy, then an overnight intensive care unit (ICU) stay with continued intubation may be necessary in high-risk patients. If deemed safe, the patient may be extubated in the operating room but should be kept under close observation in a high-dependency unit. We find that many patients can swallow liquids comfortably without aspiration within a day of surgery, but this can vary considerably among patients. In Forlì we do not routinely place a feeding tube and a liquid diet is initiated on day 1 postoperatively. It is advised that initial postoperative observation be carried out in the appropriately monitored setting. In most institutions, this would be the intensive care unit (ICU) or postanesthesia care unit rather than the typical postoperative hospital ward. Continuous pulse oximetry is recommended. The patient should have suction available at all times at the bedside and be closely monitored for signs of bleeding. Postoperative intravenous steroids can help to reduce nausea, airway edema, and pain from the inflammatory response. It is advisable to continue oral steroids on a tapering dose after discharge. Narcotics are used with caution, and close observation of respiratory rate and level of consciousness is strongly recommended postoperatively for any OSAHS surgical procedures. Elastomeric pump has also proved to be very useful.

The length of stay can vary considerably. Tracheotomy by itself necessitates a hospital stay of a few days. Other determinants include the presence or absence of other concurrent OSAHS procedures (e.g., ESP, BRP), general patient health, comorbidities, pain control, and swallowing ability. In Forlì, the average hospital stay is 5 days. Patients are followed closely after discharge. Diet is normalized as healing progresses, and formal therapist-directed swallowing therapy is rarely needed (< 5% of cases). Postoperative polysomnography is performed once healing is complete, usually at least 6 months afterward.

Following all head and neck procedures, we monitor our cases with a pain profile, swallowing profile, voice profile, and quality of life modification survey after surgery. The average pain reported in the first week is summarized in **Fig. 8.10**. As measured by means of a visual analogue scale (VAS), the average pain scored low in the 3-day window after the surgery. As expected, the pain was higher after multilevel procedures. In a pilot group of cases, the change in the voice quality was measured by means of a targeted questionnaire (V-RQOL), as reported in **Fig. 8.11**. No significant impairment was registered. In many cases the patient described a perceived improvement in the quality of voice, with reduction of the "hot potato" voice typically encountered in case of huge tongue base lymphatic hypertrophy.

A more detailed analysis was carried out for the surgical impact on swallowing. In a pilot study it was evident that the MD Anderson Dysphagia Inventory could measure a minimal short-term impact on the swallowing function (**Fig. 8.12**).

More recently one additional retrospective study was carried out on a selected group of patients who were followed by postoperative gastrographing fluoroscopy and chest X-ray; it showed minimal incidence of aspiration and other associated chest problems during the first week after surgery. A complete swallowing normalization was registered after 3 months (**Fig. 8.13**). A significant improvement in quality of life was also demonstrated as measured by the SF-36 questionnaire (**Fig. 8.14**).

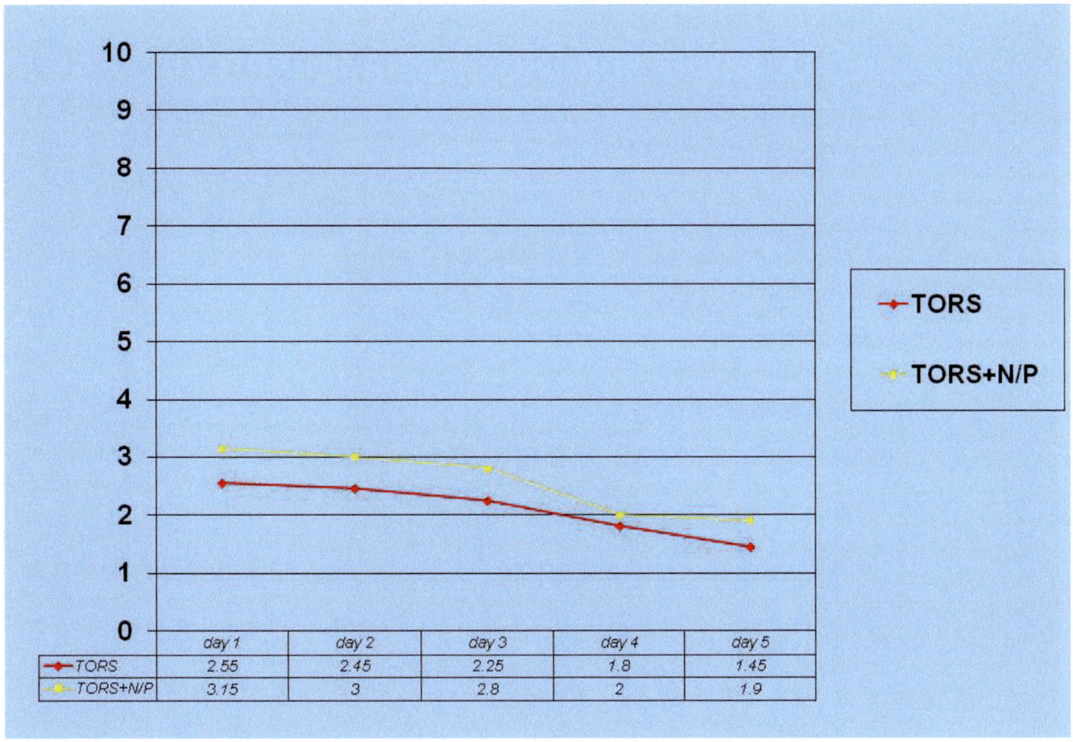

Fig. 8.10 Day 1 to day 5 graph of postoperative pain as measured by a visual analogue scale (VAS): 0 = no pain, 10 = maximum pain. The average level of standalone transoral robotic surgery (TORS; *red line*) pain proved to be inferior to the average level of postoperative pain in multilevel transoral robotic surgery procedures, including nose and palate (TORS+N/P; *yellow line*). The use of a continuous elastomeric pump for morphine release is our first line of pain relief.

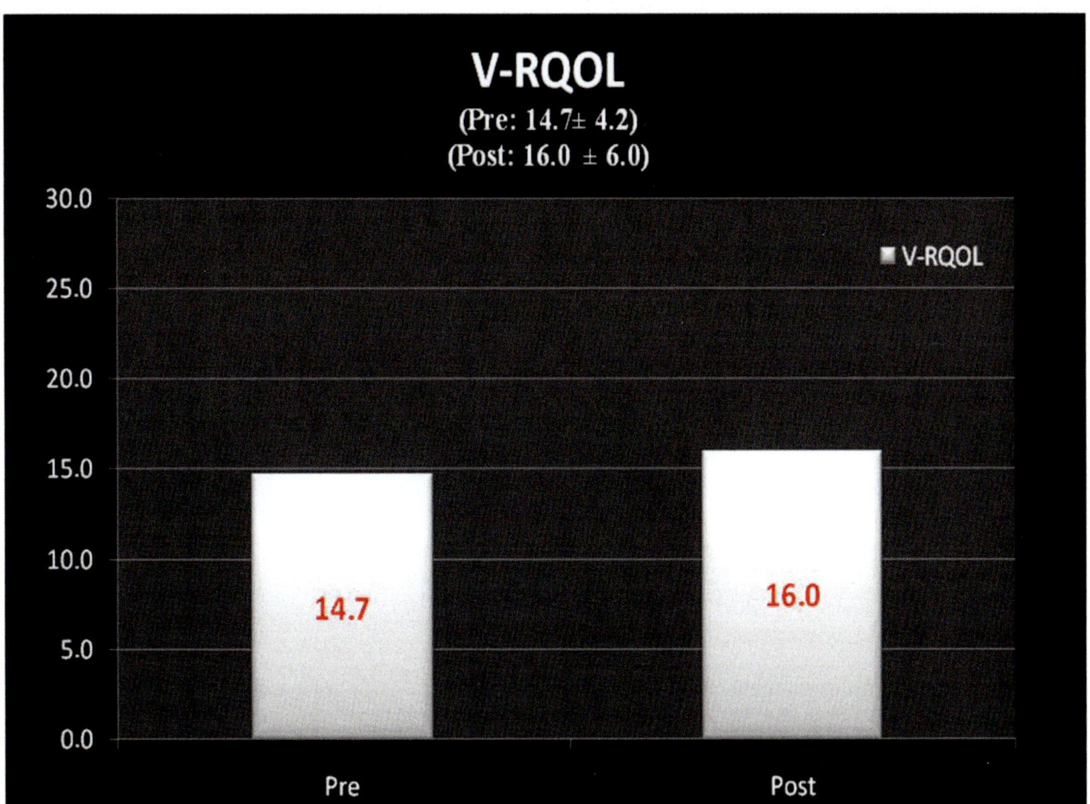

Fig. 8.11 Voice-Related Quality of Life (V-RQOL) score before and after surgery. No significant change or worsening was registered. (Data from Hogikyan ND, Sethuraman G. Validation of an instrument to measure voice-related quality of life (V-RQOL). J Voice 1999;13:557–569.)

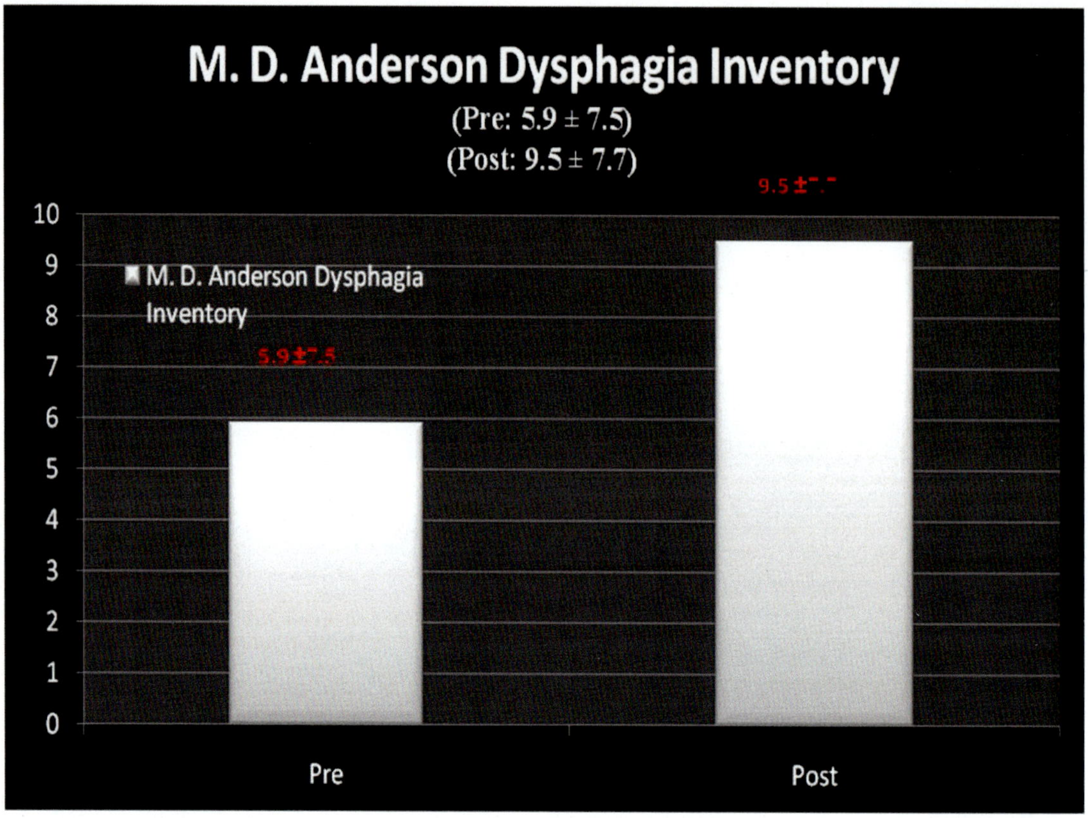

Fig. 8.12 MD Anderson Dysphagia Inventory score before and after surgery. (Data from Schindler A, Borghi E, Tiddia C, Ginocchio D, Felisati G, Ottaviani F. Adaptation and validation of the Italian MD Anderson Dysphagia Inventory (MDADI). Rev Laryngol Otol Rhinol (Bord) 2008;129(2):97–100.)

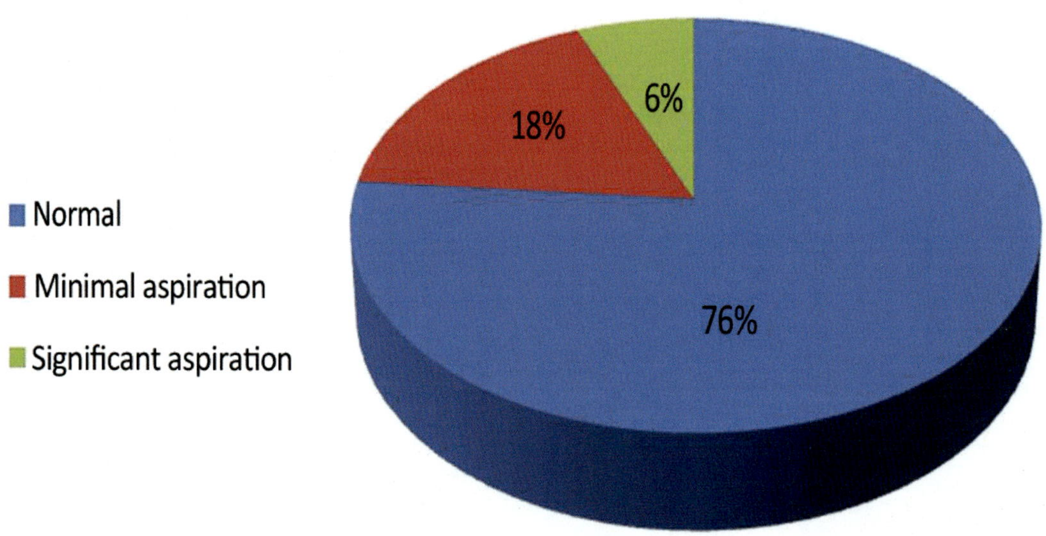

Fig. 8.13 Aspiration severity distribution (no aspiration, minimal aspiration, significant aspiration) in the studied group.

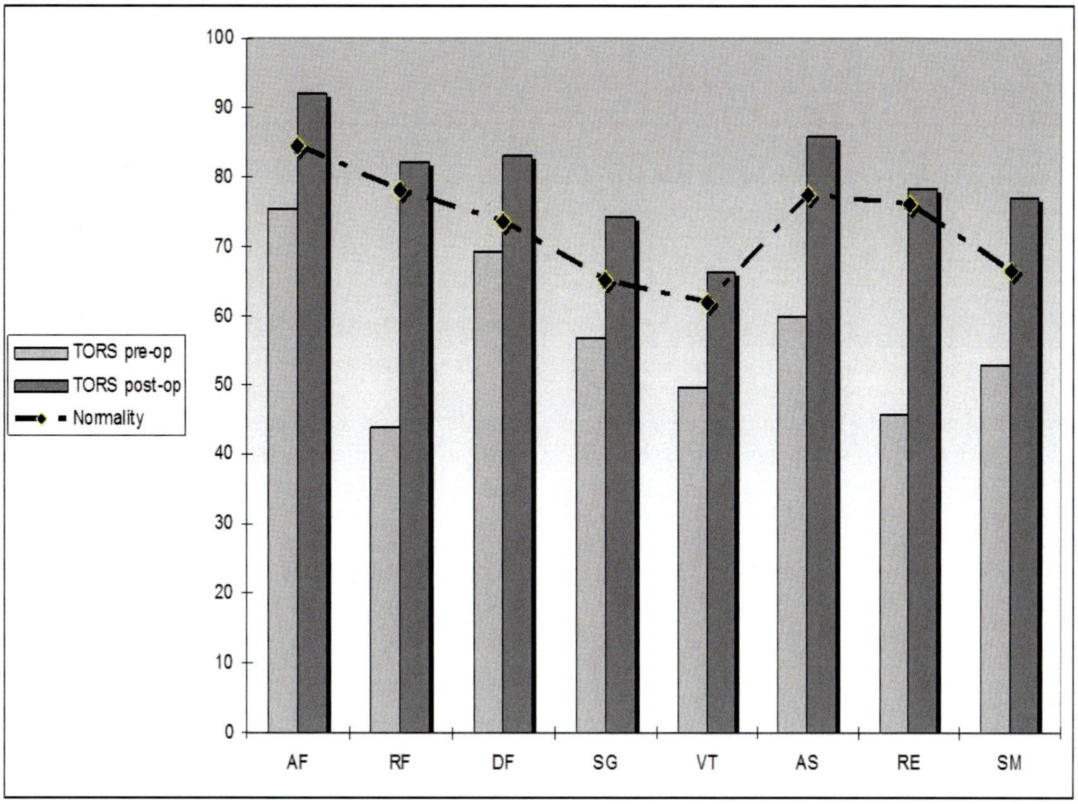

Fig. 8.14 SF-36 score modification after transoral robotic surgery (TORS) for obstructive sleep apnea. (Data from Apolone G, Mosconi P. The Italian SF-36 Health Survey: translation, validation and norming. J Clin Epidemiol 1998;51(11):1025–1036.)

■ Complications

Complications can be divided into intra- and postoperative complications and are listed here. For a detailed description of the encountered complications, see Chapter 9.

Intraoperative complications:

- Intraoperative bleeding
- Posterior wall injury/burning
- Teeth injury (teeth damage by instruments)
- One camera failure (two-dimensional vision instead of 3D)
- Pharyngeal edema

Postoperative complications:

- Late self-limited bleeding
- Bleeding requiring surgical revision
- Transient hypogeusia
- Pneumonia
- Pneumothorax

■ Outcomes

The results from our institution have been published in various reports between 2010 and 2014. The first published data on TORS for sleep apnea was in 2010 when Vicini et al evaluated the feasibility, tolerability, and efficacy of tongue base management by means of TORS in patients suffering from OSAHS primarily related to hypertrophy of the tongue base.[21,26] Seventeen patients with a minimum follow-up of 3 months were evaluated. Ten patients (mean preoperative AHI, 38.3 ± 23.5 SD) were included in the study. The postoperative polysomnographic results significantly dropped when compared to preoperative scores (mean postoperative AHI, 20.6 ± 17.3 SD), and the functional results (pain, swallowing, and quality of life) were very encouraging. Most complications were minor. This first publication showed that TORS was both feasible and effective in the management of tongue base hypertrophy causing OSAHS.

In 2014, in an enlarged and multicenter study, Vicini et al tried to create benchmarks for evaluating clinical outcomes and complications of TORS in a multicenter setting. The results of 243 patients with OSAHS from seven different academic centers treated with TORS between 2008 and 2012 were analyzed.[24] The average hospitalization was 3.5 days. The mean patient age was 50 ± 12 years, the average BMI at the time of the procedure was 28.53 ± 3.87, and the majority of the patients were men (81%). The mean preoperative and postoperative AHIs were 43.0 ± 22.6 and 17.9 ± 18.4, respectively ($p < 0.001$). The mean preoperative and postoperative ESS scores were 12.34 ± 5.19 and 5.7 ± 3.49, respectively ($p < 0.001$). The mean pre- and postoperative lowest O_2 saturations were 79.5% ± 8.77% and 83.9% ± 6.38%, respectively ($p < 0.001$). **Table 8.2** summarizes all the quoted data. Patients undergoing TORS as part of a multilevel approach for the treatment of OSAHS proved to have a reasonable expectation of success with minimal long-term morbidity.

Fig. 8.15 graphically summarizes the AHI improvement as registered in four successive series of our revised cases.

Table 8.2 Summary of data

	Preoperative mean	Postoperative mean	p value	
Body mass index	28.53	28.49	Not significant, $p = 0.0554$	Wilcoxon matched pairs signed ranks test
Apnea hypopnea index	43.21	17.54	< 0.001	Paired T-test
Lowest O_2	79.5	83.9	< 0.001	Wilcoxon matched pairs signed ranks test
Epworth Sleepiness Scale	12.5	5.78	< 0.001	Paired T-test

The progressive rise of preoperative AHI from series 1 to series 4 is related to the increased confidence with the technique—more severe cases were selected as experience increased. The reduced postoperative AHIs from series 1 to series 3 express the basic learning curve of the group. The better outcome in series 4 compared to series 1 to 3 is strongly related to the introduction of ESP for palate surgery instead of UPPP.

Fig. 8.16 shows the outcome summary for a group of 107 patients operated on in Forlì and revised within July 2012. It should be stressed that the palate and tonsil score of the group according to Friedman classification was relatively low. It means that the main obstruction was in the SGSG area and the final outcome strictly reflects the SGSG surgery more than the palate one. The average amount of BOT resected tissue was 12.71 mL. All the cardiorespiratory and the neuropsychiatric improvements proved to be statistically significant.

In 2012 Lin et al evaluated the efficacy of standalone BOT resection via TORS in the treatment of OSAHS.[23] Twelve patients who underwent BOT resection alone were included in this study. The median age for these was 48.5 (range, 19–64) and included nine women and three men. The mean AHI was 43.9 ± 41.1 preoperatively and 17.6 ± 16.2 postoperatively. This difference in AHI was statistically significant ($p = 0.007$) and reflected an average AHI reduction of 56.2% ± 28.3%. Statistically significant reductions in daytime somnolence level, as measured by EPP (13.7 ± 5.2 preoperatively vs. 6.4 ± 4.5 postoperatively; $p < 0.001$), and snoring intensity, as reported by a bed partner using a VAS (8.6 ± 1.2 preoperatively vs. 4.2 ± 1.9 postoperatively; $p < 0.001$), were achieved. There was no statistically significant difference between the preoperative and postoperative BMI (34.5 ± 7.3 vs. 33.5 ± 6.7; $p = 0.296$) or minimum oxygen saturation (83.3% ± 5.5% vs. 84.0% ± 6.4%; $p = 0.680$). This was

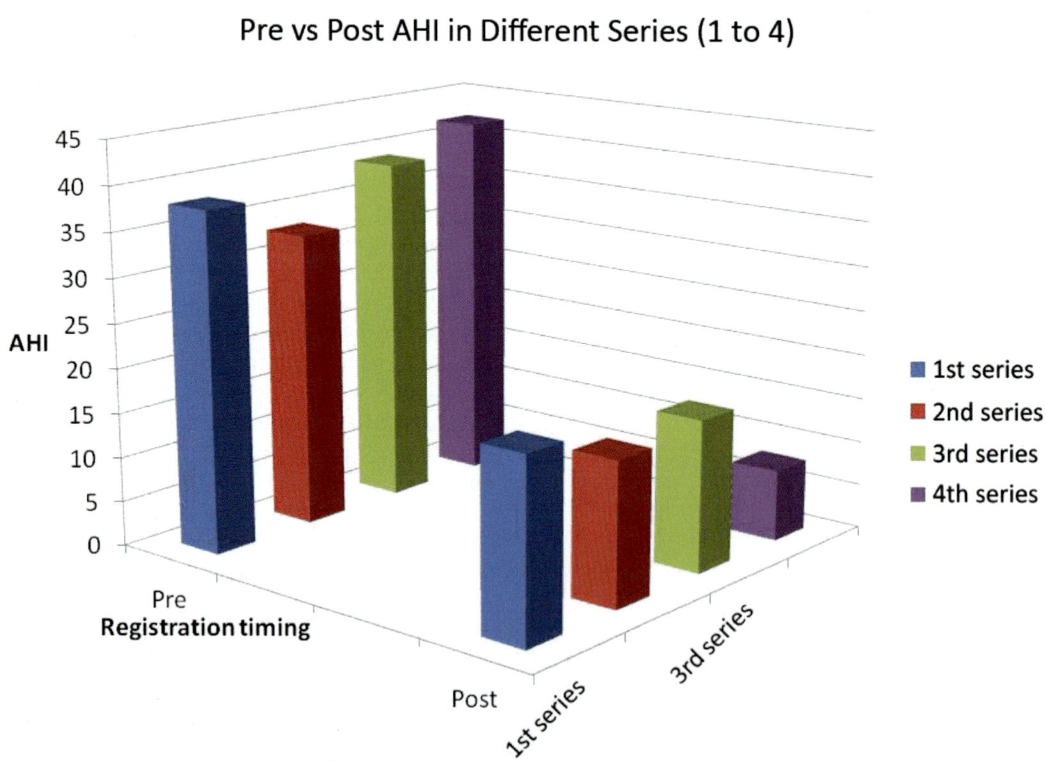

Fig. 8.15 This graph reports the pre- and postoperative apnea-hypopnea index (AHI) changing in a set of four different revised series of transoral robotic surgery for obstructive sleep apnea hypopnea syndrome patients. On the left is the first series; on the right, the last series. It is very evident that the last one is the best in terms of significant AHI reduction.

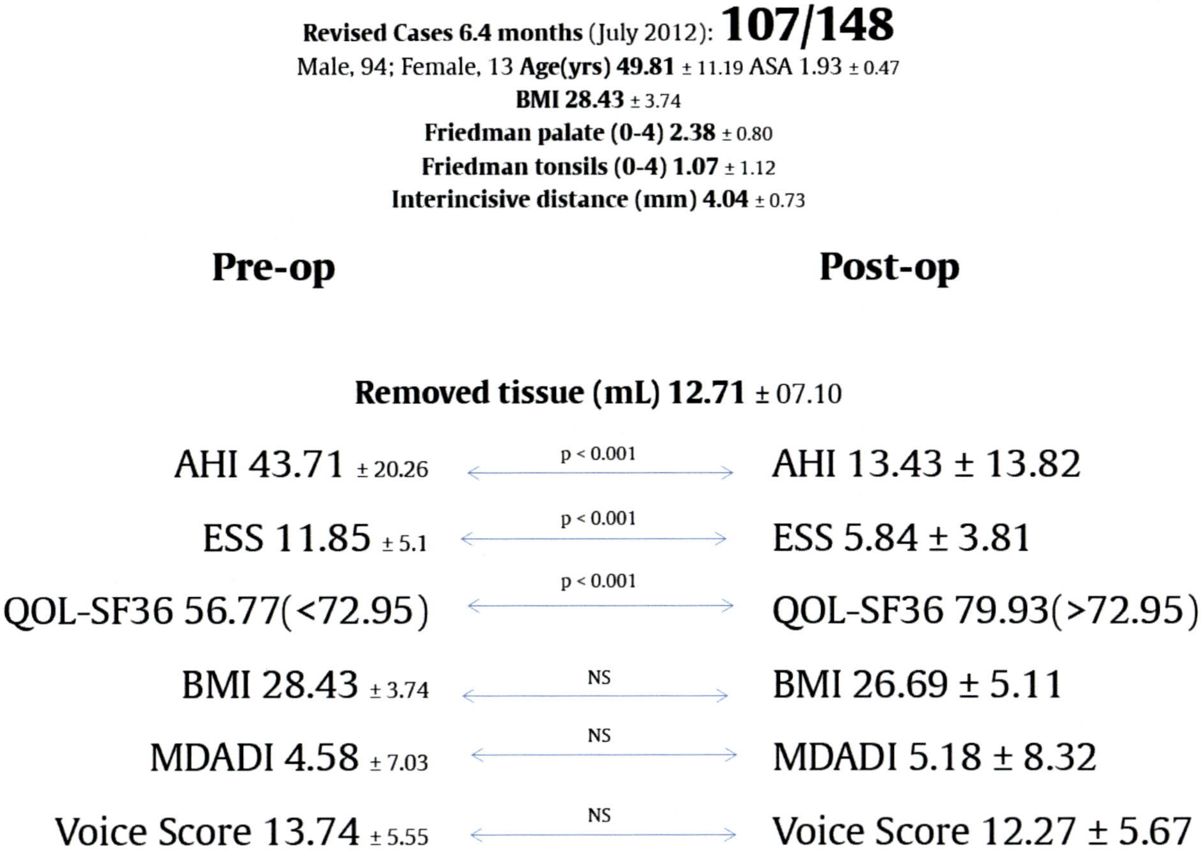

Fig. 8.16 An outcome summary for a group of 107 patients. ASA, American Society of Anesthesiologists score; BMI, body mass index; AHI, apnea-hypopnea index; ESS, Epworth Sleepiness Scale; QOL-SF36, Quality of Life Short Form 36; MDADI, MD Anderson Dysphagia Inventory; NS, not statistically significant.

the first study looking at the use of TORS to address obstruction at the level of BOT only and was not confounded by surgical alterations at other levels of the upper airway. This preliminary result on the use of BOT resection via TORS for the treatment of patients with OSAHS was encouraging and warrants further investigations.

In 2014 Lin et al reviewed their experience with TORS for BOT reduction either alone or as part of multilevel strategy in the treatment OSAHS in order to identify clinical characteristics that may be associated with surgical response. Between June 2010 and May 2014, BOT reduction via TORS ± partial epiglottectomy ± uvulopalatopharyngoplasty were performed on 72 patients with OSAHS. Thirty-nine patients (15 women and 24 men) with complete preoperative and postoperative clinical information including polysomnograms were included in the study. Mean AHI was 43.9 ± 32.3 preoperatively and 21.9 ± 23.5 postoperatively and reflected a statistically significant ($p < 0.001$) AHI reduction of 50.9% ± 38.1%. Statistically significant reduction in daytime somnolence, as measured by ESS (15.6 ± 5.4 preoperatively vs. 5.7 ± 4.3 postoperatively; $p < 0.001$), was also achieved. No statistically significant difference was found between preoperative and postoperative BMI (32.9 ± 7.0 vs. 32.4 ± 7.3; $p = 0.270$). Surgical response, as defined by > 50% reduction in AHI and final AHI < 15 with resolution of daytime somnolence, was achieved in 21 patients (53.8%). Clinical characteristics found to be significantly different between the responders and nonresponders were BMI, AHI, and lateral velopharyngeal collapse. Patients with BMI < 30, AHI < 60, or absence of lateral velopharyngeal collapse had excellent surgical response rates of 88.2%, 67.9%, or 66.7%, respectively.

In 2014 Toh et al in Singapore investigated the effectiveness of combined palatal surgery and TORS tongue base reduction with partial epiglottidectomy in the treatment of OSAHS. Twenty patients with complete preoperative and postoperative overnight polysomnograms were evaluated for surgical success and cure, according to traditional surgical criteria, and for subjective outcome measures (snoring and satisfaction on VAS and ESS) as well as complications. Traditional cure (AHI < 5) was achieved in 7 of 20 patients (35%), traditional success (AHI < 20 [> 50% reduction in AHI]) was achieved in another 11 patients (55%), and failure was observed in 2 patients (10%). Subjective improvements in snoring, satisfaction, and ESS score were observed. Improvement in mean (SD) ESS score and snoring loudness on VAS were statistically significant, from 12.4 (2.87) to 6.4 (1.43) and 8.7 (0.8) to 3.5 (1.7), respectively ($p < 0.001$ for both). None of the patients needed postoperative tracheostomy. Recorded complications included tonsillar fossa bleeding, pain, temporary dysgeusia, numbness of the tongue, and temporary dysphagia. TORS for tongue base reduction and partial epiglottidectomy for moderate to severe OSA proved to be effective in Asian patients for whom positive airway pressure treatment had failed.

A special mention is deserved of the Friedman et al study published in 2012, in which the authors aimed to assess the feasibility of performing an original robotically assisted partial midline glossectomy without tracheotomy and to assess efficacy by comparing OSAHS outcomes with those of established techniques.[22] Forty consecutive patients underwent TORS for OSAHS between October 2010 and June 2011 and were followed up with regard to complications, morbidity, and subjective and objective outcomes. Data from 27 of these patients who underwent concomitant z-palatoplasty with 6-month follow-up were compared with those of two matched cohorts of patients who underwent either radiofrequency (radiofrequency base-of-tongue reduction [RFBOT]) or coblation (submucosal minimally invasive lingual excision [SMILE]) reduction of the tongue base and z-palatoplasty. No major bleeding or airway complications were observed. Postoperative pain and length of admission were similar between groups. All groups saw ESS and snore score improvement. Patients undergoing robot-assisted surgery took longer than their SMILE and RFBOT counterparts to tolerate normal diet and longer than RFBOT patients to resume normal activity.

AHI reduction averaged 60.5% ± 24.9% for TORS versus 37.0% ± 51.6% ($p = 0.042$) and 32.0% ± 43.3% ($p = 0.012$) for SMILE and RFBOT, respectively. Only the robotic group achieved statistically significant improvement in minimum oxygen saturation. Surgical cure rate for TORS (66.7%) was significant compared with RFBOT (20.8%; $p = 0.001$) but not compared with SMILE (45.5%; $p = 0.135$). Robotically assisted partial glossectomy feasibility without the need for tracheotomy was proved. This technique resulted in greater AHI reduction but increased morbidity compared with the other techniques studied.

■ Future Directions and Conclusion

In the last 7 years, TORS has been shown to be a safe and effective surgical option for addressing BOT and SG obstruction in OSAHS patients. The most critical issue of this approach has proven to be surgical exposure in the well-known disproportionate anatomy of many OSAHS patients (limited mouth opening, very big oral tongue, micrognathia, stiff neck, etc.). The development of new and more effective mouth gags and blades is currently being undertaken, and this will hopefully allow for easier and wider exposure of the surgical fields. One new soon to be commercially available blade design has been devised with a V-shape notch in the midline in order to allow an additional midline resection of the oral tongue in cases of extreme macroglossia. In the future, the implementation of new types of barbed sutures may help the surgeon not only in palate area, but also in suturing and sustaining the tongue base after the conventional resection step. Under evaluation is the possibility to suspend the residual tongue base to the chin with special devices in order to really reproduce the classic Chabolle's operation. The most important step forward, however, will be when we develop a truly reliable and comprehensive preoperative evaluation that is able to select the appropriate patient "phenotype" and address the levels of obstruction that are truly the cause of the OSAHS.

References

1. Yaggi HK, Concato J, KernanWN, et al. Obstructive sleep apnea as a risk factor for stroke and death. N Engl J Med 2005;353: 2034–2041
2. Peppard PE, Young ET, Barnet JH. Increased prevalence of sleep-disordered breathing in adults. Am J of Epidemiol 2013;177(9): 1006–1014
3. Somers VK, White DP, Amin R, et al. Sleep apnea and cardiovascular disease: an American Heart Association/American College of Cardiology Foundation scientific statement from the American Heart Association Council for High Blood Pressure Research Professional Education Committee, Council on Clinical Cardiology, Stroke Council, and Council on Cardiovascular Nursing. J Am Coll Cardiol 2008;52(8):686–717
4. Shamsuzzaman AS, Gersh BJ, Somers VK. Obstructive sleep apnea: implications for cardiac and vascular disease. JAMA 2003;290(14):1906–1914
5. Peppard PE, Young T, Palta M, et al. Prospective study of the association between sleep-disordered breathing and hypertension. N Engl J Med 2000;342(19):1378–1384
6. Yaffe K, Laffan AM, Harrison SL, et al. Sleep-disordered breathing, hypoxia, and risk of mild cognitive impairment and dementia in older women. JAMA 2011;306(6):613–619
7. Kim HC, Young T, Matthews CG, et al. Sleep-disordered breathing and neuropsychological deficits. A population-based study. Am J Respir Crit Care Med 1997;156(6):1813–1819
8. Baldwin CM, Griffith KA, Nieto FJ, et al. The association of sleep-disordered breathing and sleep symptoms with quality of life in the Sleep Heart Health Study. Sleep 2001;24(1):96–105
9. Peppard PE, Szklo-Coxe M, Hla KM, et al. Longitudinal association of sleep-related breathing disorder and depression. Arch Intern Med 2006;166(16):1709–1715
10. Kezirian EJ. Nonresponders to pharyngeal surgery for obstructive sleep apnea: insights from drug-induced sleep endoscopy. Otolaryngol Head Neck Surg 2011;121:1320–1326
11. Fujita S, Woodson BT, Clark JL, Wittig R. Laser midline glossectomy (MLG). Laryngoscope 1991;101(8):805–809
12. Woodson BT, Fujita S. Clinical experience with lingualplasty as part of the treatment of severe obstructive sleep apnea. Otolaryngol Head Neck Surg 1992;107(1):40–48
13. Djupesland G, Schrader H, Lyberg T, Refsum H, Lilleas F, Godlibsen OB. Palatopharyngoglossopexy in the treatment of patients with obstructive sleep apnea. Acta Otolaryngol 1992;112 (suppl 492):50–54
14. Mickelson SA, Rosenthal L. Midline glossectomy and epiglottidectomy for obstructive sleep apnea syndrome. Laryngoscope 1997;107(5):614–619
15. Powell NB, Riley RW, Guilleminault C. Radiofrequency tongue base reduction in sleep-disordered breathing: a pilot study. Otolaryngol Head Neck Surg 1999;120(5):656–664
16. Chabolle F, Wagner I, Blumen MB, Séquert C, Fleury B, De Dieuleveult T. Tongue base reduction with hyoepiglottoplasty: a treatment for severe obstructive sleep apnea. Laryngoscope 1999;109(8):1273–1280
17. Senders CW, Strong EB. The surgical treatment of obstructive sleep apnea. Clin Rev Allergy Immunol 2003;25(3):213–220
18. Blumen MB, Coquille F, Rocchicioli C, Mellot F, Chabolle F. Radiofrequency tongue reduction through a cervical approach: a pilot study. Laryngoscope 2006;116(10):1887–1893
19. Vicini C, Frassineti S, La Pietra MG, De Vito A, Dallan I, Canzi P. Tongue base reduction with thyro-hyoido-pexy (TBRTHP) vs. tongue base reduction with hyo-epiglottoplasty (TBRHE)

in mild-severe OSAHS adult treatment: preliminary findings from a prospective randomised trial. Acta Otorhinolaryngol Ital 2010;30(3):144–148

20. Friedman M, Soans R, Gurpinar B, Lin HC, Joseph N. Evaluation of submucosal minimally invasive lingual excision technique for treatment of obstructive sleep apnea/hypopnea syndrome. Otolaryngol Head Neck Surg 2008;139(3):378–384
21. Vicini C, Dallan I, Canzi P, Frassineti S, La Pietra MG, Montevecchi F. Transoral robotic tongue base resection in obstructive sleep apnoea-hypopnoea syndrome: a preliminary report. ORL J Otorhinolaryngol Relat Spec 2010;72(1):22–27
22. Friedman M, Hamilton C, Samuelson CG, Kelley K, Taylor D, Pearson-Chauhan K, et al. Transoral robotic glossectomy for the treatment of obstructive sleep apnea-hypopnea syndrome. Otolaryngol Head Neck Surg 2012;146(5):854–862
23. Lin HS, Rowley JA, Badr MS, Folbe AJ, Yoo GH, Victor L, et al. Transoral robotic surgery for treatment of obstructive sleep apnea-hypopnea syndrome. Laryngoscope 2013;123(7):1811–1816
24. Vicini C, Montevecchi F, Campanini A, Dallan I, Hoff P, Matthew E, et al. Clinical outcomes and complications associated with TORS for OSAHS in 243 patients. A benchmark for evaluating an emerging surgical technology in a targeted application for benign disease. ORL 2014;76(2):63–69
25. Moore EJ, Janus J, Kasperbauer J. Transoral robotic surgery of the oropharynx: clinical and anatomic considerations. Clin Anat 2012;25(1):135–141
26. Vicini C, Dallan I, Canzi P, Frassineti S, Nacci A, Seccia V, et al. Transoral robotic surgery of the tongue base in obstructive sleep apnea-hypopnea syndrome: anatomic considerations and clinical experience. Head Neck 2012;34(1):15–22
27. Lee JM, Weinstein GS, O'Malley BW Jr, Thaler ER. Transoral robot-assisted lingual tonsillectomy and uvulopalatopharyngoplasty for obstructive sleep apnea. Ann Otol Rhinol Laryngol 2012;121(10):635–639
28. Vicini C, Montevecchi F, Magnuson, JS. Robotic surgery for obstructive sleep apnea. Curr Otorhinolaryngol Rep 2013;1:130–136
29. Vicini C, Montevecchi F, Tenti G, Canzi P, Dallan I, Huntley T. Transoral robotic surgery: tongue base reduction and supraglottoplasty for obstructive sleep apnea. Operat Tech Otolaryngol Head Neck Surg 2012;23(1):45–47
30. Vicini C, Montevecchi F, Tenti G, Canzi P, Dallan I, Thaler E. Tongue Base Reduction (TBR) and SupraGlottoPlasty (SGP) for Obstructive Sleep Apnea in: Transoral Robotic Surgery (TORS). San Diego, CA: Plural Publishing, Inc.; 2011: Chapter 12
31. Vicini C, Montevecchi F, Tenti G, Dallan I, Huntley T. Robotic Surgery for OSAHS: Transoral Robotic Tongue Base Reduction and Supraglottoplasty for OSAHS in Advanced Surgical Techniques in Snoring and Obstructive Sleep Apnea. San Diego, CA: Plural Publishing, Inc.; 2013: Chapter 29
32. Vicini C, Dallan I, Canzi P, Frassineti S, La Pietra MG, Montevecchi F. Transoral robotic tongue base resection in obstructive sleep apnoea-hypopnoea syndrome: a preliminary report. ORL J Otorhinolaryngol Relat Spec 2010;72(1):22–27
33. Dallan I, Seccia V, Faggioni L, Castelnuovo P, Montevecchi F, Casani AP, Tschabitscher M, Vicini C. Anatomical landmarks for transoral robotic tongue base surgery: comparison between endoscopic, external and radiological perspectives. Surg Radiol Anat 2013;35(1):3–10
34. Dallan I, Seccia V, Muscatello L, Lenzi R, Castelnuovo P, Bignami M, Montevecchi F, Tschabitscher M, Vicini C. Transoral endoscopic anatomy of the parapharyngeal space: a step-by-step logical approach with surgical considerations. Head Neck 2011;33(4):557–561
35. Vicini C, Montevecchi F, Pang K, Bahgat A, Dallan I, Frassineti S, Campanini A. Combined transoral robotic tongue base surgery and palate surgery in obstructive sleep apnea-hypopnea syndrome: expansion sphincter pharyngoplasty versus uvulopalatopharyngoplasty. Head Neck 2014;36(1):77–83

9 The Prevention and Management of Complications of Robotic Sleep Surgery

Filippo Montevecchi, Julia A. Crawford, Susan K. Sebastian, and Claudio A. Vicini

Introduction

Obstructive sleep apnea hypopnea syndrome (OSAHS) is a growing clinical concern, as it is the most prevalent sleep disorder in the adult population, affecting 11.4% of men and 4.7% of women. While the gold standard treatment for OSAHS remains continuous positive airway pressure (CPAP), for those patients who are unable to tolerate this treatment there needs to be another option. The first robotic OSAHS surgery was performed in 2008 and the first series outlining surgical affects was published in 2010.[1] To date, an estimated 600 transoral robotic surgeries (TORS) for OSAHS have been performed worldwide and a multicenter retrospective analysis of results and complications from seven academic centers is currently awaiting publication.[2] The purpose of this chapter is to analyze the intraoperative, perioperative, and postoperative complications that may occur during TORS for OSAHS.

Preoperative Considerations

Before undergoing any surgical intervention for OSAHS, patients should have a thorough anaesthetic assessment to identify and manage those who are at high risk secondary to medical comorbidities. There is a long list of illnesses associated with OSAHS including treatment-resistant hypertension, dysrhythmias, pulmonary hypertension, obesity, and metabolic syndrome.[3,4] These conditions need to be optimized before surgical intervention is considered. OSAHS, as a disorder in itself, is associated with an increased perioperative risk and postoperative surgical complications and this risk needs to also be considered prior to any intervention. Additionally, TORS for OSAHS is a body mass index (BMI)-sensitive procedure.[5] In patients with BMI > 30, the expected success rate decreases in accordance with an increasing BMI. Patients may benefit from a medically assisted weight loss program prior to any surgical intervention.

An important issue to consider in OSAHS surgery is the airway itself. In sleep apnea surgery, an already difficult airway can be further compromised by edema and bleeding. Difficult intubation facilities must be accessible and an endoscopic assisted intubation will often be necessary (**Figs. 9.1** and **9.2**).[6,7]

Re-intubation for postoperative edema or bleeding can be very difficult and the need for a tracheostomy should be considered whenever required. In the authors' department (ENT Department, Morgagni-Pierantoni Hospital, Forlì, Italy), we recommend an elective tracheostomy for severe OSAHS cases especially if multilevel surgery is undertaken.[8,9] Mild to moderate OSAHS cases who are having limited surgery, have reasonably good airway anatomy, and have limited medical comorbidities do not need a routine tracheostomy. However, each patient is discussed on a case-by-case scenario with the surgical and anaesthetic team before a final decision is reached. An additional and very important advantage in having a tracheostomy is that there is no tube obstructing the surgical view. This can be a significant advantage in a very narrow pharynx.

A study comparing conventional versus percutaneous tracheostomy is currently being conducted in our institution. Preliminary unpublished data favor percutaneous tracheostomy over conventional tracheostomy. This outcome is based on percutaneous tracheostomy being less aggressive, more aesthetic, and easy to perform out of the operating room in the patient's preparation area prior to commencing the surgery.

Intraoperative Complications

An understanding of transoral anatomy is essential for avoiding intraoperative complications especially that of damage to the neurovascular bundle. During the TORS resection, magnification of up to 10× combined with a three-dimensional (3D) image allows excellent visualization for identification of vessels and nerves. After the initial step of removal of the lingual tonsils from the base of tongue, additional muscle resection may be required to obtain an adequate anteroposterior sized airway and this should be done carefully under sufficiently high magnification. It is important to adjust the robotic scope appropriately, zooming in and out, to maintain this magnification. It is of paramount importance to use the tongue base midline as the point of reference to minimize risk to the hypoglossal nerve, lingual artery, and lingual neural branches. Due to the inherent anatomical variability of the tongue base and tissue distortion from tongue retraction and mouth gag placement, precise localization of these structures is not possible. Thus, an understanding of their anatomical course and landmarks is especially important.

Anatomical Consideration

The lingual artery arises from the external carotid artery at the level of the hyoid bone. It courses lateral to the middle

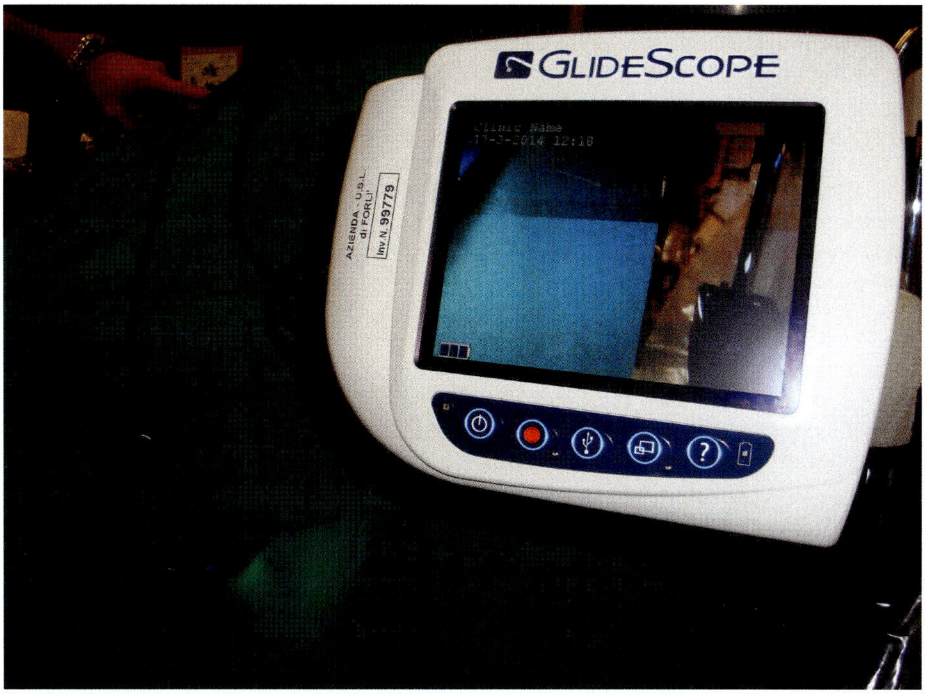

Fig. 9.1 GlideScope monitor (Verathon Inc.) available for difficult intubation.

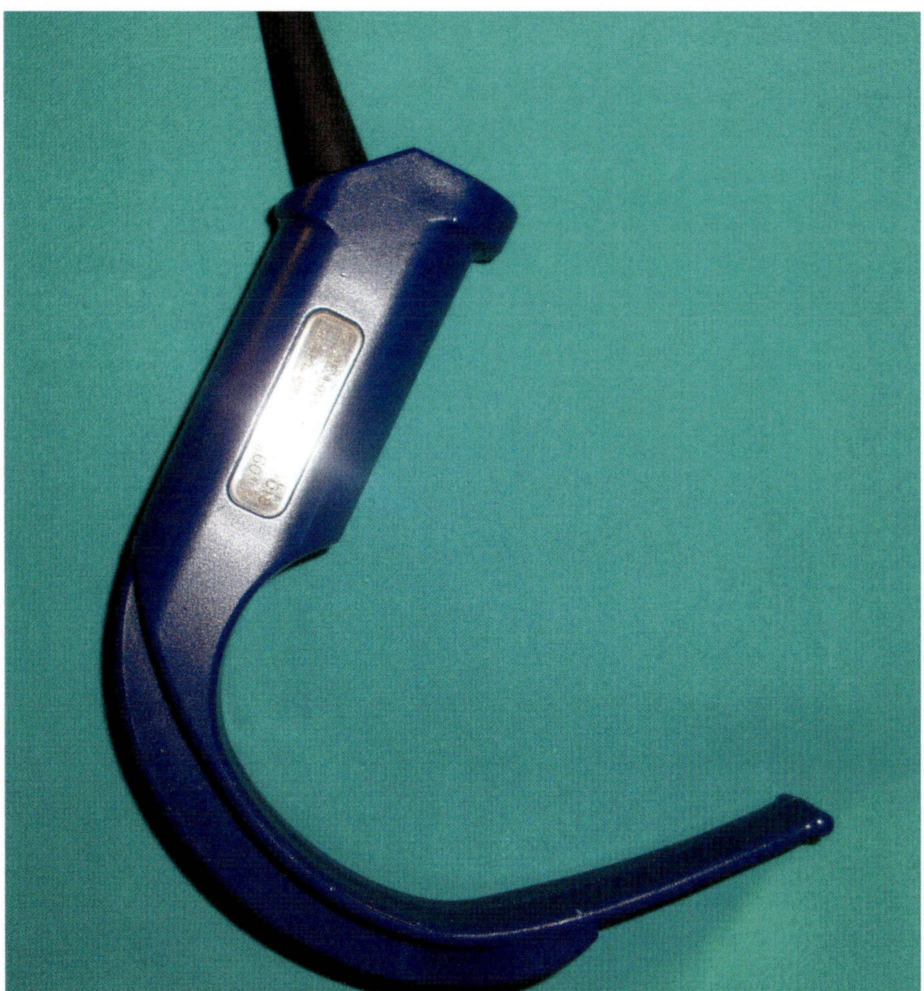

Fig. 9.2 GlideScope blade (Verathon Inc.) available for difficult intubation.

constrictor muscle where it is crossed by the hypoglossal nerve, and then it passes deep to the hyoglossus muscle where it runs on the superior surface of the hyoid bone. It is in this location that it is vulnerable to injury during transoral base of tongue surgery. The lingual artery then gives off a suprahyoid branch, a dorsal lingual artery that passes to the dorsum of the tongue, the sublingual artery, and the arteria profunda linguae that passes between the genioglossus muscle and the inferior intrinsic tongue musculature. These arteries anastomose richly with their partners from the opposite side. The tongue is drained by lingual veins that pass to the internal jugular vein directly or via the facial and retromandibular veins.

The tongue receives motor supply from the hypoglossal nerve. The hypoglossal nerve emanates from the hypoglossal canal and descends behind the internal carotid artery and the glossopharyngeal nerve and vagus nerve. It then passes between the internal carotid artery and internal jugular vein, runs in front of the vagus nerve, and loops in front of the internal and external carotid artery and lingual artery. A small branch of the occipital artery feeding the sternocleidomastoid muscle crosses over the hypoglossal nerve just below the posterior belly of the digastric muscle. The nerve then passes over the hyoglossus muscle and runs along the superior border of the hyoid bone, deep to the digastric and mylohyoid muscles. It is here that the nerve is at most risk during transoral base of tongue surgery. The hypoglossal nerve divides into terminal branches that continue between the mylohyoid and genioglossus muscles. The posterior tongue receives predominant sensory innervation by the lingual branch of the glossopharyngeal nerve for both afferent sensation and taste.[10,11,12,13,14]

Bleeding/Hemostasis

A vessel clip applier (**Fig. 9.3**) and an insulated bipolar forceps should be readily available throughout the surgery. The bipolar forceps needs to have an angled tip to achieve adequate access (**Figs. 9.4** and **9.5**). This can allow the bedside assistant to manage intraoperative bleeding. As a 30-degree upward facing scope is utilized during the procedure, all the nonrobotic instruments should be angled, especially the suction devices that are used to suction smoke, blood, and provide counter traction (**Fig. 9.6**).

At the end of the procedure the wound is inspected carefully for hemostasis, and cautery or vessel clips are used as needed for persistent bleeding. A surface tissue hemostatic agent such as Tisseel fibrin sealant (Baxter Healthcare Corp.) can be applied in a thin layer, which some clinicians feel may also help with postoperative discomfort. The tongue and airway are inspected for edema at the end of the procedure to assess the possibility of an early tube removal or the necessity of a prolonged intubation or tracheostomy.

Intraoral Trauma

An important intraoperative complication is dental or mouth trauma. To avoid damage to the teeth, the upper dental arch is protected with either a standard rubber teeth guard or a custom guard fabricated in the operating room from Aquaplast. To avoid trauma to the oral cavity and oropharynx mucosa the robotic instruments must be inserted under direct vision initially and then via the slave screen when it is no longer possible to visualize them transorally.

Technical Complications

Some common complications with the robotics arms can occur during surgery. One of these is an inverted movement of the instrument during the console joystick movement. If this occurs, when the surgeon feels the inverted movement, the dissection should be stopped and the instruments replaced in the robotic

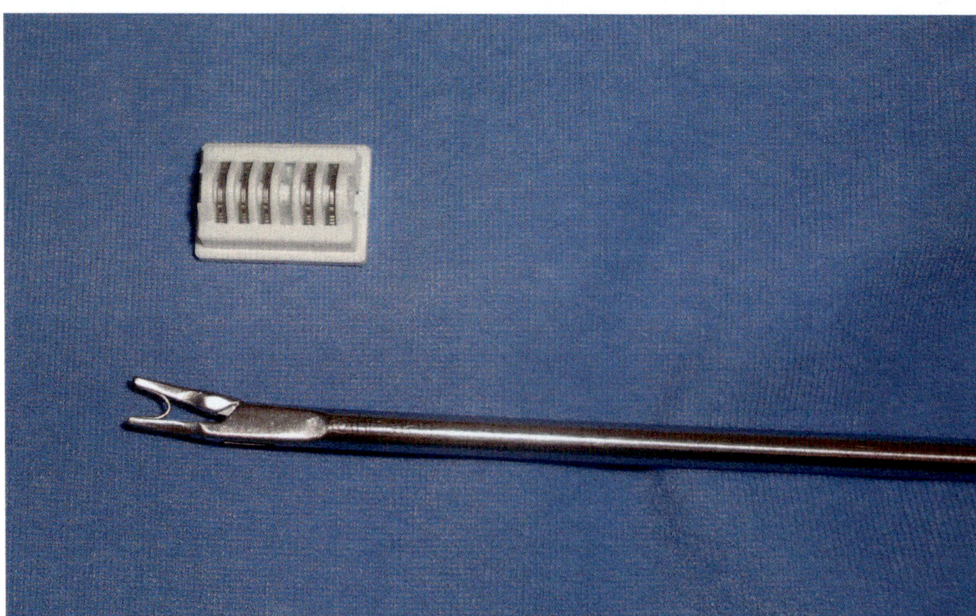

Fig. 9.3 Vessel clip applier (Karl Storz) and medium clips (Ethicon).

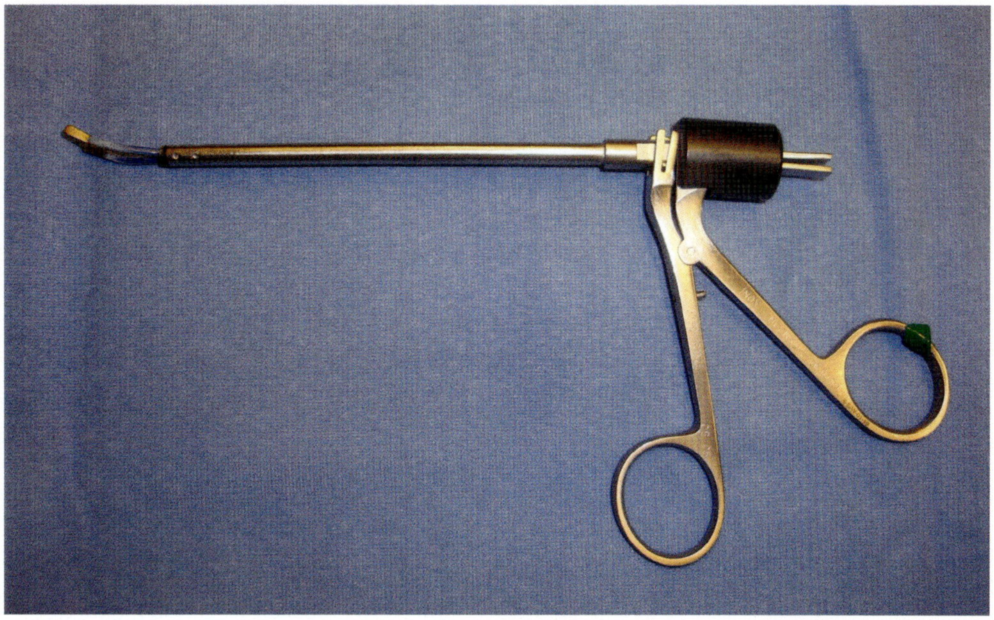

Fig. 9.4 Dessi nasal bipolar forceps (MicroFrance-Medtronic).

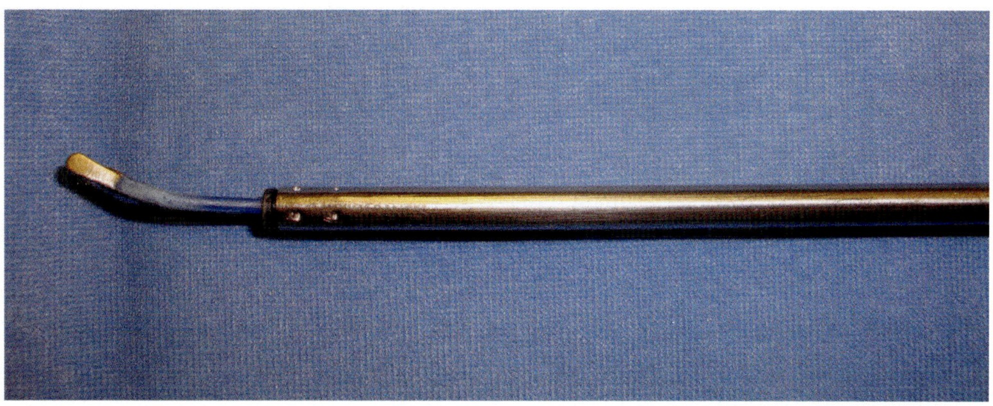

Fig. 9.5 Detail of nasal bipolar forceps (MicroFrance-Medtronic) with angled tip to achieve adequate access.

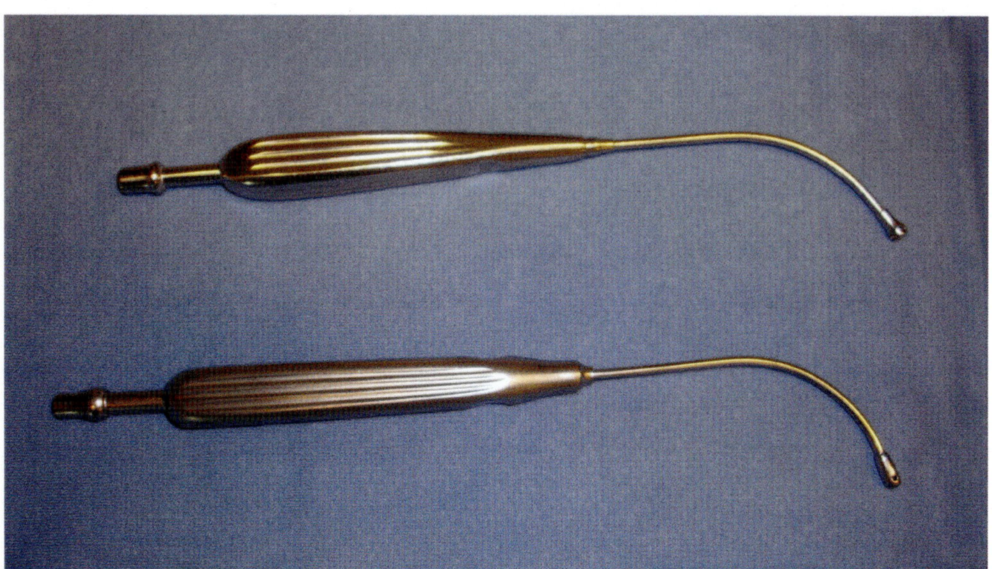

Fig. 9.6 Pinchon suction devices that are used to suction smoke and blood and provide counter traction (Lawton, code 160274, and Medicon, code 098508).

and arm. This way, the robot will be allowed to recognize the instrument once again. This may need to be repeated several times.

Another possible occurrence is failure of one of the two robotic cameras. The primary surgeon can continue to perform the procedure, however, it will be in two dimensions instead of 3D. During this technical complication the surgery may be more difficult as the primary surgeon will not have the same depth perception as with the 3D camera.

■ Immediate Postoperative Complications

The immediate postoperative period is crucial to avoid serious complications; the patient should be monitored carefully in a high acuity nursing setting. Intravenous steroids are given to minimize lingual edema and nausea. Intravenous broad-spectrum antibiotics are infused pre- and postoperatively as per hospital protocol or surgeon preference to avoid possible infections.

If the patient did not undergo tracheostomy as the initial step in the operative procedure, then the patient should have a prolonged postoperative intubation either in recovery or in an intensive care setting. This is done to avoid laryngospasm that may result from aspiration of saliva or blood. In an already difficult airway, re-intubation is made even more difficult due to postoperative edema, bleeding, and modified anatomy. Prior to removal of the endotracheal tube, we check the airway with a flexible endoscope. This optimizes the timing of tube removal and is usually a few hours after the surgery.

As detailed previously, for severe OSAHS cases with a narrow mouth opening, a covering tracheostomy is strongly recommended for postoperative ventilation assistance, especially if multilevel surgery has been performed. One more key reason for performing a planned tracheostomy is the degree of difficulty of re-intubation if the patient develops postsurgical airway edema or postoperative bleeding.

The first postoperative night, the patient should be monitored in a high-acuity setting. In most institutions this would be in an intensive care or high-dependency unit rather than the typical postoperative hospital ward. The patient should have continuous pulse oximetry and suction should be available at all times by the bedside. The patient should be watched closely for bleeding and respiratory depression.

The authors find that many patients can swallow liquids comfortably without aspiration within a day of surgery, but this can vary considerably between patients. In the authors' institution, we routinely do not insert a feeding tube and a liquid diet is started on postoperative day 1. We also continue oral steroids after discharge on a tapering dose. Narcotics are used as needed but this must be in the context of close observation of respiratory rate and level of consciousness, as recommended postoperatively for other OSAHS surgical procedures.

The length of stay can vary considerably depending upon a number of variables and surgeon comfort level. Tracheostomy by itself necessitates a multi-day hospital stay. Other determinants include the extent of surgery, comorbidities, pain control, and swallowing ability. In the United States, a patient is discharged on the first postoperative day. In Europe, however, a longer hospitalization of 3 to 5 days is followed.

■ Delayed Postoperative Complications

Patients are followed closely after discharge. Diet is normalized as the healing progresses and formal therapist-directed swallowing therapy is rarely needed. Most patients will resume a normal diet within 1 month of surgery. Patients who have undergone multilevel surgery may need more time than patients who have had only one site treated.

In case of delayed postoperative bleeding, if conservative measures fail, a suspension laryngoscope should be used to achieve an operative view of the base of tongue (**Fig. 9.7**). It is unlikely that a view of the bleeding area will be achieved with a tonsil gag. Typically a suction monopolar diathermy device is then used for hemostasis (**Fig. 9.8**).

Another important and difficult to manage long-term complication is that of synechia formation or stenosis of the orohypopharynx following TORS. If a good exposure is not achieved at the time of TORS and there is not sufficient space between tongue base–epiglottis and the posterior pharyngeal wall, it is possible to injure the mucosa of the posterior and lateral oropharyngeal walls through the use of monopolar cautery. This circumferential damage could produce a concentric keloid in the first months after surgery (**Fig. 9.9**). This complication may necessitate a long-term tracheostomy and gastrostomy tube. To avoid a concentric scar, especially in patients where a palate surgery is performed, 1–2 mm of intact mucosa should be left between the palatine tonsil fossa and the tongue base. This is a devastating complication, so prevention is the best strategy.

■ Conclusion

The adverse events recorded as part of a multicentric study (seven centers in Europe and the United States) are summarized in **Table 9.1**.[2] In 243 cases so far there is a 0.0% mortality rate and a 20.5% morbidity rate, and most of the morbidities are minor and short-term. The most common patient complaint was a transient and mild hypogeusia (14.2%), which recovered within 8 months in all the patients. Bleeding was the second most common complication (5% of the procedures). In most of the cases (2.9%) late postoperative bleeding was self-limited and did not require operative intervention. Only 1.7% of the patients required an additional surgical procedure to control the bleeding. Finally, in 0.4% of surgeries a significant intraoperative hemorrhage was reported. Pharyngeal scarring with minimal to mild stenosis was a late complication in 0.4% of the procedures. Transient pharyngeal edema was observed in 0.4% of patients.

Overall, our series to date shows that there is a good side effect profile for this procedure. It is generally well tolerated and

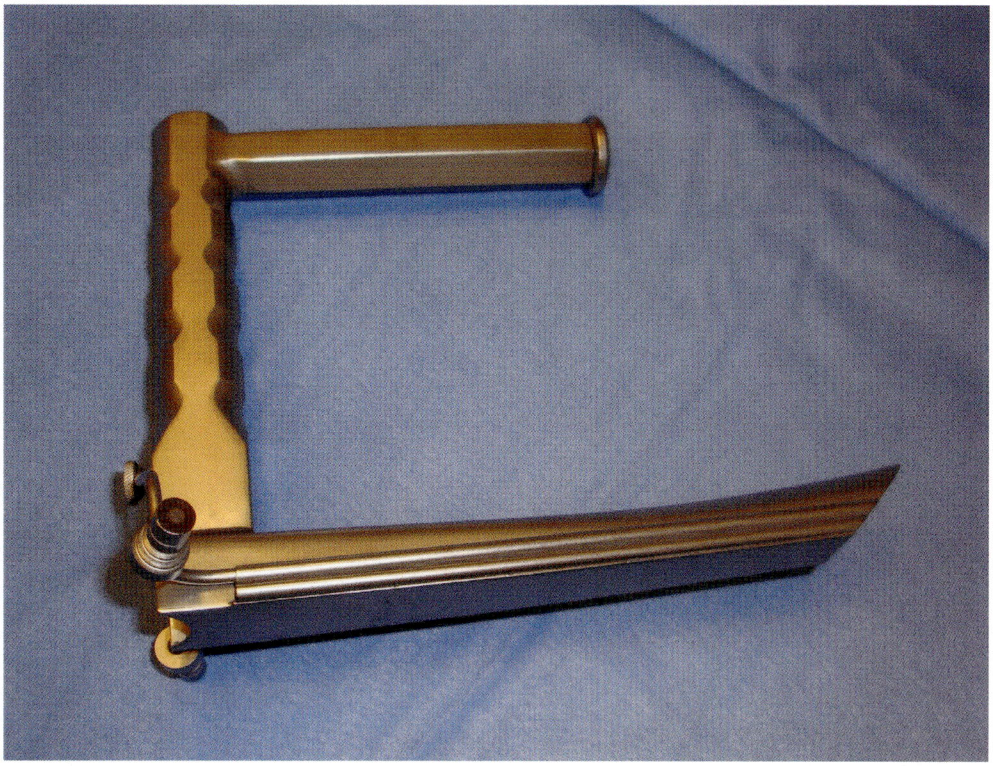

Fig. 9.7 Sataloff laryngoscope (MicroFrance-Medtronic) to achieve an operative view of the base of tongue.

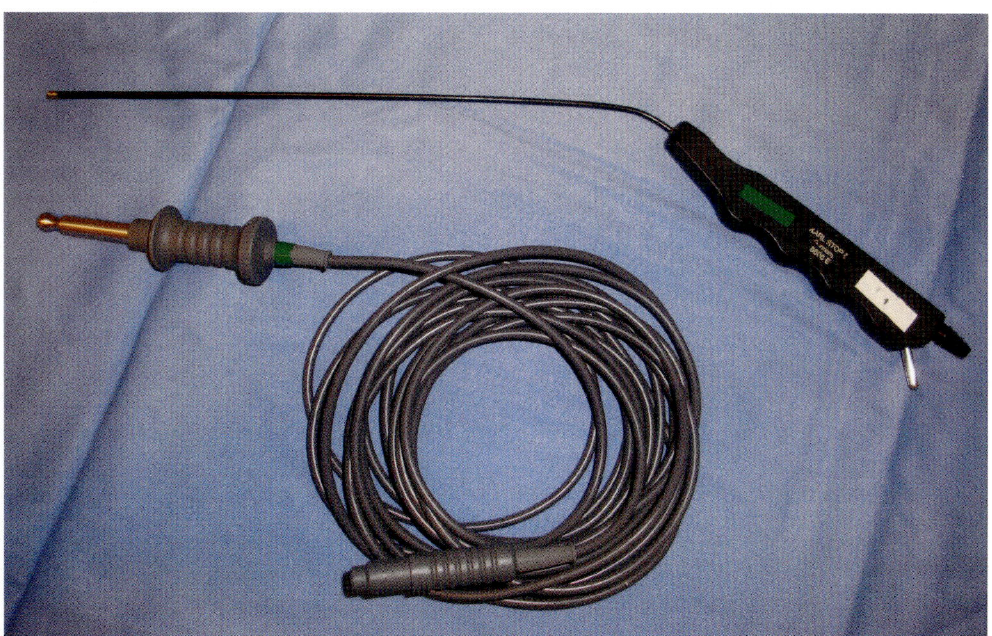

Fig. 9.8 Suction monopolar diathermy device (Karl Storz) used for hemostasis.

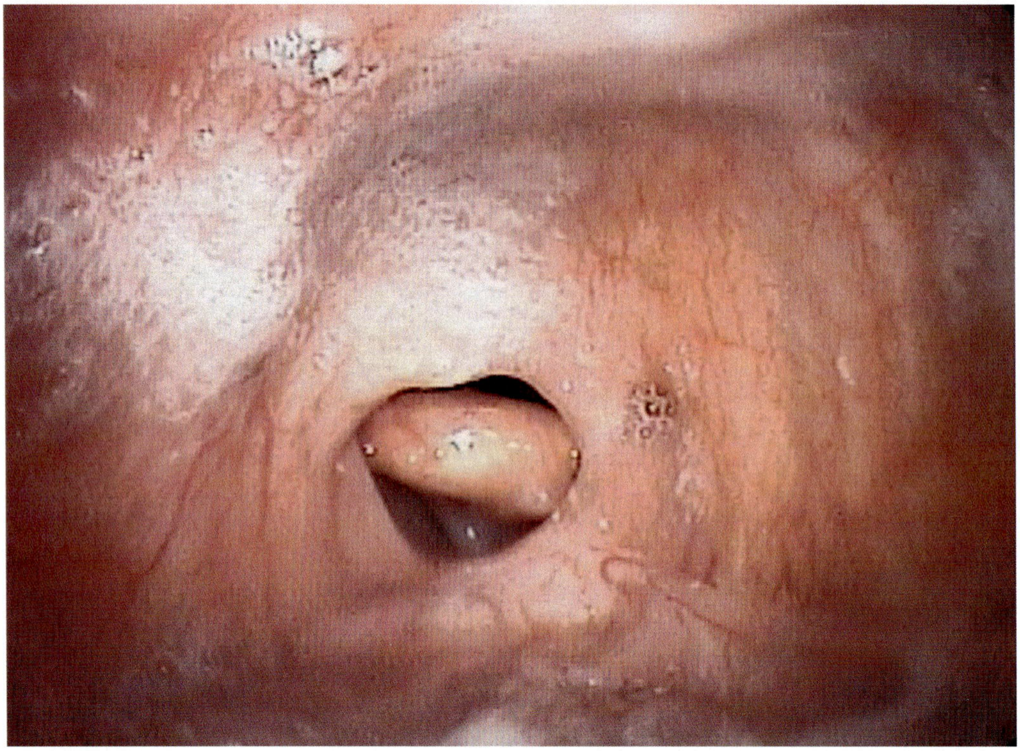

Fig. 9.9 Postoperative stenosis of the orohypopharynx due to a concentric keloid. The epiglottis tip is visible below the stenosis.

Table 9.1 Complications of robotic sleep surgery

No complication	79.5%
Transient hypogeusia	14.2%
Postoperative self-limited bleeding	2.9%
Late bleeding managed in the operating room	1.7%
Intraoperative bleeding	0.4%
Pharyngeal stenosis	0.4%
Transient globus sensation	0.4%
Transient pharyngeal edema	0.4%

complications are limited in number and severity; however, no deaths or definite severe impairments were registered.

References

1. Vicini C, Dallan I, Canzi P, Frassineti S, La Pietra MG, Montevecchi F. Transoral robotic tongue base resection in obstructive sleep apnoea-hypopnoea syndrome: a preliminary report. ORL J Otorhinolaryngol Relat Spec 2010;72(1):22–27
2. Vicini C, Montevecchi F, Campanini A, et al. Clinical outcomes and complications associated with TORS for OSAHS. A benchmark for evaluating an emerging surgical technology in a targeted application for benign disease. ORL J Otorhinolaryngol Relat Spec 2014;76(2):63–69
3. Shahar E, Whitney CW, Redline S, et al. Sleep-disordered breathing and cardiovascular disease: cross-sectional results of the Sleep Heart Health Study. Am J Respir Crit Care Med 2001;163(1):19–25
4. Yaggi HK, Concato J, Kernan WN, Lichtman JH, Brass LM, Mohsenin V. Obstructive sleep apnea as a risk factor for stroke and death. N Engl J Med 2005;353:2034–2041
5. Vicini C, Montevecchi F, Pang K, et al. Combined transoral robotic tongue base surgery and palate surgery in obstructive sleep apnea-hypopnea syndrome: expansion sphincter pharyngoplasty versus uvulopalatopharyngoplasty. Head Neck 2014;36(1): 77–83
6. Kim JA, Lee JJ. Preoperative predictors of difficult intubation in patients with obstructive sleep apnea syndrome. Can J Anaesth 2006;53(4):393–397
7. Hillman DR, Loadsman JA, Platt PR, Eastwood PR. Obstructive sleep apnoea and anaesthesia. Sleep Med Rev 2004;8(6): 459–471
8. Sun H, Lou W, Wang L, Wu Y. Clinical significance of preoperative tracheotomy in preventing perioperative OSAHS severe complications. Lin Chuang Er Bi Yan Hou Ke Za Zhi 2005;19(9):394–395
9. Campanini A, De Vito A, Frassineti S, Vicini C. Temporary tracheotomy in the surgical treatment of obstructive sleep apnea syndrome: personal experience. Acta Otorhinolaryngol Ital 2003;23(6):474–478

10. Moore EJ, Janus J, Kasperbauer J. Transoral robotic surgery of the oropharynx: clinical and anatomic considerations. Clin Anat 2012;25(1):135–141
11. Vicini C, Dallan I, Canzi P, et al. Transoral robotic surgery of the tongue base in obstructive sleep apnea-hypopnea syndrome: anatomic considerations and clinical experience. Head Neck 2012;34(1):15–22
12. Dallan I, Seccia V, Faggioni L, et al. Anatomical landmarks for transoral robotic tongue base surgery: comparison between endoscopic, external and radiological perspectives. Surg Radiol Anat 2013;35(1):3–10
13. Lauretano AM, Li KK, Caradonna DS, Khosta RK, Fried MP. Anatomic location of the tongue base neurovascular bundle. Laryngoscope 1997;107(8):1057–1059
14. Sequert C, Lestang P, Baglin AC, Wagner I, Ferron JM, Chabolle F. Hypoglossal nerve in its intralingual trajectory: anatomy and clinical implications. Ann Otolaryngol Chir Cervicofac 1999;116(4):207–217

10 Robotic Surgery of the Larynx

Richard V. Smith

■ The Clinical Problem

The surgical management of laryngeal disorders has been practiced for more than a century. The initial surgeries were done primarily for cancer, as the procedures were often radical, performed through an external approach, and had high complication rates. The evolution of surgery as a whole—with improved surgical techniques, antibiotic therapy, anesthetic advancements, and other advancements—has led us to an entirely different concept of laryngeal surgery since the 1960s. The open radical surgeries, total laryngectomy and its variants, have given way to open partial laryngectomies and subsequently transoral endoscopic resections for more limited lesions. Laryngeal surgery for benign disease has an extensive portfolio of minimally invasive approaches, but has few indications for transoral robotic surgery (TORS) at this time.

■ Current Standards

The current standards for the treatment of larynx cancer are largely dependent upon stage of disease and institution where the patient is treated. Early stage disease, stage I or II, is treated with either transoral laser microsurgery (TLM) or radiation therapy. Advanced disease, stage III or IV, may be treated with surgery, radiation, chemotherapy and radiation, or all three. Philosophical differences are present regarding the optimal means of therapy for the advanced stage group and often show institutional bias. Radiation has a long record of success in treating early larynx cancer, with stage-dependent results. Surgery for early stage larynx cancer has shown equivalent results between radiation and TLM.[1,2,3] Others, however, have demonstrated improved disease-specific survival with organ preservation surgery.[4] Given the comparable survival, there is a shift toward functional assessment to determine the better approach. When looked at as a group, studies of radiation and TLM show no significant difference between the two approaches for functional outcome. Advanced larynx cancer has been treated primarily with chemotherapy and radiation therapy in the United States for the past few decades, and although there is no difference in overall survival between concurrent chemotherapy and radiation, induction chemotherapy and radiation, or radiation alone, concurrent therapy has a higher rate of organ preservation.[5] Those with T4 laryngeal cancer, when examined separately, have improved survival with initial surgery.[6] It is evident, therefore, that surgery continues to play an important role in the primary management of laryngeal cancer.

This chapter focuses on the transoral robotic techniques of laryngeal surgery. The current techniques of transoral robotic partial and total laryngectomy represent waypoints along a continuum in the development of minimally invasive surgery for laryngeal cancer. The acceptance of TORS as a whole, and for the larynx in particular, has been quite rapid and is based upon little clinical data.[7,8,9] The oncologic basis for this approach comes from the results of transoral laser microsurgical resection of larynx cancer, which has an established record of success[2,10,11,12,13] and has been shown to be equivalent to open partial laryngectomy for the cure of primary laryngeal cancer.[14] TORS is simply an extension of the TLM technique.

There is debate among head and neck surgeons and laryngologists regarding which transoral modality is superior. Some argue that TLM is superior, since there are many options for instrumentation, including a large variety of endoscopes, many microlaryngeal instruments, and readily accessible lasers to assist in dissection and resection. In addition, the TLM technique purposefully divides the tumor to better assess the intraoperative resection and margin status. Others feel the three-dimensional HD visualization provided by the surgical robot, the tremor scaling, and the fact that the tumor can often be resected in toto, with planned transection of the tumor tissue avoided, make TORS a more preferable modality. Increasing experience with TORS techniques leads to decreased complication rates and decreased hospitalization.[15] In addition, TORS management of oropharynx and supraglottic cancers has been shown to result in better short- and long-term swallowing function when compared to chemoradiotherapy.[16] This chapter focuses primarily on TORS supraglottic partial laryngectomy, with some discussion of TORS total laryngectomy and cordectomy. Other laryngeal TORS techniques have been reported, including benign lesion excision and supracricoid partial laryngectomy,[17] but are not extensively discussed here.

■ Treatment Goals

As with any oncologic surgery, the main goal of treatment is to cure the patient of their cancer. A secondary, although equally important, goal in larynx cancer patients is maximization of their function and quality of life. Successful achievement of cure and function is aided by TORS partial laryngectomy. Negative margin transoral supraglottic laryngectomy, with selective neck dissection, provides cure rates equivalent to chemoradiotherapy and can avoid the use of adjuvant radiation. This can result in excellent swallowing and speech function while maintaining excellent cure rates.

The overall goals remain the same for primary TORS laryngeal surgery or salvage surgery: tumor eradication with maintenance of the laryngeal functions (i.e., speaking, swallowing, and breathing). The outcomes and complications are different in the two scenarios, with wound healing issues and functional sequelae being more significant in the salvage setting. Inadequate swallowing is more common in the salvage group, due to delayed healing, and, although rarely required in a primary setting, tracheotomy may be required during the perioperative and healing phase in salvage surgery. Previously irradiated laryngeal tissues have a higher propensity for edema of the residual tissue, which will nearly always resolve over time. In either primary or salvage TORS for laryngeal cancer, swallowing and airway function are excellent in the majority of patients.

Preoperative Planning and Special Equipment

Preoperative planning for any tumor resection is critical. For partial or total laryngectomy anatomical imaging is usually required, with the exception of T1 and select T2 glottic tumors. Standard imaging would include a contrast computed tomography (CT) scan to evaluate the thyroid and cricoid cartilages, the pre-epiglottic and paraglottic spaces, and the cervical lymph nodes. Positron emission tomography (PET)/CT is increasingly being used at the time of diagnostic imaging and can help identify disease laterally in the neck in the absence of radiographically positive adenopathy on anatomical imaging. As with all head and neck cancer patients, a frank discussion with the patient and his/her family of all available treatment modalities is critically important. Evaluation by the appropriate nonsurgical specialists with prospective presentation at a tumor board is also an important part of the treatment plan.

Special equipment is required for this type of surgery. In addition to the da Vinci surgical robot (Intuitive Surgical, Inc.), multiple robotic instruments are important to maximize operative success. Although other robotic platforms have been reported (**Table 10.1**), this chapter focuses on the use of the da Vinci system. The surgical arms should include a Maryland forceps, Schertel forceps, and Teflon-coated blade tip electrocautery. A CO_2 fiber laser (or another type of fiber laser) is advantageous when performing TORS on the larynx. The surgical arms should be 5-mm instruments and the endoscope 12 mm if possible. If transoral suturing is planned, 8-mm needle drivers should be used in both arms, as the distal tip of the 8-mm robotic arm articulates in a much shorter radius, facilitating suturing in a confined space. The bedside assistant is responsible for the management of significant hemorrhage from vessels such as the superior laryngeal artery. A laparoscopic articulating clip applier is used for significant vessels, while the robotic cautery or a suction cautery will control the majority of any intraoperative bleeding. The small or medium clip applier may be used, at the discretion of the surgeon. The vasculature is often in predictable locations[21] and the transoral surgeon must possess a detailed anatomical knowledge pertinent to the approach. Laparoscopic peanuts and the Hurd retractor are also very useful adjuvants for tissue retraction. Finally, the Feyh-Kastenbauer (FK) retractor system (Gyrus Medical Inc.) is required to maximize exposure options during the surgery. The Crowe-Davis and Dingman mouth gags may also be useful. There have been recent descriptions of customized phonosurgical tips for the da Vinci robot and enhancements to the retractor system,[18] which could significantly enhance current operative techniques.

Benefits and Drawbacks of Robotic Laryngeal Surgery

Appropriate patient selection is critical for TORS laryngeal surgery, taking into account features of the tumor and patient. As is the case with TLM, appropriate patient motivation is paramount, as there will always be a temporary compromise of swallowing following supraglottic partial laryngectomy. Adequate

Table 10.1 Robotic laryngeal systems

Device	Patient Use	Endoscope	Instruments	Advantages	Limitations
da Vinci	Yes	12 mm 0-degree 12 mm 30-degree 8.5 mm 0-degree 8.5 mm 30-degree	8 and 5 mm	3D HD image FDA approved	No haptic feedback Cost
da Vinci[18]	No	See above	Sickle knife Angled pick Spatula Microlaryngeal elevator	Fine instruments mirroring current instruments	Custom made
AESOP[19]	Yes	Standard rigid telescopes – 0, 30, 70, and 120 degrees	All commercially available TLM instruments	Endoscopic scope holder Voice activated	Standard telescope without 3D
Highly Flexible Robot[20]	No	Fiberoptic	Flexible grasper and cautery	Not "line of site" Standard retractors	Limited quality visualization and instruments

Abbreviations: 3D, three-dimensional; FDA, U.S. Food and Drug Administration; HD, high-definition; TLM, transoral laser microsurgery.

pulmonary reserve is required to tolerate small amounts of temporary aspiration. Additionally, poorly controlled diabetes can impair wound healing after partial laryngectomy.[22] When TORS is used for salvage surgery, one can expect delayed healing and potentially worse functional outcomes. Functional deficits in these patients may be related to prolonged edema or laryngopharyngeal fibrosis from the radiation therapy, which impedes normal laryngeal elevation and pharyngeal contraction with swallowing.

Tumor stage and extent are important considerations. Supraglottic tumors, T1–T4a, may be considered for transoral resection. Supraglottic laryngectomy can be a technically demanding procedure, so those new to the technique should confine themselves to T1 or T2 tumors. Once a surgeon is more facile, larger tumors can be considered. Neither pre-epiglottic space involvement nor tongue base involvement are contraindications to TORS resection, provided the exposure is adequate. Extension into the paraglottic area with vocal fold immobility is a relative contraindication to a TORS supraglottic at this time if the spatula electrocautery is the active source for the dissection. The spread of current into the glottis area may result in bilateral vocal fold immobility and the need for a permanent tracheotomy. In fact, in the authors' opinion, any TORS glottic surgery should be avoided if the spatula electrocautery is used. The development of laser carrying fibers and manipulators for the robotic arms will facilitate the development and expansion of glottic surgery with TORS. Special consideration should also be undertaken in cases of salvage partial laryngectomy. In addition to poor healing, the tissue planes relied upon for margin assessment are much less obvious and soft tissue edema can affect the interaction of the cautery and the tissue, complicating the procedure and the outcomes.

Equipment and anatomical factors are equally important for TORS laryngeal surgery. Current retractor systems have been, for the most part, developed for TLM and not for TORS. The instrumentation required, two 5-mm instruments and a 12-mm telescope, are much more bulky than the TLM instruments. Consequently, instrument conflicts become more significant as one proceeds into the distal pharynx or larynx, as the space becomes more constrained and the instruments begin to cone down. Therefore, maximal mouth opening is essential, precluding the surgery in cases of trismus. Additionally, full dentition, particularly the presence of maxillary central incisors, can significantly impede exposure. Anterior laryngeal positioning also provides a challenge to adequate exposure, although TORS is less limited in that regard than TLM. A narrow posterior mandibular arch also inhibits exposure of the larynx. Adequate exposure is the most important technical feature and a variety of retractors should be available for every case to maximize exposure. The minimum retractor complement should include a Crowe-Davis and FK retractor system. Multiple blades may be required for any given procedure and several may need to be assessed before the optimal exposure is obtained.

■ Procedures

Positioning

As with any surgical procedure, proper patient and equipment positioning is important. This topic is thoroughly discussed in Chapter 4 of this book. There are several issues pertinent to laryngeal surgery that merit additional note. For larynx surgery a shoulder roll is generally not necessary. Routine use will often limit the anteroposterior exposure of the larynx, further limiting an already narrowed surgical field. It is frequently helpful to place a suture transversely through the anterior midline tongue to facilitate exposure by tongue traction. Care must be taken to avoid compression of the tongue between the teeth and the retractor blade during the surgery, either anteriorly or laterally. Lateral compression of the tongue is a particular problem with laryngeal robotic surgery as eccentric positioning of the retractor blades, with significant anterior tilt, may be required for exposure. For most laryngeal TORS procedures, the 30-degree endoscope is used facing up. The tip of endoscope should be placed as far from the operative field as possible to minimize instrument conflicts. Resections will use 5-mm instruments and often start with the Schertel grasper (supraglottic procedures) or the Maryland grasper (glottic procedures) in the nondominant hand and the spatula Bovie or laser fiber in the dominant hand.

Supraglottic Laryngectomy

The dissection for a supraglottic laryngectomy begins superiorly, in all cases, after adequate exposure and visualization has been confirmed. The main limitations are usually in the anteroposterior exposure of the larynx, due to either radiation changes or anatomical features of the patient. The technical description that follows is that of a complete supraglottic laryngectomy. The extent of the dissection will depend upon the extent and location of the tumor. An example is presented in **Video 10.1**, in which a complete TORS supraglottic laryngectomy is performed with the CO_2 laser.

The dissection will be initiated either at the anterior aspect of the vallecula or the lateral aspect of the pharyngoepiglottic fold. This dissection should be carried to the inner surface of the hyoid to facilitate complete removal of the pre-epiglottic space (**Fig. 10.1**). The superior laryngeal vascular bundle is predictably encountered fairly early in the dissection of the lateral pharyngoepiglottic fold. These vessels should be taken prospectively and controlled with 5-mm vascular clips employing a laparoscopic clip applier (**Fig. 10.2**). If the vessel is transected before it is clipped, it should be stabilized with the robotic forceps and subsequently clipped. It should not be managed with cautery. The dissection proceeds anteriorly and laterally to resect the pre-epiglottic space in continuity with the tumor. The aryepiglottic folds are then transected superior and lateral to the arytenoid, incising obliquely to transect the posterior vestibular fold and enter the ventricle (**Fig. 10.3**).

The transection continues anteriorly at the ventricular apex until the petiole and anterior commissure are encountered. The pre-epiglottic dissection is connected to the transection inferior to the epiglottic petiole to allow removal of the specimen. If necessary, division of the specimen into quadrants is performed to improve exposure and visualization of the dissection planes. Hemostasis is obtained and the area irrigated. Margins can be taken as necessary to assess the adequacy of resection. Dissection into the inferior paraglottic space may result in immobility of the ipsilateral vocal fold due to scar fixation. This should not be undertaken with electrocautery. Use of a laser

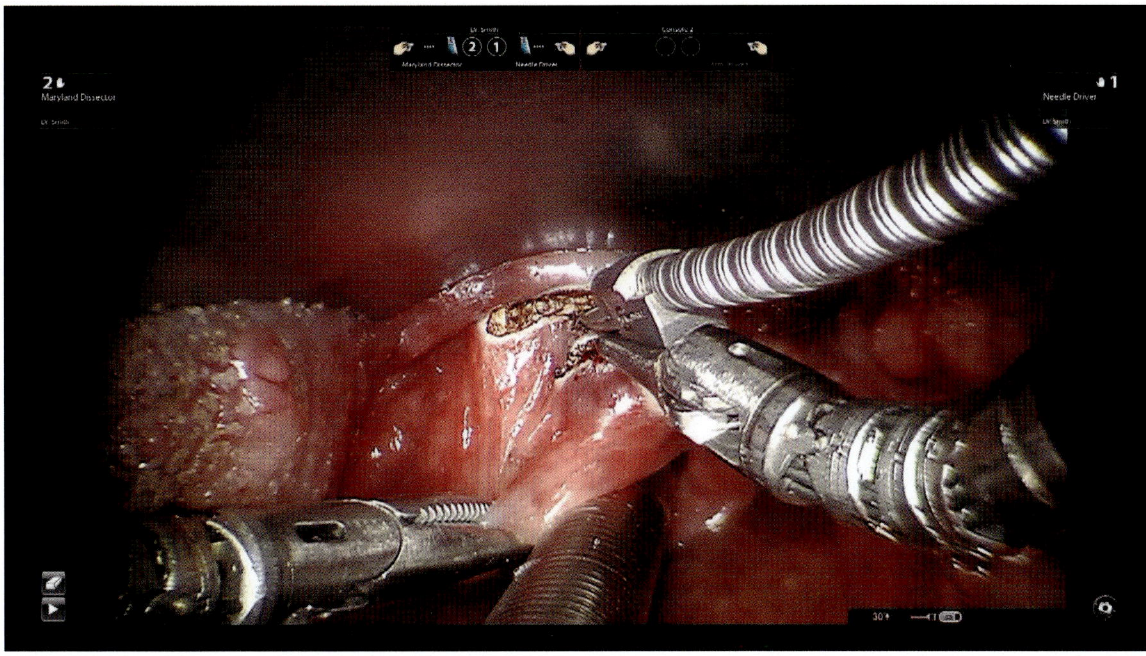

Fig. 10.1 Anterior vallecular incision with a CO_2 laser just behind the hyoid.

fiber may allow a limited paraglottic resection as required, but should be avoided bilaterally. An arytenoid may be resected if necessary oncologically, but should be avoided if possible as postoperative swallowing function will be compromised. Local flap reconstruction should be considered in such cases. The details of total supraglottic resection are also well described by Dziegielewski and Ozer.[23]

Variations on the above procedure should be undertaken based upon the extent of the tumor. Unlike the lessons from open horizontal supraglottic laryngectomy, where total supraglottic removal was necessary to minimize the need for a feeding tube or a tracheotomy tube for edematous airway obstruction, transoral supraglottic laryngectomy is a tumor-based surgery with an appropriate but limited margin, usually less than 5 mm. This means as much normal tissue as possible should be retained to provide intact mucosal sensory function to aid in swallowing and airway protection. An example of this may be seen in **Video 10.2**, which demonstrates a partial supraglottic resection of the infrahyoid epiglottis for a T1 squamous cell carcinoma. In contrast, when performed in a salvage setting, tissue planes are more poorly defined and margins may be obscured (**Video 10.3**), necessitating a liberal use of intraoperative frozen sections.

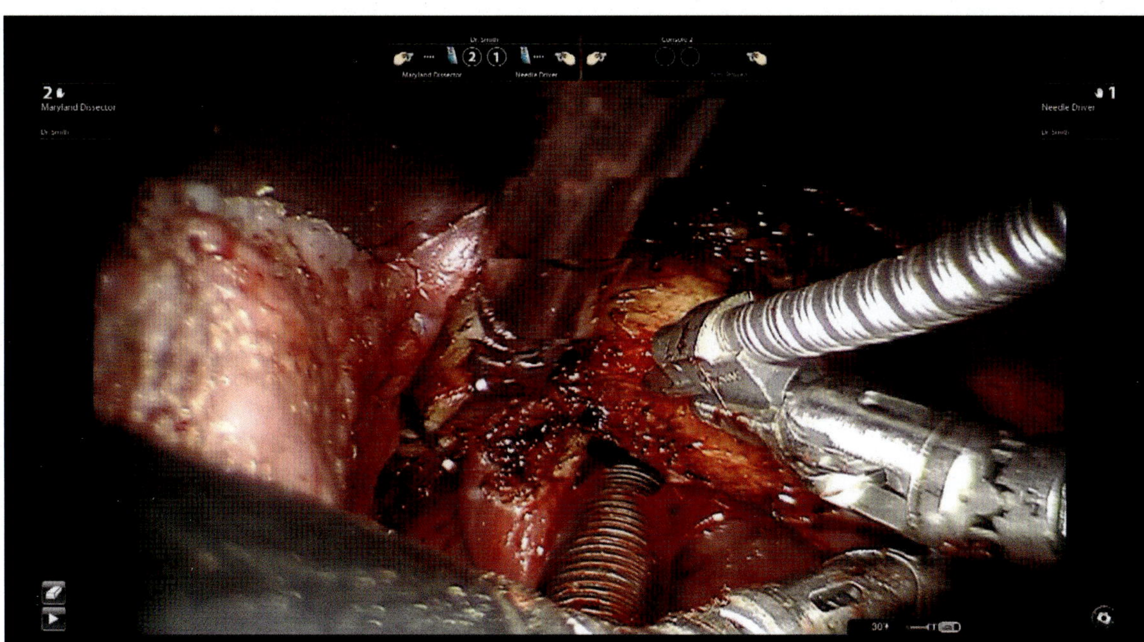

Fig. 10.2 Left lateral superior laryngeal vessels with vascular clips.

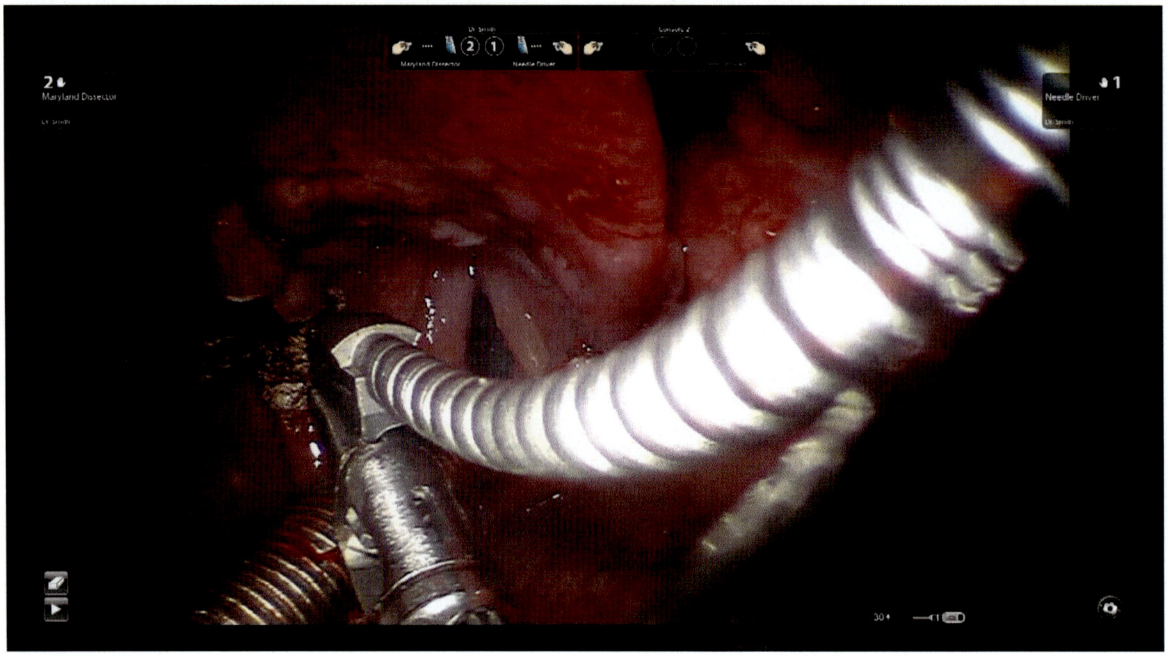

Fig. 10.3 Oblique laser incision from the superior aspect of the arytenoid extending into the left false vocal fold.

Cordectomy

TORS cordectomy has been reported by several authors. The procedure is similar to standard TLM techniques, with the notable exception being the operative instruments. The robotic Maryland forceps and spatula cautery are the instruments that have been described. The lesion is grasped and medialized while the cautery device incises the peripheral and deep tissue planes to facilitate resection. This dissection can be taken laterally to the inner thyroid perichondrium, encompassing the paraglottic space, and resect the anterior commissure tendon as well. En bloc resection is the norm with this technique. Cautery is used, as necessary, for hemostasis. As reported, many patients underwent adjuvant tracheotomy to secure the airway from edema following the resection.

Total Laryngectomy

TORS total laryngectomy is a procedure in evolution and limited case series have been published. Its use has been primarily in salvage laryngectomy cases not requiring concurrent neck dissection. Careful patient selection is required as the exposure considerations are more pertinent to this procedure given the dissection deeper within the pharynx. This is a technically demanding procedure and should not be considered if the surgeon is not experienced in transoral tumor surgery. **Video 10.4** demonstrates the technique.

The procedure begins with a transcutaneous approach to the trachea to secure the airway under local anesthesia. The stomal incision is outlined between the cricoid cartilage and suprasternal notch, the skin of the stomal site is excised, and dissection of the pretracheal tissue is completed with division of the thyroid isthmus (**Fig. 10.4**). The anterior trachea is exposed from the cricoid to the fourth tracheal ring and the trachea is entered between the second and third rings. An anode endotracheal tube is placed and general endotracheal anesthesia initiated, after which paratracheal dissection, either uni- or bilateral, is completed through the stomal opening (**Fig. 10.5**). The posterior wall of the trachea is then incised and the posterior tissues are mobilized superiorly, separating the remaining superior trachea from the esophagus. The anterior half of the trachea is then matured to the inferior stomal incision and the remainder of the procedure (**Fig. 10.6**), with the exception of closing the superior half of the stoma and insertion of a closed suction drain, is completed transorally.

The resection begins by incising the lateral pharyngoepiglottic fold and anterior vallecula in the standard fashion used for endoscopic supraglottic laryngectomy. The hyoid bone is dissected free from the pre-epiglottic tissues, maintaining the integrity of the fascial compartment containing the pre-epiglottic fat (**Fig. 10.7**) and this plane of dissection is continued inferiorly to expose the superior border of the thyroid cartilage. Once identified, the thyroid ala is mobilized posteriorly, leaving the outer thyroid perichondrium intact (**Fig. 10.8**).

The anterior pyriform sinus mucosa is incised and the lateral pyriform mucosa is mobilized. Transection of the superior laryngeal suspensory ligament facilitates access to the constrictor muscles, which are then dissected. The muscles are then sharply divided, along with the remaining fascia separating the intraoral dissection from the stomal dissection (**Fig. 10.9**). At this point the only area preventing removal of the larynx is the postcricoid area. The postcricoid mucosal cut is made under direct transoral visualization, providing appropriate margins for the tumor, and the remainder of the specimen is dissected (**Fig. 10.10**). The larynx is then fully mobilized and removed transorally (**Fig. 10.11**).

(text continued on page 109)

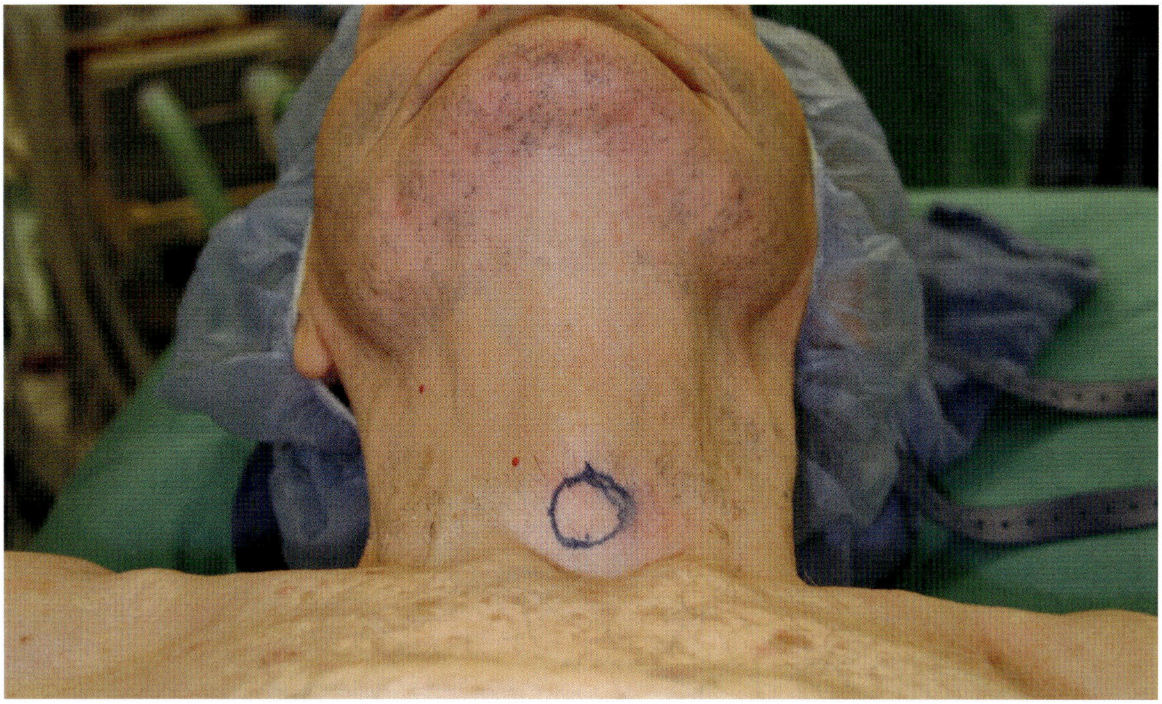

Fig. 10.4 Incision marked out in area of planned final stoma.

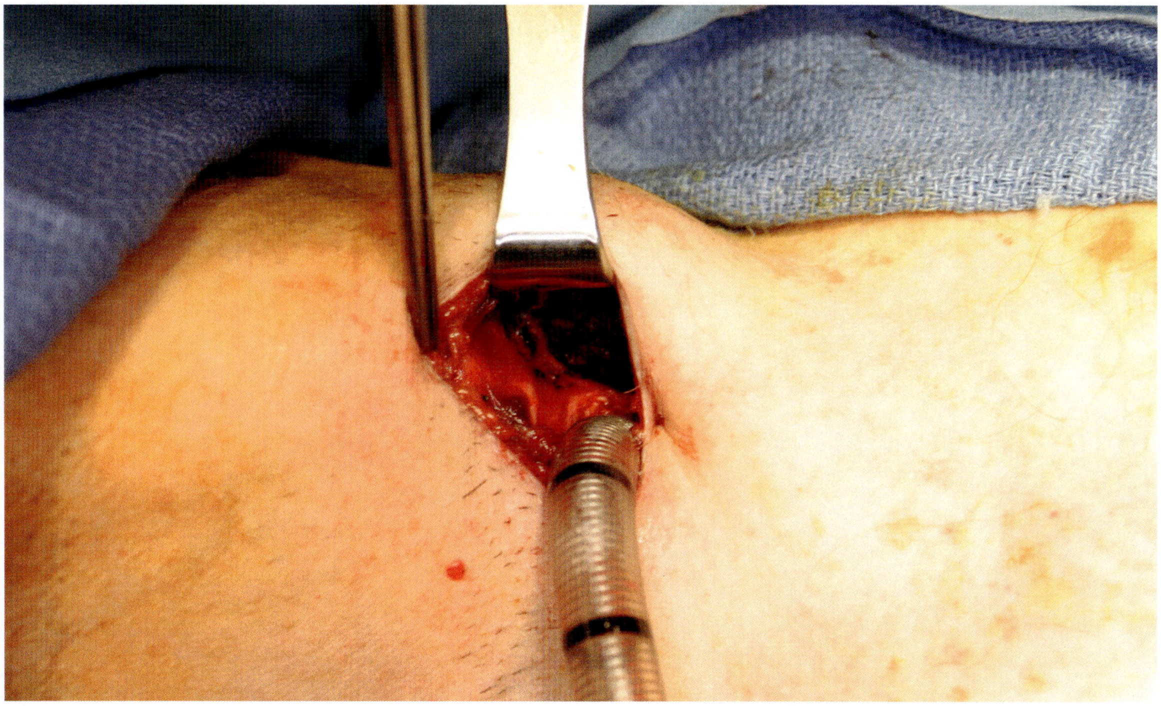

Fig. 10.5 View of the left paratracheal area following the left level VI dissection.

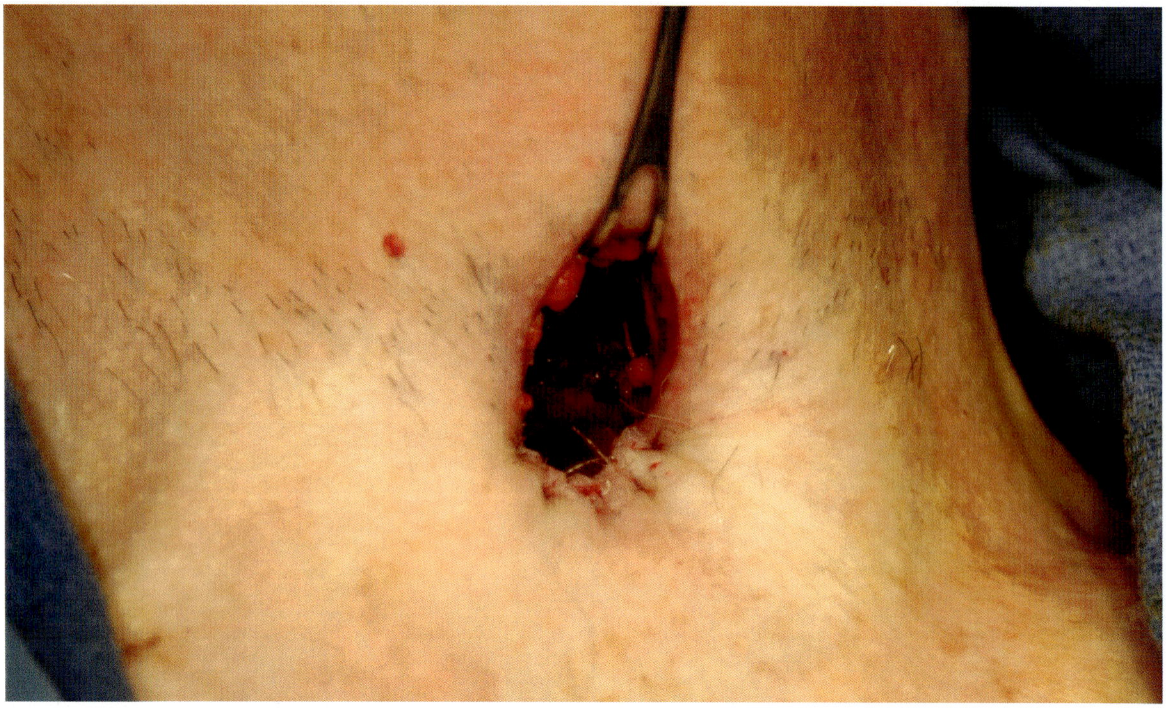

Fig. 10.6 The inferior stoma is matured with Monocryl sutures.

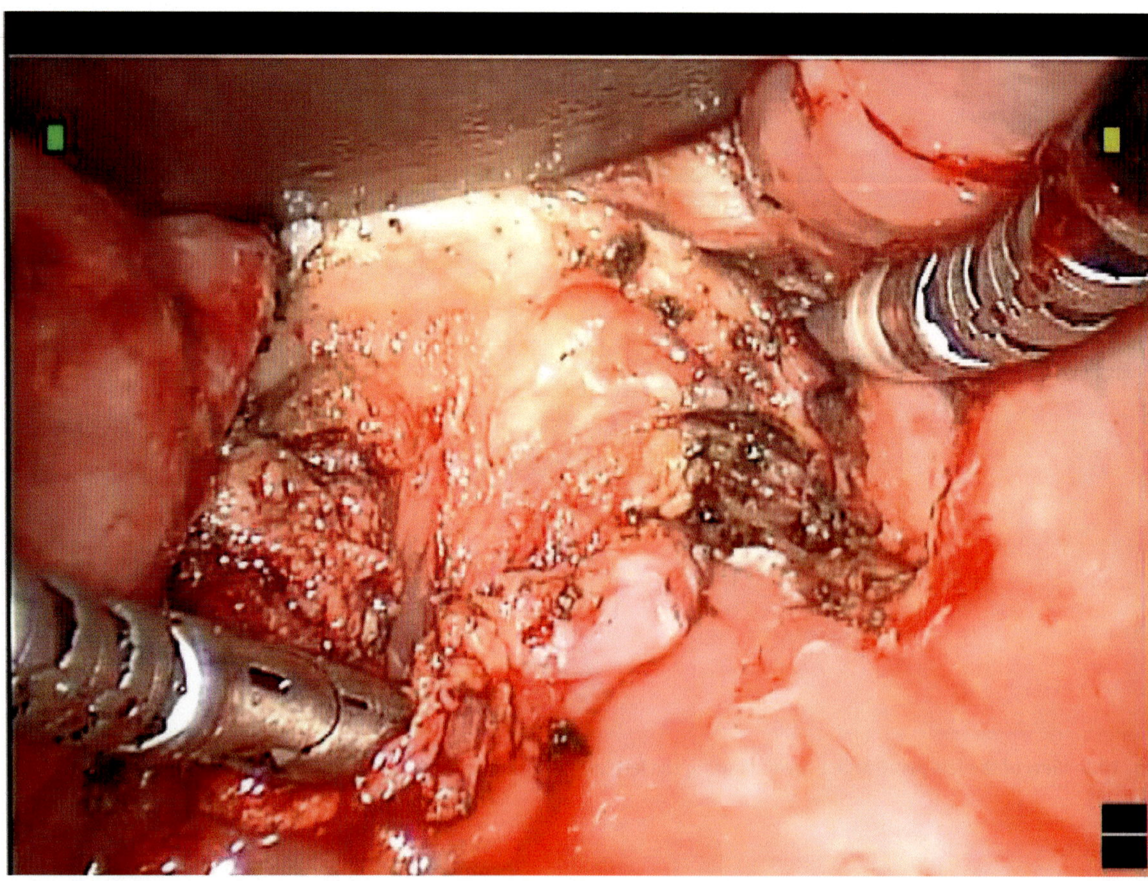

Fig. 10.7 The anterior vallecular incision is complete and carried down to the posterior aspect of the hyoid bone while maintaining the integrity of the pre-epiglottic fat pad.

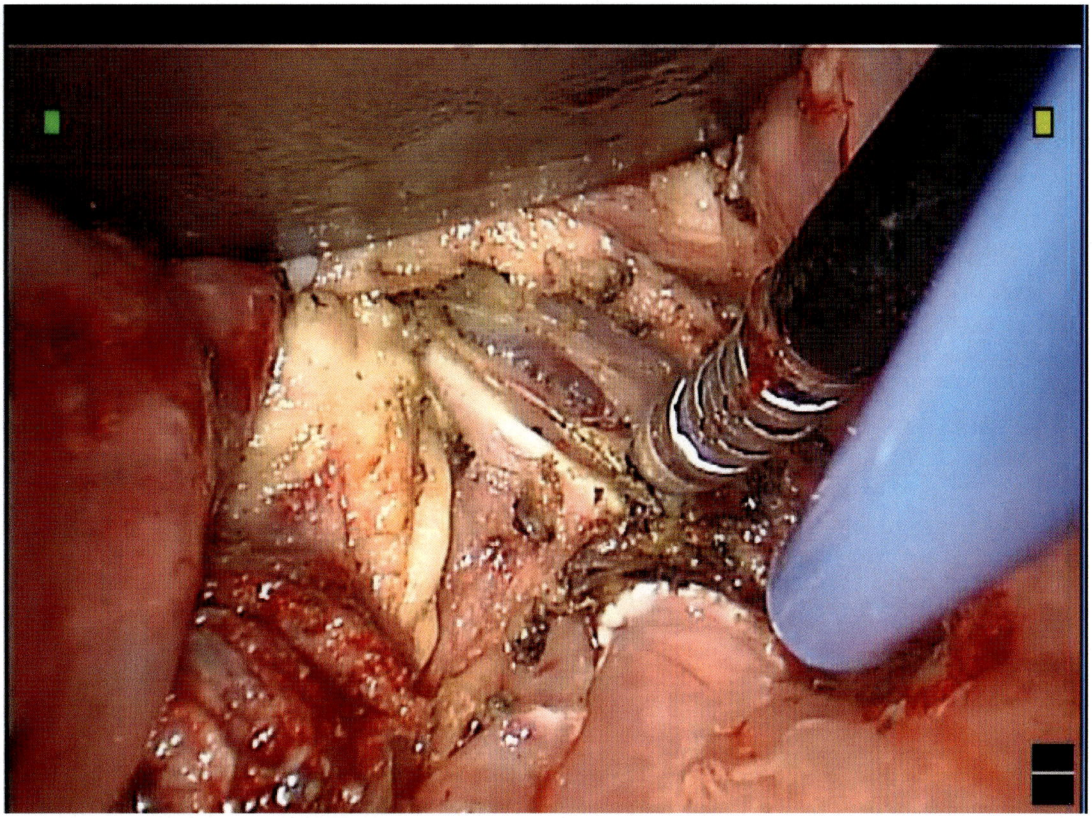

Fig. 10.8 The right thyroid ala is visualized and dissection carried out anteriorly.

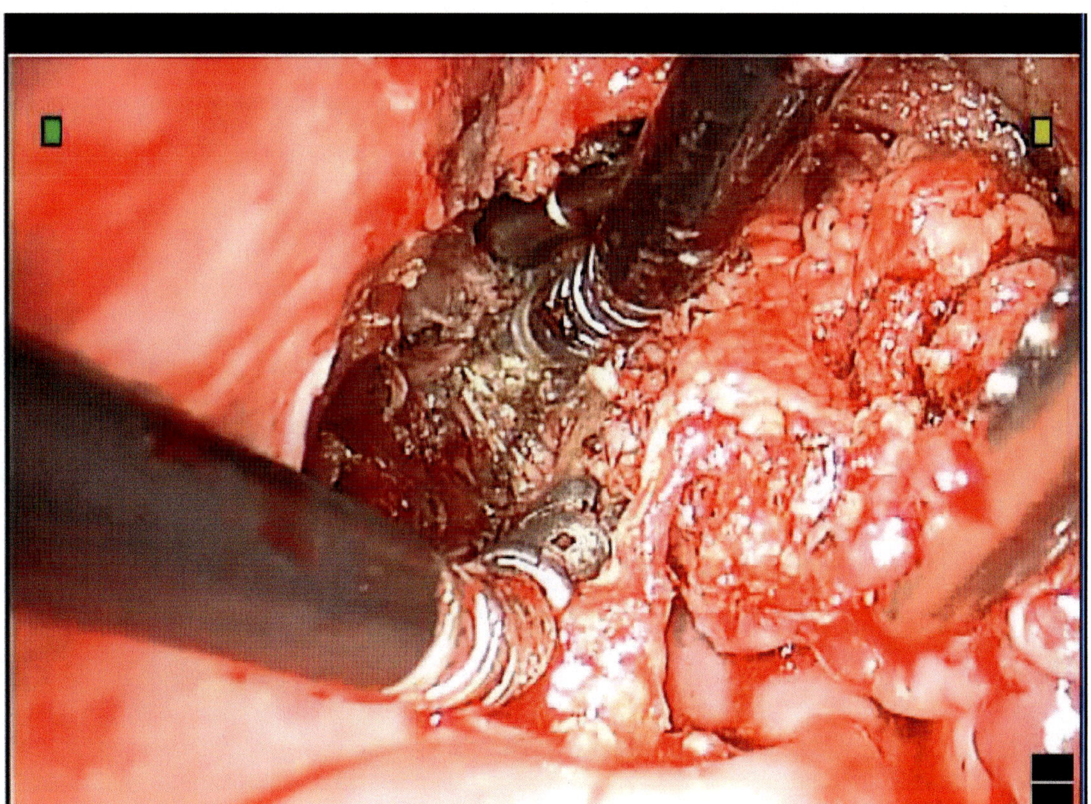

Fig. 10.9 The left strap muscles are being divided as they attached to the thyroid ala on the oblique line.

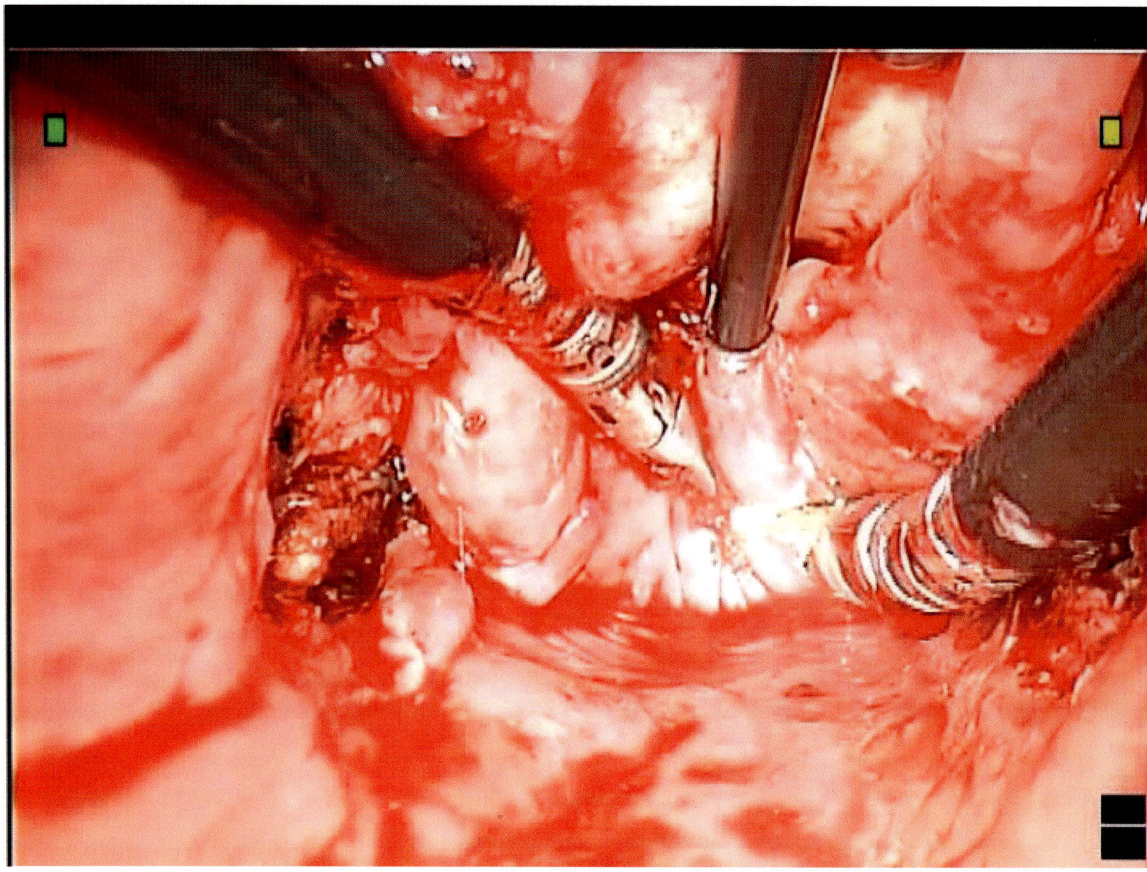

Fig. 10.10 The postcricoid mucosa is being incised from right to left under direct visualization.

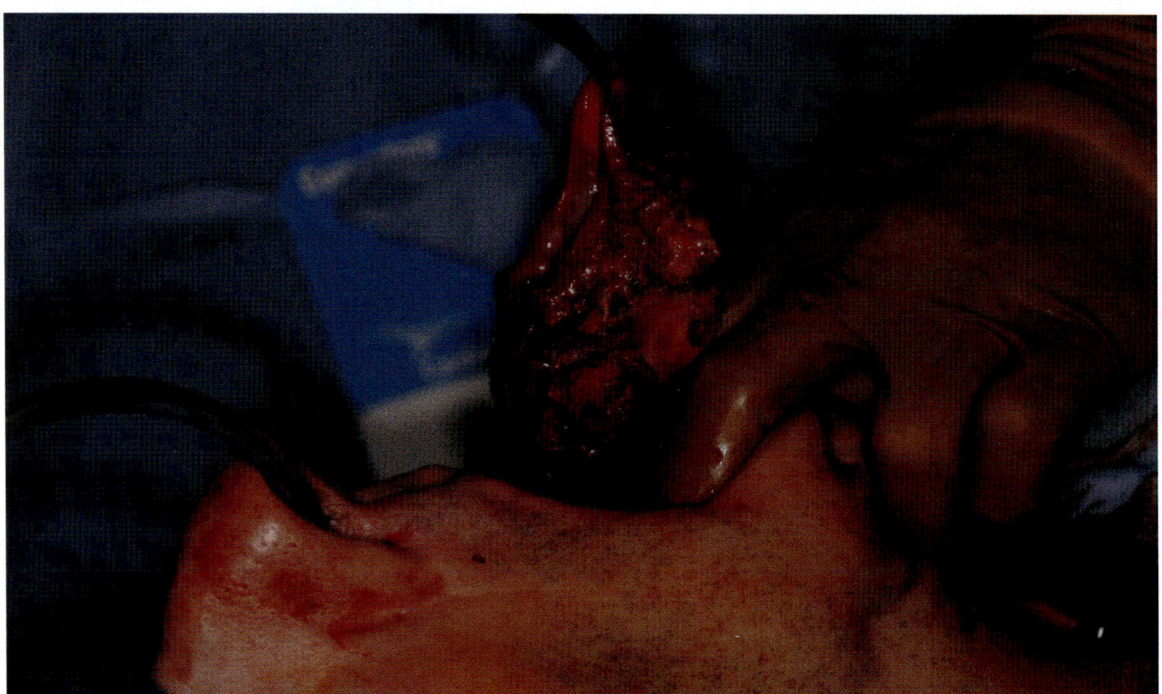

Fig. 10.11 The larynx is removed transorally.

Closure of the wound is then performed. All surfaces are irrigated and hemostasis is assured, after which the mucosal incision is then closed with several running 3-0 Vicryl sutures. The pharynx is closed primarily with a single horizontal suture line. However, since the integrity of the strap muscles is maintained, if the mucosa was not sufficient to close to itself primarily, the inferior and lateral mucosal surfaces could be closed to the strap muscles in a U-shaped configuration, allowing the central component to heal, as is currently the standard for endoscopic resections. The area is again irrigated and inspected from the stoma to confirm a watertight closure. A suction drain is then placed through a separate stab incision into the external compartment and the stomal suturing is completed to finish the procedure (**Fig. 10.12**). The technique of robotic total laryngectomy is well illustrated by Smith.[24]

■ Complications

The potential complications of this surgery can be broken down into those related to the robot and those related to the tumor removal. Standard complications apply to the tumor removal and include bleeding, airway compromise, swallowing dysfunction, and fistula. Hemorrhage is the most feared of the complications since these patients usually do not have a tracheotomy in place and a significant, acute bleeding episode could obstruct the airway in addition to hemodynamic changes. The most effective management of a postoperative hemorrhage is prevention and avoiding perioperative antithrombotic medications.[25] A detailed understanding of the vascular anatomy,[21] from "inside to out," is critical for successful transoral laryngeal supraglottic or total laryngectomy. The large vessels should be prospectively identified and must be clipped, not cauterized, to minimize the risk of a significant postoperative hemorrhage. A recent survey of TORS surgeons noted hemorrhage to be the most common complication of TORS (3.1%) and all patients who died following TORS did so from hemorrhage.[26]

Airway compromise is rarely an issue after the tumor has been removed, unless there is a significant amount of redundant and edematous tissue left in place following the resection. This should be managed at the time of the resection and is more likely in a previously irradiated patient. Aspiration and swallowing abnormalities are the norm following supraglottic laryngectomy and all patients should have a formal swallowing evaluation, with maneuvers, prior to initiating oral feeding. Fistula is uncommon and would be most likely if concurrent extensive neck dissection is performed; if noted intraoperatively, a fistula should be managed with local tissue coverage. Lingual or hypoglossal nerve injury has been reported in 1.6% of patients,[26] and unusual complications, such as skin necrosis from transoral dissection of the subcutaneous tissues,[27] have also been reported. Complications related to the robot are very uncommon and include dental injury, mucosal laceration, and device malfunction. These can be avoided by careful placement of the robotic arms and focused attention of the bedside assistant. Device malfunction is very unlikely, but backup robotic arms should be available.

■ Postprocedural Care and Recovery

The same postoperative care used for open or TLM procedures is employed for TORS supraglottic or total laryngectomy. For supraglottic laryngectomy, postoperative humidification, proton pump inhibitors, antibiotics, and cervical wound care are used. As noted above, initial nasogastric feeding is used, followed by a careful

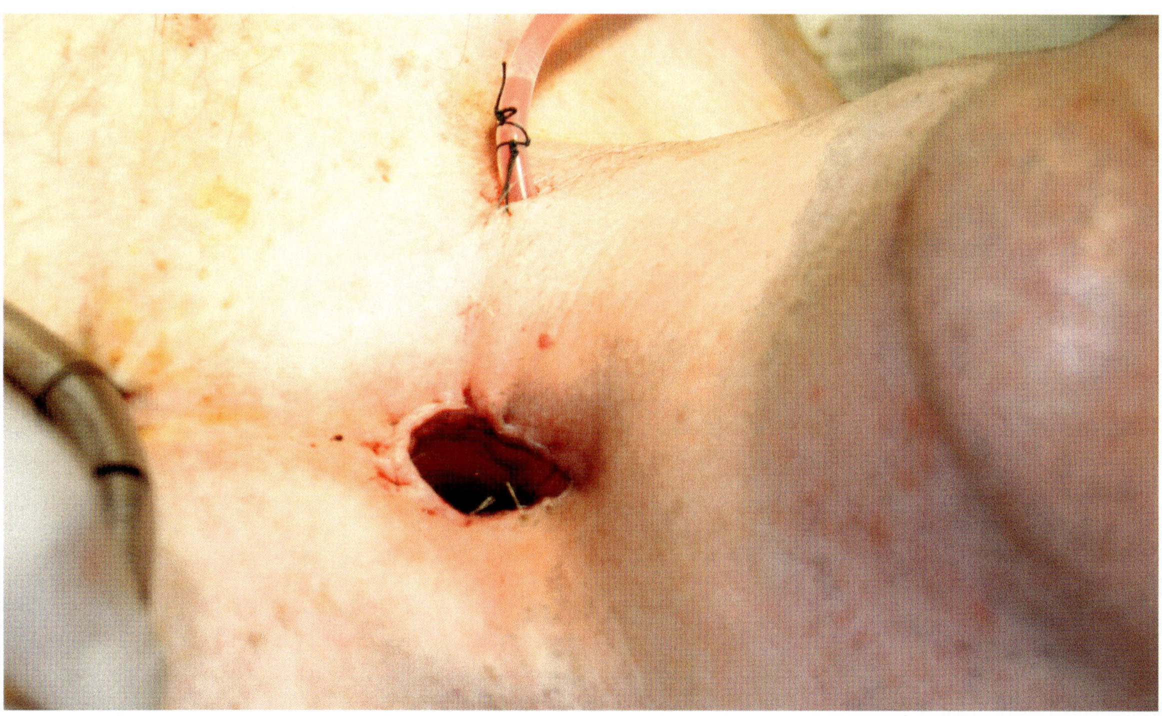

Fig. 10.12 The stoma is completely matured and a suction drain has been placed from the right lower neck.

assessment of swallowing by a speech/swallowing therapist. The initiation of oral intake should be supervised and employ whichever swallowing maneuvers are effective. Early postoperative resumption of oral intake is expected in the majority of these patients. Care for the total laryngectomy patient is not different than an open total laryngectomy, consisting of nasogastric feeding, stomal care, humidification, antibiotics, and cervical wound care.

■ Outcomes and Clinical Results in the Literature

Given its relative infancy, there are limited long-term data on the oncologic results of TORS. Most studies have presented varied primary sites, predominantly oropharynx, and have discussed complication and safety issues, short-term quality of life, and short-term oncologic results. Functional results have focused on swallowing function and tracheotomy rates. In a study for the University of Alabama involving 29 of 36 patients undergoing successful TORS for head and neck cancer, 10 patients had laryngeal cancer.[28] Seven of the 10 patients had a successful resection, and 4 of those 7 were extubated at the completion of the procedure. The remainder had planned intubation (two patients) or emergent reintubation (one patient), and all were subsequently successfully extubated. In contrast, however, six of the seven patients required prolonged tube feeding. Park et al recently reviewed their experience with 141 patients managed with TORS and included 36 patients with laryngeal cancer.[29] Unlike other series, the majority of their laryngeal patients (n = 26) had glottic cancers. All patients who had cancer underwent tracheotomy, regardless of tumor site. Specific results on decannulation and swallowing function were not presented, but presumably all were ultimately decannulated and resumed oral feeding. The 2-year disease-free survival for the entire cohort was 91%, with that of the laryngeal cancer patients not reported. An earlier analysis by the same group that looked specifically at laryngeal and hypopharyngeal cancers noted that all five laryngeal patients were decannulated by postoperative day 8 and resumed oral feeding by postoperative day 7.[30]

Transoral robotic laryngeal surgery has been limited by several factors. The current retractor systems more easily expose the oropharynx, instrument conflicts increase the farther the lesion is from the oral opening, and the limited instrumentation further complicates the procedure. Glottic surgery was first described in a canine model,[31] and has subsequently been reported in humans.[29,32] Most surgeons have been hesitant to perform glottic surgery in the absence of an integrated robotic laser instrument, fearing the potential collateral damage from monopolar electrocautery. Kayhan first reported a series of 10 patients undergoing TORS cordectomy with electrocautery.[32] All were stage T1 and achieved negative margins; nine were extubated immediately postoperatively and began oral alimentation the day of the surgery. One required a temporary tracheotomy and nasogastric tube. The 26 glottic cancer patients reported by Park all underwent cordectomy with the monopolar electrocautery as well.[29] Lallemant et al included 13 patients with early glottic carcinoma and TORS cordectomy in their series, reporting positive margins in 23%, tracheotomy in 8%, and gastrostomy in 23%.[33] The results of these series are presented in **Table 10.2**. The variability of results, when compared with TLM, is an important consideration in the indication for this approach. Voice results and larynx function have not been reported in either series, so comparison with TLM approaches and radiation therapy voice results cannot be performed. One must remain concerned about vocal function in the absence of a laser. This may soon change as laser couplers have been developed by several companies, including Lumenis and Omniguide.[34,35]

There are still technical limitations that authors have sought to resolve. De Virgilio and associates have described their techniques to optimize laryngeal and hypopharyngeal exposure during TORS.[36] This was based upon TORS for 22 hypopharyngeal cancers, 19 glottic cancers, and 7 supraglottic cancers. They recommend the following: (1) trial the FK retractor system and 30-degree telescope for exposure during the initial diagnostic laryngoscopy; (2) employ intraoperative muscle relaxants; (3) routinely perform tracheotomy before the TORS; (4) use the 30-degree robotic endoscope positioned as far from the operative site as feasible; (5) position the 30-degree scope at the posterior pharyngeal wall at an acute angle; (6) retract the tongue anteriorly; and (7) perform an ipsilateral epiglottectomy for pyriform sinus lesions. Their exposure outcomes were mixed, with 4 laryngeal patients deemed “good” exposure, 21 “fair,” and 1 “poor.” Those with hypopharyngeal cancers more frequently had poor or fair exposure. Unlike open cases, the current instrumentation for TORS laryngeal surgery continues to impact procedures.

The majority of TORS laryngeal resection reports have been for supraglottic tumors. The functional and oncologic results are presented in **Table 10.3**. Initial descriptions were published by Solares and Strome[43] who performed one TORS supraglottic

Table 10.2 Results of transoral robotic glottic cancer surgery

Author	Patients (n)	Initial T1/T2	Positive margins	Perioperative tracheotomy	Gastrostomy	Complications	Adjuvant therapy	2-year DSS
Lallemant[33]	13	12/1	3	1	3	PTX, bleed	0	NA
Kayhan[32]	10	10/0	0	1	0	Trach, edema	0	NA
Park[30]	2	1/1	1	2	0	None	1	NA

Note: This table represents current publications describing glottic TORS.
Abbreviations: DSS, disease-specific survival; NA, not available; PTX, pneumothorax.

Table 10.3 Results of transoral robotic resection for supraglottic cancer

Author	Patients (n)	Initial T1/T2 (%)	Positive margins (%)	Perioperative tracheotomy (%)	Gastrostomy (%)	Complications	Adjuvant therapy (%)	2-year DSS (%)
Weinstein 2007[37]	3	67	0	NA	0 *	None	33	NA
Ozer 2012[38]	13	85	0	0	8	None	15	NA
Olsen 2012[39]	9	78	0	78	44	1 supraglottic stenosis	67	88
Park 2013[40]	16	75	12	100 #	0	None	50	91
Mendelsohn 2013[41]	18	72	0	0	0	5 – not specified	50	100
Lallemant 2013[42]	10	100	20	30	0 *	1 bleed	40	100
Oysu[43] 2013	3	100	NA	0	0	None	67	NA

Note: This table represents current publications describing supraglottic TORS. Several publications were omitted due to either low numbers of successful surgeries or patients already included in the series listed.
Abbreviations: DSS, disease-specific survival; NA, not available; *, routine use of prolonged nasogastric tubes; #, routine use of perioperative tracheotomy, all patients decannulated.

laryngectomy in three patients, while Weinstein and O'Malley reported their series of three successful TORS supraglottic laryngectomies.[37] TORS supraglottic laryngectomy came about at a time when TLM supraglottic partial laryngectomy gained oncologic acceptance among many head and neck surgeons. Therefore, several centers began employing this technique, feeling that the three-dimensional visualization, angled view and working space, and relative ease of surgical technique make this a desirable alternative to TLM supraglottic laryngectomy. The feasibility of TORS supraglottic laryngectomy was assessed by Alon et al.[28] They used this technique in seven patients with T1–3 lesions using the FK retractor with the laryngeal blade. Four of their patients received tracheotomy, which remained in place for a range of 4 days to permanent and five patients had prolonged tube feedings. Two had gastrostomies (time not reported) and three had prolonged nasogastric tubes (38 to 56 days). Two of their patients, both with N2 neck disease, underwent adjuvant radiotherapy, both of whom had gastrostomy tubes and one of whom had the permanent tracheotomy tube. The follow-up was too brief to evaluate survival.

Subsequent studies have presented larger, but still small, patient series and have shown good results. Interestingly, however, there is a significant institutional bias to the use of tracheotomy and/or gastrostomy tubes. The Korean group seems to be the only group routinely performing tracheotomy[40] and, in general, most surgeons see these techniques as a way to avoid routine tracheotomy and feeding tube placement, both of which have a negative impact on quality of life. Functional recovery is excellent, with some authors instituting oral feeding on postoperative day 1.[38] Tumor stage has been predominantly early stage disease, T1 or T2, but T3 lesions, based upon pre-epiglottic extension, are also amenable to this technique. Mendelsohn has found tumor stage to be an important predictor of functional recovery, with early T stage (pT1/pT2) having a statistically significant earlier return to swallowing, both liquids and solids, than late T stage (pT3/T4).[41] This is intuitive, given larger surgical defects and greater sacrifice of compensatory structures in that situation. Female gender, simultaneous neck dissection, and vocal fold hypomobility were also found to have significance.

Survival data have been limited as the technique has only recently been employed. The mean follow-up for all series has been under 3 years, significantly limiting the generalizability of the oncologic results. Mendelsohn et al have reported 2-year outcomes in their 18 patients with a mean follow-up of 28 months.[41] Their locoregional control, disease-specific survival, and overall survival were 83%, 100%, and 89%, respectively. Three patients recurred in the neck, one of whom only had a sentinel node biopsy, and there were four distant failures. Half of their patients received adjuvant chemotherapy and radiation therapy for advanced neck disease. In a study of 16 patients with a mean follow-up of 20 months, Park et al reported a 2-year disease-free survival rate of 91%, although only 2 patients enrolled had a follow-up of more than 20 months.[40] Half of their patients underwent adjuvant therapy as well, 19% with radiation only (for pT3 disease) and 31% with chemotherapy and radiation (two for positive margins and three for extracapsular nodal spread). They also compared their TORS supraglottic laryngectomy patients to a matched cohort of open supraglottic laryngectomy patients and found earlier decannulation, earlier oral feeding, and shorter hospitalization in the TORS group.

There has been wide variability in the application of adjuvant therapy. Most often the adjuvant therapy is used for advanced nodal disease, rather than positive margins. In our center we shield the central structures from full-dose radiotherapy in order to maximize pharyngeal and laryngeal function. The use of adjuvant therapy, however, is not without consequence, as functional complications following TORS, either prolonged tracheotomy or gastrostomy, are often present only in this treatment group.[39] The goal of surgical therapy in these patients should be avoidance of adjuvant therapy if at all possible, using the TORS and neck dissection as unimodality therapy. This has been shown to be possible with TLM and should be so for TORS as well. If adjuvant therapy is known to be necessary at the onset, one must carefully assess the benefits and risks of adding surgery to the treatment plan.

Transoral robotic total laryngectomy is a new extension of this operative modality. Only two series of patients have been reported thus far, but the results are promising.[44,45] Salvage surgery is the main indication for this procedure at this time and access remains the limiting factor. The pliability of laryngeal and pharyngeal structures is often decreased following the chemotherapy and radiation and the pharyngeal operative field is often reduced from local tissue contracture, fibrosis, and stenosis. Of particular concern for this procedure is the placement of a tracheotomy prior to the procedure. Low tracheotomy has a detrimental effect on the TORS total laryngectomy and should be carefully assessed preoperatively.[44] Dowthwaite and colleagues recommend exposure with the FK retractor at the time of tumor endoscopy to maximize the opportunity for TORS laryngectomy success.[45] The challenging exposure is often inferiorly in the pyriform sinus and postcricoid region. This can be managed with a slight extension of the stomal incision, in conjunction with the transoral robotic incisions, to complete a more difficult total laryngectomy with a hybrid approach, still employing minimally invasive techniques. Although it is a technically challenging procedure, TORS total laryngectomy holds the advantage of limited tissue manipulation during a narrow field laryngectomy in the recurrence setting. This may reduce fistula rates and minimize stricture, given maintenance of the surrounding structures. Its success is also predicated upon the ability to limit lateral neck dissection in these patients, addressing level VI during the TORS laryngectomy, and leaving levels II–IV intact.[46,47] At this time the exact indications for this procedure are unclear, but as more surgeons use this technique, those indications should become more defined.

■ Future Directions and Conclusion

TORS laryngeal surgery is an effective and safe method to manage laryngeal cancer in the primary and salvage setting. The challenges are related to equipment and patient-specific anatomical access. If a TLM approach is appropriate for a given supraglottic tumor, it is most likely that a TORS approach will be appropriate as well. The magnified angled view, facile instrument motion, and ability to suture deep within the pharynx are benefits of this approach, whereas instrumentation and access are limitations. Instrumentation and access can be expected to improve with the development of new robots and retractors designed for TORS. As more surgeons gain experience with this technique some of these limitations may be eliminated. The concept of transoral partial laryngectomy has been well validated through the use of TLM techniques and there is no reason to assume the results will be any different for TORS, provided the surgeon adheres to the standard principles of transoral resection (TORS or TLM).

References

1. Lee HS, Chun B-G, Kim SW, Kim ST, Oh JH, Hong JC, Lee KD. Transoral laser microsurgery for early glottic cancer as a one-stage single-modality therapy. Laryngoscope 2013;123:2670–2674
2. Gallo A, de Vincentiis M, Manciocco V, Simonelli M, Fiorella ML, Shah JP. CO_2 laser cordectomy for early-stage glottic carcinoma: a long-term follow-up of 156 cases. Laryngoscope 2002;112: 370–374
3. Motta G, Esposito E, Testa D, Iovine R, Motta S. CO_2 laser treatment of supraglottic cancer. Head Neck 2004;26:442–446
4. Arshad H, Jayaprakash V, Gupta V, et al. Survival differences between organ preservation surgery and definitive radiotherapy in early supraglottic squamous cell carcinoma. Otolaryngol Head Neck Surg 2014;150:237–244
5. Forastiere AA, Zhang Q, Weber RS, et al. Long-term results of RTOG 91-11: a comparison of three nonsurgical treatments strategies to preserve the larynx in patients with locally advanced larynx cancer. J Clin Oncol 2012;31:845–852
6. Gourin CG, Conger BT, Sheils C, Bilodeau PA, Coleman TA, Porubsky ES. The effect of treatment on survival in patients with advanced laryngeal carcinoma. Laryngoscope 2009;119:1312–1317
7. Ceruse P, Lallemant B, Moriniere S, et al. Transoral minimally invasive robotic surgery for carcinoma of the pharynx and the larynx: a new approach. Anti-Cancer Drugs 2011;22:591–595
8. Genden EM, O'Malley BW, Weinstein GS, et al. Transoral robotic surgery: role in management of upper aerodigestive tract tumors. Head Neck 2010;34:886–893
9. Hans S, Badoual C, Gorphe P, Brasnu D. Transoral robotic surgery for head and neck carcinomas. Eur Arch Otorhinolaryngol 2012;269: 1979–1984
10. Motta G, Esposito E, Motta S, Tartaro G, Testa D. CO_2 laser surgery in the treatment of glottis cancer. Head Neck 2005;27:566–574
11. Peretti G, Piazza C, Cocco D, et al. Transoral CO2 laser treatment for Tis-T3 glottic cancer: the University of Brescia experience on 595 patients. Head Neck 2010;32:977–983
12. Iro H, Waldfahrer F, Altendorf-Hofmann A, Weidenbecher M, Sauer R, Steiner W. Transoral laser surgery of supraglottic cancer: follow-up of 141 patients. Arch Otolaryngol Head Neck Surg 1998;124: 1245–1250
13. Bussu F, Almadori G, De Corso E, et al. Endoscopic horizontal partial laryngectomy by CO_2 laser in the management of supraglottic squamous cell carcinoma. Head Neck 2009;31:1196–1206
14. Mantsopoulos K, Psychogios G, Koch M, Zenk J, Waldfahrer F, Iro H. Comparison of differnet surgical approaches in T2 glottic cancer. Head Neck 2012;34:73–77
15. White HN, Frederick J, Zimmerman T, Carroll WR, Magnuson JS. Learning curve for transoral robotic surgery: A 4 year analysis. JAMA Otolaryngol Head Neck Surg 2013;139:564–567
16. More YI, Tsue TT, Girod DA, Harbison J, Sykes KJ, Williams C, Shnayder Y. Functional swallowing outcomes following transoral robotic surgery vs primary chemoradiotherapy in patients with advanced-stage oropharynx and supraglottis cancers. JAMA Otolaryngol Head Neck Surg 2013;139:43–48
17. Vural E, Tulunay-Ugur OE, Suen JY. Transoral robotic supracricoid partial laryngectomy with cartilaginous framework preservation. J Robotic Surg 2010;6:363–366

18. Lalich IJ, Olsen SM, Ekborn DC. Robotic microlaryngeal surgery: feasibility using a newly designed retractor and instrumentation. Laryngoscope 2014;124:1624–1630
19. Alessandrini M, De Padova A, Napolitano B, Cmillo A, Bruno E. The AESOP robot system for video-assisted rigid endoscopic laryngosurgery. Eur Arch Otorhinolaryngol 2008;265:1121–1123
20. Rivera-Serrano CM, Johnson P, Zubiate B, Kuenzler R, Choset H, Zenati M, Tully S, Duvvuri U. A transoral highly flexible robot: novel technology and application. Laryngoscope 2012;122:1067–1071
21. Goyal N, Yoo F, Setabutr D, Goldenberg D. Surgical anatomy of the supraglottic larynx using the da Vinci robot. Head Neck 2014; 36(8):1126–1131
22. Vilaseca-Gonzalez I, Bernal-Sprekelsen M, Blanch-Alejandro J-L, Moragas-Lluis M. Complications in transoral CO_2 laser surgery for carcinoma of the larynx and hypopharynx. Head Neck 2003;25: 382–388
23. Dziegielewski PT, Ozer E. Transoral robotic surgery: supraglottic laryngectomy. Operative Tech Otolaryngol 2013;24:86–91
24. Smith RV. Transoral robotic total laryngectomy. Operative Tech Otolaryngol 2013;24:92–98
25. Asher SA, White HN, Kejner AE, Rosenthal EL, Carroll WR, Magnuson JS. Hemorrhage after transoral robotic-assisted surgery. Otolaryngol Head Neck Surg 2013;149:112–117
26. Chia SH, Gross ND, Richmon JD. Surgeon experience and complications with transoral robotic surgery (TORS). Otolaryngol Head Neck Surg 2013;149:885–892
27. Alon EE, Kasperbauer JL, Olsen KD, Moore EJ. Feasibility of transoral robotic-assisted supraglottic laryngectomy. Head Neck 2012;34: 225–229
28. Boudreaux BA, Rosenthal EL, Magnuson JS, Newman JR, Desmond RA, Clemons L, Carroll WR. Robot-assisted surgery for upper aerodigestive tract neoplasms. Arch Otolaryngol Head Neck Surg 2009;135:397–401
29. Park YM, Kim WS, Byeon HK, De Virgilio A, Lee SY, Kim S-H. Clinical outcomes of transoral robotic surgery for head and neck tumors. Ann Otol Rhinol Laryngol 2013;122:73–84
30. Park YM, Lee WJ, Lee JG, Lee WS, Choi EC, Chung SM, Kim S-H. Transoral robotic surgery (TORS) in laryngeal and hypopharyngeal cancer. J Laparoendosc Adv Surg Tech A 2009;19:361–368
31. O'Malley BW, Weinstein GS, Hockstein NG. Transoral robotic surgery (TORS): glottic microsurgery in a canine model. J Voice 2006;20:263–268
32. Kayhan FT, Kaya KH, Sayin I. Transoral robotic cordectomy for early glottic carcinoma. Ann Otol Rhinol Laryngol 2012;121: 497–502
33. Lallemant B, Chambon G, Garrel R, et al. Transoral robotic surgery for treatment of T1-T2 carcinoma of the larynx: preliminary study. Laryngoscope 2013;123:2485–2490
34. Remacle M, Matar N, Lawson G, Bachy V, Delos M, Nollevaux M-C. Combining a new CO_2 laser wave guide with transoral robotic surgery: a feasibility on four patients with malignant tumors. Eur Arch Otorhinolaryngol 2010;269:1833–1837
35. Desai SC, Sung C-K, Jang DW, Genden EM. Transoral robotic surgery using a carbon dioxide flexible laser for tumors of the upper aerodigestive tract. Laryngoscope 2008;118:2187–2189
36. De Virgilio A, Park YM, Kim WS, Baek SJ, Kim S-H. How to optimize laryngeal and hypopharyngeal exposure in transoral robotic surgery. Auris Nasus Larynx 2013;40:312–319
37. Weinstein GS, O'Malley BW, Snyder W, Hockstein NG. Transoral robotic surgery: supraglottic partial laryngectomy. Ann Otol Rhinol Laryngol 2007;116:19–23
38. Ozer E, Alvarez B, Kakarala K, Durmus K, Tecknos TN, Carrau RL. Clinical outcomes of transoral robotic supraglottic laryngectomy. Head Neck 2013;35:1158–1161
39. Olsen SM, Moore EJ, Koch CA, Price DL, Kasperbauer JL, Olsen KD. Transoral robotic surgery for supraglottic squamous cell carcinoma. Am J Otolaryngol 2012;33:379–384
40. Park YM, Kim WS, Byeon HK, Lee SY, Kim S-H. Surgical techniques and treatment outcomes of transoral robotic supraglottic partial laryngectomy. Laryngoscope 2013;123:670–677
41. Mendelsohn AH, Remacle M, Van Der Vorst S, Bachy V, Lawson G. Outcomes following transoral robotic surgery: supraglottic laryngectomy. Laryngoscope 2012;123:208–214
42. Oysu C, Sahin-Yilmaz A. En bloc resection of epiglottic tumors with transoral robotic approach – preliminary results. Int J Med Robotics Comput Assist Surg 2013;9:477–479
43. Solares CA, Strome M. Transoral robot-assisted CO_2 laser supraglottic laryngectomy: experimental and clinical data. Laryngoscope 2007;117:817–820
44. Smith RV, Schiff BA, Sarta C, Hans S, Brasnu D. Transoral robotic total laryngectomy. Laryngoscope 2012;123:678–682
45. Dowthwaite S, Nichols AC, Yoo J, et al. Transoral robotic total laryngectomy: report of 3 cases. Head Neck 2013;35:E338–342.
46. Koss SL, Russell MD, Leem TH, Schiff BA, Smith RV. Occult nodal disease in patients with failed laryngeal preservation undergoing surgical salvage. Laryngoscope 2014;124:421–428
47. Basheeth N, O'Leary G, Sheahan P. Elective neck dissection for N0 neck during salvage total laryngectomy: findings, complications, and oncological outcome. JAMA Otolaryngol Head Neck Surg 2013;139:790–796

11 Robotic Surgery of the Hypopharynx

Brett A. Miles

Introduction

Transoral robotic surgery (TORS) has transformed the treatment of head and neck cancer, specifically for malignant lesions of the oropharyngeal region. Advances in minimally invasive surgery including the TORS approach have allowed surgeons to perform oncologic sound resections of tumors while decreasing treatment-related morbidity and improving quality of life.[1,2] Recent investigations have shown that TORS is a safe procedure and can provide favorable clinical outcomes with respect to traditional surgical approaches and offers improved functional outcomes compared to traditional concurrent chemoradiotherapy in many cases. These investigations have also noted several advantages relative to traditional transmandibular approaches, which include faster recovery of swallowing and vocal function, decreased need for reconstruction, decreased incidence in aspiration pneumonia, and decreased length of hospitalization.[3,4]

Robotic systems currently employed by head and urologic and cardiac surgeons pioneered neck surgeons and with recent instrumentation advances these systems have been adapted for head and neck surgery. Current TORS applications in the head and neck include lesions of the laryngopharyngeal subsites including the base of tongue, tonsillar fossa, palate, and posterior pharynx. However, patients who present with hypopharyngeal lesions represent a special situation in TORS due to issues related to current instrumentation and surgical access. This chapter reviews aspects of hypopharyngeal malignancy and robotic surgical applications related to this challenging patient population.

Background

Hypopharyngeal squamous cell carcinoma (HSCC) is a relatively rare (3–5% all of head and neck squamous cell carcinomas [SCCs]) but aggressive malignancy associated with a poor survival and often presents at an advanced stage.[5] The vast majority of these malignancies are smoking-related malignancies and previous data indicate that pyriform sinus HSCC accounts for more than 85% of hypopharynx SCC.[6] In addition to 90% of patients presenting with a significant smoking history, approximately 50% present with an associated rate of alcohol abuse.[7,8] With this risk factor profile it is hardly surprising that the rate of synchronous lesions in this subset of patients approaches 8%.[7] Of particular concern is that due to a lack of significant symptoms in early stage disease, or the fact that symptoms may be confused for more benign clinical entities such as sore throat and reflux, over 50% of patients present with advanced, stage 4 disease.[8] Advanced stage at presentation is also a function of the lymphatic drainage accompanying the hypopharynx, which contributes to a rate of ipsilateral nodal disease in the range of 60 to 80%.[9] Up to 40% of patients with HSCC present with contralateral nodal metastasis.[10] In the clinically negative neck, the rate of occult ipsilateral and contralateral neck disease can be as high as 36% and 27%, respectively.[8,10]

The summary of this data is that HSCC is associated with a poor prognosis. Of nearly 3,000 hypopharyngeal SCC diagnosed from 1980–1985 and 1990–1992, the 5-year disease-specific survival was 63.1%, 57.5%, 41.8%, and 22% for stages I, II, III, and IV, respectively.[7] Despite significant advances in surgical therapies, chemotherapeutic options, and radiation technology, the overall prognosis in HSSC has not significantly improved.[11]

Current Standard Treatment of Hypopharyngeal Squamous Cell Carcinoma

The paradigms in treatment of HSCC have undergone significant change over the last decades. In the 1940s radiation therapy was the primary modality of treatment for HSCC, until it was replaced in the 1950s and 1960s with surgical management, primarily in the form of laryngopharyngectomy.[12,13,14] In the 1970s conservation surgery was developed and a variety of surgical techniques evolved to avoid the functional devastation of radical surgery for HSCC.[15,16,17] Surgical resection, radiation therapy, or a combination of these modalities was considered standard of care until the introduction of platinum-based chemotherapeutics in the 1980s. Significant functional disturbances began to be evaluated and strategies to avoid complications were developed.[15,18,19,20,21] During this period of time, chemoradiotherapy protocols originally applied to laryngeal SCC were adopted for hypopharyngeal lesions.[22,23,24] For the next 20 years the treatment trend revolved around organ preservation, mostly applied from the experience gained in laryngeal carcinoma. Concurrent chemoradiotherapy gained significant momentum as the primary modality of treatment for hypopharynx carcinoma and remains the current standard in many institutions presently. As opposed with the case of laryngeal carcinoma, the quality of evidence to support this treatment modality in the hypopharynx is somewhat questionable. We have continued to see poor survival rates and significant functional disturbances regardless of whether surgical or nonsurgical "organ-sparing" approaches are utilized. In 1996 a randomized controlled trial of hypopharynx carcinoma that included a surgical arm was performed. Induction chemotherapy followed by radiation therapy (in responders) was compared with surgery followed by postoperative radiation therapy. This study found no significant difference in survival or recurrence; however, a larger percentage of patients in the induction arm retained a functioning larynx.[22] Interestingly, all patients in the surgical arm had total laryngectomy with partial pharyngectomy. A trial designed currently would likely involve minimally invasive robotic or endoscopic resection when feasible; however, it would be difficult to obtain a survival difference with minimally invasive techniques for HSCC given that total laryngectomy did not appear to improve survival in this initial investigation. Nevertheless, this work has not been performed to date.

While there have been technical improvements in partial laryngopharyngectomy including combined suprahyoid and lateral pharyngectomy, as well as pedicled and free myocutaneous reconstructive techniques, laryngopharyngectomy with reconstruction remains associated with a significant functional impairment and has not been shown to improve survival for HCSS. In the situation of advanced disease, including infiltrating tumors with significant cartilage involvement, initial radical surgery followed by adjuvant therapy, as opposed to concurrent chemoradiotherapy, is generally advocated,[23,25,26] but remains controversial.[27] Furthermore, combined chemotherapy and radiation therapy increase toxicity to the aerodigestive tract and are associated with a likely underreported rate of detrimental effects on swallowing function.[28] The current treatment "standards" are further complicated by reviewing the results of concurrent chemotherapy versus induction chemotherapy.[24,29,30] The data on induction chemotherapy in HSCC are unclear at best and even in laryngeal SCC, which has been investigated more thoroughly, the literature suggests that as concurrent chemotherapy became the more common treatment for larynx carcinoma, the associated overall survival decreased.[31,32] However, contrary results were found in similar European trials.[33] This summary of data is that HSCC remains a very difficult disease to treat with poor outcomes, and that currently no standard therapy exists, although multimodality strategies are generally preferred. It should also be noted that traditional open surgical approaches have declined over time due to the increased use of nonsurgical strategies and minimally invasive techniques.[34]

■ Minimally Invasive Surgical Management of Hypopharynx Cancer

Transoral Laser Microsurgery

Over the past four decades, the field of head and neck surgery has witnessed significant advancements in minimally invasive surgical techniques. In the 1970s, transoral endoscopic laser microsurgery (TLM) was developed and soon thereafter was applied to the treatment of hypopharynx SCC; TLM continues to be used in many centers currently.[35,36,37,38] TLM has been shown to provide equivalent oncologic outcomes to both open surgery and organ-preserving concurrent chemoradiation therapy protocols with a low rate of postoperative morbidity in HSCC.[39,40] The advantage of TLM is the ability to gain exposure to the hypopharynx, without the need to disrupt the laryngeal framework and the inherent functional impairment associated with those traditional transcervical or transmandibular approaches. Furthermore, healing is accomplished by secondary intention, negating a bulky reconstruction.[39,41,42] TLM continues to provide excellent outcomes, is a well-established, minimally invasive technique, and offers some advantages when dealing with hypopharyngeal lesions, including more robust instrumentation for surgical access when compared with current robotic instrumentation and advantages related to laser surgery including decreased margin cautery artifact.[38]

Transoral Robotic Surgery

Despite the advantages of TLM, the recent development of transoral robotic surgery (TORS) offers an additional technique that has provided equivalent locoregional control without the collateral functional impairment of traditional surgery.[2,24,43,44] TORS techniques offer a solution to some of the limitations associated with TLM including line of sight issues related to the microscope and technical challenges related to training and margin orientation.[35,45] The inherent advantages of robotic assisted surgery, in terms of improved tissue manipulation and visualization as well as relative degrees of freedom, have provided a potentially superior technique in the treatment of hypopharynx SCC.[11,43,45]

TORS for has been very successful in applications related to the upper aerodigestive tract malignancies in terms of completeness of resection and postoperative morbidity.[3,46] Certainly, the greatest challenge in the application of TORS to treatment of the larynx and hypopharynx is access, with up to 25% of carefully selected patients having difficult exposure.[43,47,48] However, this issue is currently the topic of several investigations and a variety of techniques can be utilized to overcome this issue. Park et al performed a preliminary investigation evaluating TORS for HSCC, which was a prospective case series that included 10 patients with T1 or T2 pyriform sinus or posterior pharyngeal wall SCC treated successfully. All patients had clear margins without significant perioperative complications. Patients received prophylactic intraoperative tracheotomy with an average time to decannulation of 6.3 days, and a return of swallowing function within 8.3 days after surgery. This investigation suggested that TORS hypopharyngectomy was a feasible option with favorable morbidity.[11] In a larger prospective study of 23 patients with hypopharynx SCC, designed to determine oncologic outcomes, the 3-year overall survival and disease-free survival of 89% and 84%, respectively, compared favorably to both open surgical techniques and concurrent chemotherapy strategies. Functional outcomes of voice and swallow were objectively assessed with favorable results.[45] While these series are limited by surgical selection bias, they indicate that TORS is a feasible and valid oncologic option for HSCC. Other investigations have confirmed the utility of TORS for hypopharyngeal surgery.[43,44,49,50]

Preoperative Evaluation

Oncologic Feasibility

When considering a patient for surgical management of hypopharyngeal SCC the initial evaluation is critical for success from an oncologic and technical standpoint. Several issues in addition to the traditional workup for hypopharyngeal malignancy present when considering a minimally invasive surgical approach. After complete physical examination, fiberoptic examination, and evaluation of the appropriate imaging studies, the first issue to address is the validity of a surgical approach. While some cases may be amenable to surgical approaches, if the initial workup and staging indicate high oncologic risk, and the patient will require concurrent chemoradiotherapy, a surgical approach is rarely warranted unless significant dose reductions or functional benefits are realized with the surgical plan. Advanced nodal disease with high risk for distant metastasis may dictate a nonsurgical approach. Performing minimally invasive surgery for HSCC followed by postsurgical concurrent chemoradiation at curative doses is not supported by the current literature from an oncologic standpoint and is more likely to worsen posttreatment functional results. This of course is a very individualized decision-making process, which should occur in the setting of the multidisciplinary tumor board.

Technical Feasibility

Once the decision has been made that the patient will benefit from an oncologic or functional standpoint with a minimally invasive surgical approach, other issues regarding the technical feasibility of surgery are considered. The feasibility of transoral robotic supraglottic laryngectomy has been assessed by several groups and one center has shown that it can be performed safely with appropriate surgical margins and excellent functional outcomes.[43,44,45,48] However, each group has commented that inadequate transoral exposure is the critical issue hindering the performance of the procedure. In many patients, the ability to gain appropriate exposure to the lesion often dictates which patients can undergo TORS, rather than oncologic considerations alone. Suboptimal exposure leads to increased operative times, greater risk of surgical complications, and the possibility of inadequate surgical resection margins. The patient should be carefully evaluated for issues related to surgical access. Body habitus and anatomic considerations are evaluated in a systematic fashion. Obesity, a short neck, large shoulders, and issues related to cervical flexibility such as severe kyphosis/degenerative cervical spine disease may all preclude a surgical approach. While these factors are important for all transoral minimally invasive procedures, they are particularly important for hypopharyngeal surgery given the issues with access in this region. Previous cervical spine surgery, radiation therapy, and arthritis may all create access issues that would prevent the surgeon from accessing the lesion adequately.

In addition, evaluation of interincisal distance (normal 40–50 mm), mouth opening, tongue size, previous surgery in the oral cavity and oropharynx, and issues related to temporomandibular joint arthrosis/ankylosis also require recognition. Anatomic features such as a retrognathic mandible, macroglossia, and small oral aperture limit the ability to provide an adequate surgical port to introduce the endoscopic camera and instrument arms. Recent data have indicated that the size of the base of tongue and the epiglottis was a major problem in exposure for the hypopharynx and larynx.[50] Surgical or radiation-related trismus may not allow appropriate access for minimally invasive surgical approaches. In these cases, nonsurgical modalities may be utilized, or in the salvage situations alternative surgical approaches may be entertained. It is critical that the surgeon evaluating the patient recognize these issues prior to embarking on a transoral surgical approach for obvious reasons. Objective evaluation of specific data may be applied in order to predict problematic patients when transoral surgery is considered. These variables include an interincisal distance < 40 mm, neck circumference > 40 cm, hyomental and sternomental distance less than 6.05 and 13.9 cm, respectively, as well as Mallampati scores > 3.[51] Furthermore, the size of the tongue and tongue base should be assessed and have been shown to predict patients with difficult access during TORS of hypopharynx SCC.[48]

Surgical Feasibility of Resection

At this point factors related to the primary tumor should be considered to determine if the lesion is amenable to the transoral robotic approach. Fiberoptic examination of the lesion is critical for the surgeon to assess the mucosal surface and extent of disease as well as the current function standpoint in terms of airway management and swallowing/aspiration. Imaging studies including high-resolution computed tomography (CT) and positron emission tomography (PET)-CT should be carefully evaluated to determine surgical feasibility. Magnetic resonance imaging (MRI) is especially helpful when dealing with submucosal spread and areas difficult to evaluate on CT scan such as the pyriform sinus and supraglottic structures. Preoperative staging was not designed to determine surgical feasibility but may offer a guideline for consideration. T1–T3 supraglottic, pyriform sinus, and posterior pharyngeal wall lesions as potential candidates for TORS provide at least one intact arytenoid with normal vocal cord mobility. However, we exclude lesions with significant posterior cricoid involvement or those that involve the apex of the pyriform sinus or with vocal cord fixation. Previous data indicate that pyriform sinus HSCC accounts for more than 85% of hypopharynx SCC.[6] Lesions with medial and lateral pyriform involvement are usually managed with nonsurgical strategies. Advanced stage disease such as T4 lesions and lesions with thyroid cartilage, prevertebral fascia, or carotid artery invasion are usually poor candidates for minimally invasive approaches such as transoral robotic resection.

The importance of panendoscopy cannot be overstated in this population. In addition to obtaining tissue diagnosis, a preoperative panendoscopy provides an opportunity to determine eligibility for TORS and is highly recommended.[48] The larynx and hypopharynx are carefully examined to determine arytenoid mobility and to characterize the tumor in terms of size, subsite involvement, and lateral extension. Often the depth of the pyriform sinus requires direct laryngoscopy for a complete evaluation of mucosal disease and recognition of lateral mucosal extension. Panendoscopy also serves as the perfect platform to determine transoral surgical exposure in patients who are being considered for TORS. The FK retractor (Gyrus Medical, Inc.) can be placed at this time and exposure can be assessed. In particular, "good exposure" is defined as full vision of the supraglottis and an unfolded pyriform sinus; "fair vision" is defined as full vision of the supraglottis and a folded pyriform; and "poor vision" is defined as a limited view of the supraglottis and folded pyriform sinuses.[48]

■ Description of Procedure

Anesthetic Considerations

Nontraumatic nasotracheal intubation is essential to maintain the anatomic delineation of the primary malignancy and prevent unwarranted edema. At our institution, we often prefer an awake fiberoptic nasotracheal intubation in conjunction with topical and local anesthetic administration. A laser safe endotracheal tube is preferred to reduce the risk of airway fire when either the laser or cautery is used adjacent to the glottis. General anesthesia is then induced and an appropriate dose of induction dexamethasone is administered to limit laryngeal edema and postoperative nausea. In addition, expired $FiO_2 < 30\%$ is preferred if physiologically feasible. An appropriate dose of muscle relaxant is essential to optimize surgical access for the retractor system. In rare situations where tracheotomy is indicated, tracheotomy at the first or second intercartilaginous space is performed prophylactically prior to the TORS resection in order to optimize visualization. The decision to extubate/decannulate depends on a variety of factors including extent of surgical resection, degree of edema, history of radiation therapy, and anatomic factors related to the patient's anatomy.[52]

Operating Room Setup

The operating room and da Vinci robotic system (Intuitive Surgical, Inc.) are set up in the standard fashion, which has been described in detail in the literature.[52,53,54] Briefly, the foot of the da Vinci robotic system is positioned at approximately 30 degrees to the surgical bed, in order to optimize access of the robotic arms for the surgical field. The 30-degree endoscope is calibrated and balanced. While there is evidence CO_2 laser causes less thermal damage and associated edema to adjacent structures when compared to monopolar cautery, our data indicate both techniques have equivalent results.[3] A foam doughnut is placed under the patient's head without a shoulder roll (**Fig. 11.1**).

Retractor Placement

A 2-0 silk suture is placed in the anterior tongue and anterior traction is applied while an appropriate blade is inserted in the FK retractor. Often experimentation is required to determine which of the laryngeal and tongue blades should be inserted into the FK retractor to provide the most optimal exposure. It has been our experience that the tongue blade is most useful in accessing the pyriform sinuses, which is also supported at other centers.[48] Some centers have advocated the FK-WO retractor to allow a wider lateral working space, but the standard FK retractor has provided adequate exposure in most cases.[43,45,49] Sufficient anterior traction applied to the tongue suture optimizes the view of the hypopharynx. The 12-mm 30-degree endoscope is inserted face up, followed by a 5-mm instrumentation including the spatula monopolar cautery ipsilateral to the tumor and the 5-mm Maryland forceps to the contralateral side (**Fig. 11.2**).

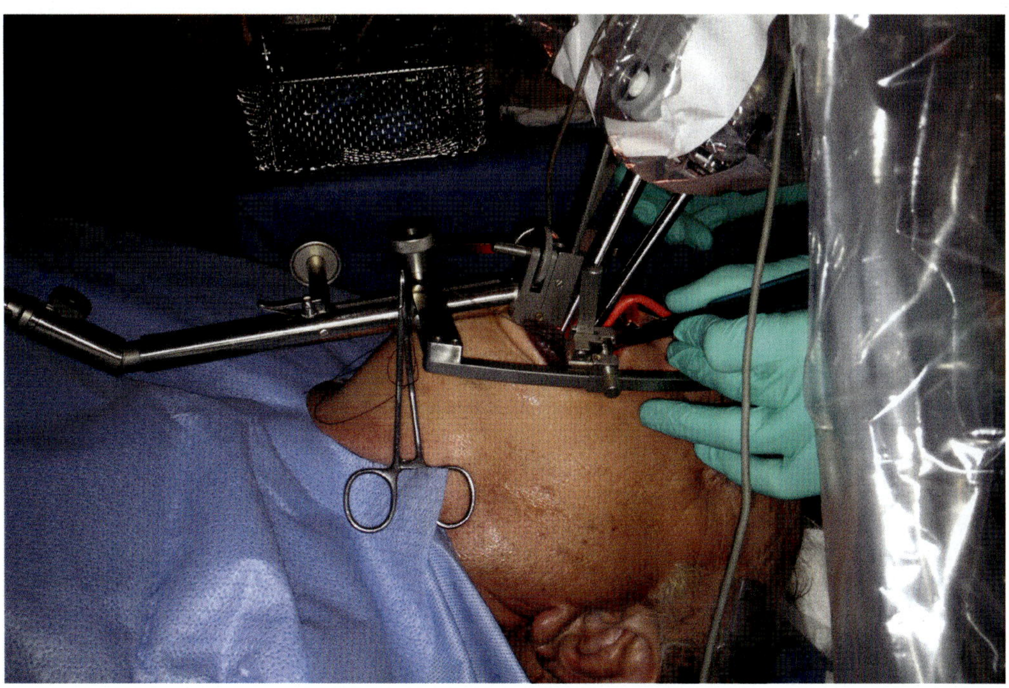

Fig. 11.1 Patient positioned for robotic surgery, retractor robotic arms positioned.

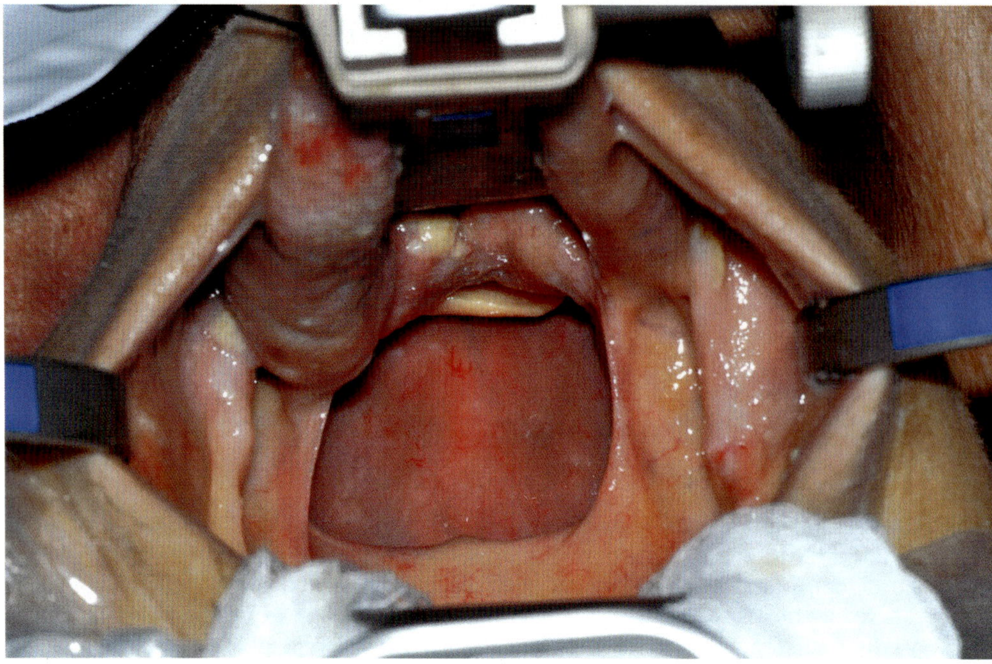

Fig. 11.2 Intraoral view of retractor setup, tongue suture in place. Note tip of epiglottis visualized.

In patients with a limited view anteriorly, manual posterior compression of the larynx can be applied to improve visualization. In select patients with an enlarged or flaccid epiglottis obstructing the surgical view, a partial ipsilateral epiglottectomy has been successfully applied to aid in visualization. This is particularly useful to access the pyriform sinus during TORS.[48] It should be noted that while the 30-degree telescope usually provides the most optimal visual field, on occasion the 0-degree telescope may be applied with laryngeal compression to obtain the necessary angle to view the lesion with a 30-degree endoscope.

Hypopharyngeal Surgery

Pyriform Sinus

The goal of transoral robotic resection of pyriform sinus tumors is to remove the tumor with appropriate oncologic margins while inflicting minimal morbidity in terms of airway and deglutition. This is achieved by performing a "cone-shaped" resection of the pyriform bounded superiorly at the vallecula and extending down to the apex of the cone just below the apex of the pyriform sinus. The resection includes the aryepiglottic fold medially and the perichondrium of the thyroid cartilage laterally for the majority of cases. The dissection is initiated medially at the anterior aryepiglottic fold and proceeds posteriorly to the depth of the sinus as indicated. Care is taken to preserve the integrity of the arytenoid and associated vocal and muscular processes that are critical for laryngeal function. The dissection is then advanced laterally along the aryepiglottic fold toward the thyroid cartilage if necessary. An incision is made laterally through the perichondrium and onto the thyroid cartilage. The perichondrium is then carefully peeled inferiorly, while the cartilage remains intact. In general the posterior margin should include the inferior constrictor muscle to provide oncologic control. When the resection requires dissection posterolaterally, careful blunt technique should be utilized to avoid injury of the great vessels. The final dissection occurs at the attachment of the apex of the pyriform sinus completing the en bloc resection (**Video 11.1**).

Posterior Pharyngeal Wall

Posterior pharyngeal wall tumors are generally less technically demanding due to improved access secondary to the vector of approach. In addition, the dissection is less anatomically complicated, especially in the situation of a midline lesion. More inferiorly located lesions in the region of the postcricoid recess do offer a challenge in terms of functional considerations due to stricture and swallowing issues related to surgery in this area. The setup is as noted above, with the exception that the 0-degree scope will often provide adequate visualization due to the posterior location of the lesion. The advantage of the robotic system is particularly appreciated during the dissection where, as opposed to the transoral laser microsurgery, the dissection plane remains in view and the wristed robotic instrumentation allows for an easier transition of the inferior incision. The dissection is initiated superiorly, where a mucosal incision is designed with appropriate surgical margins. The dissection is then carried to the level of the prevertebral fascia, which serves as the deep margin. Preoperative evaluation of imaging studies is critical to ensure that prevertebral fascia is not invaded and that an appropriate deep margin is feasible. Often contrast-enhanced MRI is required to make this determination. The appropriate plane of dissection is just anterior to the prevertebral fascia and proceeds inferiorly. Lateral incisions of appropriate width around the lesion are performed and the dissection proceeds inferiorly beyond the lesion. In general there is very little blood loss if the appropriate planes are respected; however, the prevertebral venous plexus may require cauterization for hemostasis. The lesion is circumferentially resected with adequate mucosal margins by completing the final inferior mucosal incision. Again, the wristed robotic instrumentation allows for superior access when making the final inferior mucosal incision.

Surgical Management of the Neck

This risk of cervical metastasis related to HSCC is well known. The reported incidence is greater than 20% and this mandates management of the neck in the majority of cases.[8,9] Selective neck dissection including levels II–IV is routinely advocated for patients managed surgically.[8] Bilateral selective neck dissection is warranted for any tumor crossing an approaching midline (i.e., posterior pharyngeal wall, or postcricoid recess), as well as significant tumors involving the medial wall of the pyriform sinus. Contralateral neck dissection should also be considered in patients presenting with advanced disease.[23] Retropharyngeal node basin dissection may be indicated for lesion of risk, or in salvage situations where salvage radiotherapy is not possible. Occasionally, selective level VI dissection should be considered for advanced disease.[55] The majority of neck dissections are performed simultaneously with the robotic resection. In general, this poses minimal risk, but the potential for pharyngocutaneous fistula should be born in mind. Careful inspection of the neck after neck dissection is warranted and pharyngeal methylene blue can be used in questionable cases to identify perforations, which would result in fistula formation. In general primary closure with local muscle flap rotation (infrahyoid strap, sternocleidomastoid muscle, etc.) is adequate to manage these situations. In situations of large fistula or postradiation salvage, more comprehensive reconstruction strategies may be required, although we have found this to be extremely rare in the majority of cases.

■ Postoperative Management

In general, postoperative management is routine with administration of intravenous antibiotics, pain medication, and steroids as indicated. Many patients will require nasogastric feeding tube support during the postoperative recovery for several days. This can be removed when the patient is tolerating oral intake and aspiration risk has been assessed and is reasonable. Aspiration is common in this patient population and close observation is warranted early in the postsurgical period. In cases where moderate to severe aspiration is suspected, formal swallowing evaluation is necessary and occasionally gastrostomy tube placement may be required, more commonly in postirradiation settings. Additionally, while prolonged tracheostomy dependence is rare, some patients, including previously radiated and elderly patients, may require long-term tracheostomy. It is essential to properly consent patients for this recovery period. In the case series reported to date the average times to decannulation and return to deglutition are approximately 6 and 8 days, respectively.[11]

■ Clinical Pearls

- Careful selection of patients is integral to successful oncologic and functional outcomes. Preoperative evaluation of anatomic factors impairing surgical access is critical for success.
- Placement of the FK retractor system during a diagnostic panendoscopy is extremely valuable to verify adequate exposure for robotic surgery of the hypopharynx.
- Anesthesia technique and appropriate setup are critical to avoid complications such as prolonged airway edema, bleeding, and airway fire.
- Maneuvers to improve exposure include anterior tongue suture traction, posterior laryngeal pressure, and partial epiglottectomy and retractor blade experimentation.
- Oncologic margin control is critical and is facilitated by meticulous hemostasis and specimen handling/orientation.
- A low threshold for tracheostomy is important when performing surgical resections involving the hypopharyngeal and supraglottic regions.

■ Complications

Complications related to minimally invasive surgery of the hypopharynx are generally complications associated with transoral laser/transoral robotic surgery in general. These include airway obstruction; bleeding; airway fire; damage to lips, tongue, and dentition; as well as lingual and hypoglossal nerve injuries as a result of retractor systems. Complications specific to hypopharyngeal surgery include inadvertent damage to the arytenoid complex, vocal cord paralysis, mediastinitis (rare), cervical fistula, and esophageal inlet stricture with resulting dysphagia.[43,56,57]

■ Future Directions and Conclusion

TORS of the hypopharynx is an oncologically sound approach and relatively safe according to current literature. In addition, preliminary data indicate promising function outcomes.[34,37,43,44,45,49,50] Long-term survival data are currently not available, but appear to be equivalent in selected cases. This highlights the extreme importance of careful patient selection to obtain successful oncologic and functional outcomes. Adequate exposure is a critical component of this technique that facilitates clear margins with minimal postoperative morbidity. Novel techniques have been described, such as midline mandibulotomy to improve access.[47] While this solution offers some promise, improvements in robotic technology are likely to result in systems designed for hypopharyngeal surgery to be employed, improving access and broadening surgical indications for hypopharyngeal and laryngeal robotic surgery.[58] Further prospective trials in this high-risk population will allow future surgeons to determine which patients would benefit from TORS and advances in technique and instrumentation are likely to impact this approach in the future.

References

1. Newman JG, Kuppersmith RB, O'Malley BW, Jr. Robotics and telesurgery in otolaryngology. Otolaryngol Clin North Am 2011; 44(6):1317–1331, viii
2. Iseli TA, Kulbersh BD, Iseli CE, Carroll WR, Rosenthal EL, Magnuson JS. Functional outcomes after transoral robotic surgery for head and neck cancer. Otolaryngol Head Neck Surg 2009;141(2):166–171
3. Genden EM, Desai S, Sung CK. Transoral robotic surgery for the management of head and neck cancer: a preliminary experience. Head Neck 2009;31(3):283–289
4. Weinstein GS, O'Malley BW Jr, Desai SC, Quon H. Transoral robotic surgery: does the ends justify the means? Curr Opin Otolaryngol Head Neck Surg 2009;17(2):126–131
5. Cooper JS, Porter K, Mallin K, et al. National Cancer Database report on cancer of the head and neck: 10-year update. Head Neck 2009;31(6):748–758
6. Kirchner JA. Pyriform sinus cancer: a clinical and laboratory study. Ann Otol Rhinol Laryngol 1975;84(6):793–803
7. Hoffman HT, Karnell LH, Shah JP, et al. Hypopharyngeal cancer patient care evaluation. Laryngoscope 1997;107(8):1005–1017
8. Hall SF, Groome PA, Irish J, O'Sullivan B. The natural history of patients with squamous cell carcinoma of the hypopharynx. Laryngoscope 2008;118(8):1362–1371
9. Gourin CG, Terris DJ. Carcinoma of the hypopharynx. Surg Oncol Clin North Am 2004;13(1):81–98
10. Buckley JG, MacLennan K. Cervical node metastases in laryngeal and hypopharyngeal cancer: a prospective analysis of prevalence and distribution. Head Neck 2000;22(4):380–385
11. Park YM, Kim WS, Byeon HK, De Virgilio A, Jung JS, Kim SH. Feasiblity of transoral robotic hypopharyngectomy for early-stage hypopharyngeal carcinoma. Oral Oncol 2010;46(8):597–602
12. Sisson GA. Reconstruction of the hypopharynx and cervical esophagus after radical excisional surgery. Laryngoscope 1956; 66(10):1268–1290
13. Leroux-Robert J. Indications for radical surgery, partial surgery, radiotherapy and combined surgery and radiotherapy for cancer of the larynx and hypopharynx. Ann Otol Rhinol Laryngol 1956;65(1):137–153
14. Snitman MF, Horwitz ID. Surgery of carcinoma of the hypopharynx. AMA Arch Otolaryngol 1955;62(5):493–496
15. Sessions DG, Zill R, Schwartz SL. Deglutition after conservation surgery for cancer of the larynx and hypopharynx. Otolaryngol Head Neck Surg 1979;87(6):779–796
16. Gall AM, Sessions DG, Ogura JH. Complications following surgery for cancer of the larynx and hypopharynx. Cancer 1977; 39(2):624–631
17. Schechter GL, McLarey D. Conservation surgery of the larynx and hypopharynx. Mil Med 1973;138(10):639–642
18. Stell PM. The present status of surgery in the treatment of carcinoma of the hypopharynx and cervical oesophagus. Adv Otorhinolaryngol 1988;39:120–134
19. Hirano M, Kurita S, Tanaka H. Histopathologic study of carcinoma of the hypopharynx: implications for conservation surgery. Ann Otol Rhinol Laryngol 1987;96(6):625–629
20. Bahadur S, Amatya RC, Kacher SK. Primary surgery versus radiation-failed salvage surgery in advanced carcinoma of the larynx and hypopharynx. Indian J Cancer 1986;23(2):89–93
21. Levitt SH, Beachley MC, Zimberg Y, Pastore PN, DeGiorgi LS, King ER. Combination of preoperative irradiation and surgery in the treatment of cancer of the oropharynx, hypopharynx, and larynx. Cancer 1971;27(4):759–767
22. Lefebvre JL, Chevalier D, Luboinski B, Kirkpatrick A, Collette L, Sahmoud T. Larynx preservation in pyriform sinus cancer: preliminary results of a European Organization for Research and Treatment of Cancer phase III trial. EORTC Head and Neck Cancer Cooperative Group. J Natl Cancer Inst 1996;88(13): 890–899
23. Chan JY, Wei WI. Current management strategy of hypopharyngeal carcinoma. Auris Nasus Larynx 2013;40(1):2–6
24. Lefebvre JL. Surgery for laryngopharyngeal SCC in the era of organ preservation. Clin Exp Otorhinolaryngol 2009;2(4):159–163
25. Godballe C, Jorgensen K, Hansen O, Bastholt L. Hypopharyngeal cancer: results of treatment based on radiation therapy and salvage surgery. Laryngoscope 2002;112(5):834–838
26. Kraus DH, Zelefsky MJ, Brock HA, Huo J, Harrison LB, Shah JP. Combined surgery and radiation therapy for squamous cell carcinoma of the hypopharynx. Otolaryngol Head Neck Surg 1997; 116(6 Pt 1):637–641
27. Hall SF, Groome PA, Irish J, O'Sullivan B. Radiotherapy or surgery for head and neck squamous cell cancer: establishing the baseline for hypopharyngeal carcinoma? Cancer 2009;115(24): 5711–5722
28. Levendag PC, Teguh DN, Voet P, et al. Dysphagia disorders in patients with cancer of the oropharynx are significantly affected by the radiation therapy dose to the superior and middle constrictor muscle: a dose-effect relationship. Radiother Oncol 2007; 85(1):64–73
29. Forastiere AA, Goepfert H, Maor M, et al. Concurrent chemotherapy and radiotherapy for organ preservation in advanced laryngeal cancer. N Engl J Med 2003;349(22):2091–2098
30. Forastiere AA, Zhang Q, Weber RS, et al. Long-term results of RTOG 91-11: a comparison of three nonsurgical treatment strategies to preserve the larynx in patients with locally advanced larynx cancer. J Clin Oncol 2013;31(7):845–852
31. Hoffman HT, Porter K, Karnell LH, et al. Laryngeal cancer in the United States: changes in demographics, patterns of care, and survival. Laryngoscope 2006;116(9 Pt 2 Suppl 111):1–13
32. Chen AY, Halpern M. Factors predictive of survival in advanced laryngeal cancer. Arch Otolaryngol Head Neck Surg 2007; 133(12):1270–1276
33. Arbyn M, Raifu AO, Weiderpass E, Bray F, Anttila A. Trends of cervical cancer mortality in the member states of the European Union. Eur J Cancer 2009;45(15):2640–2648
34. Takes RP, Strojan P, Silver CE, et al. Current trends in initial management of hypopharyngeal cancer: the declining use of open surgery. Head Neck 2012;34(2):270–281
35. Steiner W. [Therapy of hypopharyngeal cancer. Part III: The concept of minimally invasive therapy of cancers of the upper aerodigestive tract with special reference to hypopharyngeal cancer and trans-oral laser microsurgery]. HNO 1994;42(2): 104–112
36. Matschke RG. Experiences with laser surgery in benign and malignant findings of the oro- and hypopharynx. Adv Otorhinolaryngol 1995;49:153–157
37. Chan JY, Wei WI. Current management strategy of hypopharyngeal carcinoma. Auris Nasus Larynx 2013;40(1):2–6
38. Vilaseca I, Blanch JL, Bernal-Sprekelsen M. Transoral laser surgery for hypopharyngeal carcinomas. Curr Opin Otolaryngol Head Neck Surg 2012;20(2):97–102
39. Rudert HH, Hoft S. Transoral carbon-dioxide laser resection of hypopharyngeal carcinoma. Eur Arch Otorhinolaryngol 2003; 260(4):198–206
40. Steiner W, Ambrosch P, Hess CF, Kron M. Organ preservation by transoral laser microsurgery in piriform sinus carcinoma. Otolaryngol Head Neck Surg 2001;124(1):58–67

41. Martin A, Jackel MC, Christiansen H, Mahmoodzada M, Kron M, Steiner W. Organ preserving transoral laser microsurgery for cancer of the hypopharynx. Laryngoscope 2008;118(3):398–402
42. Bernal-Sprekelsen M, Dazert S, Sudhoff H, Blanch JL, Vilaseca I. [Complications of transoral laser surgery for malignant tumors of the larynx and hypopharynx]. Laryngorhinootologie 2009; 88(1):28–34
43. Park ES, Shum JW, Bui TG, Bell RB, Dierks EJ. Robotic surgery: a new approach to tumors of the tongue base, oropharynx, and hypopharynx. Oral Maxillofac Surg Clin North Am Feb 2013;25(1):49–59, vi
44. Ozer E, Alvarez B, Kakarala K, Durmus K, Teknos TN, Carrau RL. Clinical outcomes of transoral robotic supraglottic laryngectomy. Head Neck 2013;35(8):1158–1161
45. Park YM, Kim WS, De Virgilio A, Lee SY, Seol JH, Kim SH. Transoral robotic surgery for hypopharyngeal squamous cell carcinoma: 3-year oncologic and functional analysis. Oral Oncol 2012;48(6):560–566
46. Boudreaux BA, Rosenthal EL, Magnuson JS, et al. Robot-assisted surgery for upper aerodigestive tract neoplasms. Arch Otolaryngol Head Neck Surg 2009;135(4):397–401
47. Iloreta AM, Anderson K, Miles BA. Mandibular osteotomy for expanded transoral robotic surgery (MOTORS): a novel technique. Laryngoscope 2014;124(8):1836–1842
48. De Virgilio A, Park YM, Kim WS, Baek SJ, Kim SH. How to optimize laryngeal and hypopharyngeal exposure in transoral robotic surgery. Auris Nasus Larynx 2013;40(3):312–319
49. Lee HS, Koh MJ, Koh YW, Choi EC. Transoral robotic surgery for huge spindle cell lipoma of the hypopharynx. J Craniofac Surg 2013;24(4):1278–1279
50. De Virgilio A, Park YM, Kim WS, Baek SJ, Kim SH. How to optimize laryngeal and hypopharyngeal exposure in transoral robotic surgery. Auris Nasus Larynx 2013;40(3):312–319
51. Crosby ET, Cooper RM, Douglas MJ, et al. The unanticipated difficult airway with recommendations for management. Can J Anaesth 1998;45(8):757–776
52. Chi JJ, Mandel JE, Weinstein GS, O'Malley BW Jr. Anesthetic considerations for transoral robotic surgery. Anesthesiol Clin 2010; 28(3):411–422
53. Weinstein GS, O'Malley BW Jr, Snyder W, Hockstein NG. Transoral robotic surgery: supraglottic partial laryngectomy. Ann Otol Rhinol Laryngol 2007;116(1):19–23
54. Weinstein GS, O'Malley BW Jr, Snyder W, Sherman E, Quon H. Transoral robotic surgery: radical tonsillectomy. Arch Otolaryngol Head Neck Surg 2007;133(12):1220–1226
55. Harrison DF. Surgical pathology of hypopharyngeal neoplasms. J Laryngol Otol 1971;85(12):1215–1218
56. Yoshida K, Inoue T, Inoue T, Tanaka E, Shiomi H, Teshima T. Treatment results of radiotherapy with or without surgery for posterior pharyngeal wall cancer of oropharynx and hypopharynx: prognostic value of tumor extension. Radiat Med 2004;22(1): 30–36
57. Vilaseca-Gonzalez I, Bernal-Sprekelsen M, Blanch-Alejandro JL, Moragas-Lluis M. Complications in transoral CO2 laser surgery for carcinoma of the larynx and hypopharynx. Head Neck 2003; 25(5):382–388
58. Johnson PJ, Rivera Serrano CM, Castro M, et al. Demonstration of transoral surgery in cadaveric specimens with the medrobotics flex system. Laryngoscope 2013;123(5):1168–1172

12 Robotic Surgery of the Parapharyngeal Space

Suren Krishnan

■ Introduction

The parapharyngeal space is an intriguing compartment of the head and neck. Although it is the site of only 0.5% of all head and neck masses, the unusual pathology and proximity to vital anatomy attract the special interest of surgeons, radiologists, and pathologists.[1,2] Lesions of the parapharyngeal space may involve a wide spectrum of primary pathologies. The advent of multiplanar radiological imaging—including fine-sliced computed tomography (CT) with contrast and magnetic resonance imaging (MRI) with fat suppression sequences and gadolinium for contrast—together with histological diagnosis with fine needle aspiration cytology has improved preoperative diagnostic accuracy. This allows for a better understanding of the nature of these lesions and a better plan for the surgical approach to them.

There has been increasing interest and use of transoral robotic surgery (TORS) in the treatment of benign and malignant tumors of the oropharynx. TORS has had the approval of the U.S. Food and Drug Administration (FDA) for use in early oropharyngeal cancers and benign lesions of the head and neck since 2009. The da Vinci surgical robotic system (Intuitive Surgical, Inc.) provides three-dimensional, high-resolution visual access with magnification as well as tremor filtration and motion scaling of robotic instruments. This allows for delicate dissection and addresses previous concerns leveled against transoral approaches to the parapharyngeal space with respect to controlled dissection around vital neurovascular structures and tumor spillage.

■ Anatomy

The parapharyngeal space is classically described as an inverted pyramid-shaped potential space (**Fig. 12.1**). Its base lies superiorly at the skull base and comprises the sphenoid and temporal bones. This area includes the jugular and hypoglossal canal and the foramen lacerum. Its apex lies inferiorly at the greater cornu of the hyoid bone. It has three sides—medial, lateral, and posterior—and an anterior leading edge, which is the pterygomandibular raphe.

The medial surface is distensible and comprises the superior pharyngeal constrictor muscle, the buccopharyngeal membrane, and the pharynx. The lateral surface, which is relatively immobile, comprises the medial pterygoid muscle, the ramus of the mandible, and the deep lobe of the parotid gland. Below the level of the mandible, the lateral aspect is bordered by the fascia of the posterior belly of the digastric muscle. It has a posterior surface that is part of the prevertebral fascia, bordered by the carotid sheath posterolaterally and the retropharyngeal space posteromedially.

Two fascial condensations in the parapharyngeal space are of surgical importance. First, the parapharyngeal space is divided into two parts by the fascial condensation called the aponeurosis of Zuckerkandl and Testut (**Fig. 12.2**). This fascia joining the styloid process to the tensor veli palatini divides the parapharyngeal space into the prestyloid and poststyloid compartments. The prestyloid compartment contains adipose tissue, lymphatics, ectopic salivary gland tissue and small nerves and vessels, a small branch of the trigeminal nerve to the tensor veli palatini muscle, and branches of the ascending pharyngeal artery and pharyngeal venous plexus. It is related to the retromandibular, deep aspect of the parotid gland. The poststyloid compartment is posteromedial and contains the internal

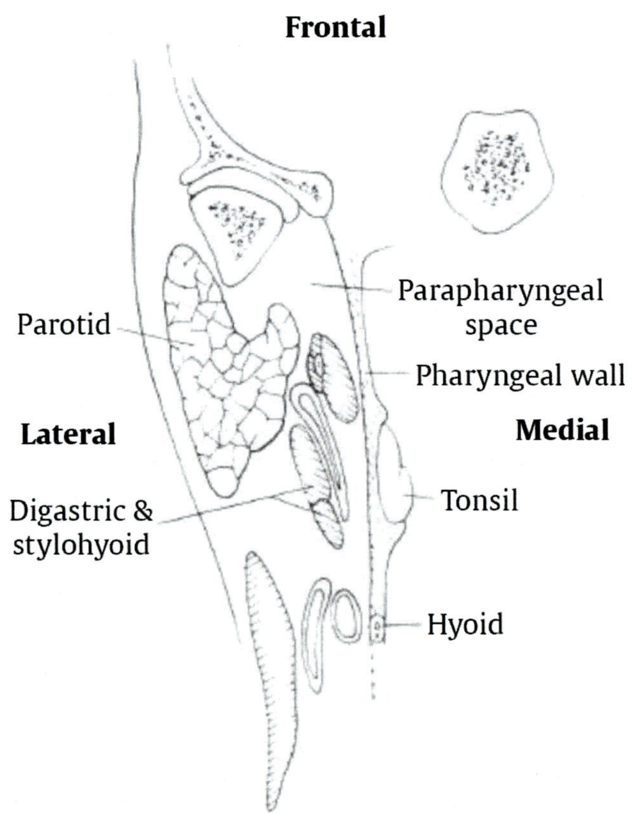

Fig. 12.1 The parapharyngeal space resembles an inverted pyramid. (Used with permission from Olsen KD. Tumors of the parapharyngeal space. Laryngoscope 1994;104(5 Pt 2 Suppl 63):2. Courtesy of the Mayo Clinic, Rochester, Minnesota.)

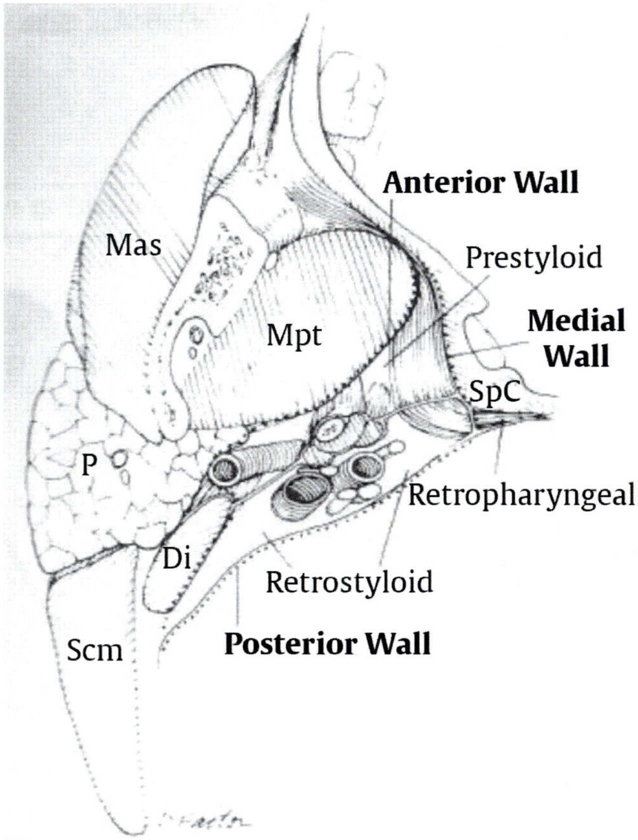

Fig. 12.2 Prestyloid and poststyloid (retrostyloid) compartments separated by condensation of fascia—the aponeurosis of Zuckerkandl and Testut. Mas, masseter muscle; Mpt, medial pterygoid muscle; SpC, splenius capitis muscle; P, parotid gland; Di, digastric muscle; Scm, sternocleidomastoid muscle. (Used with permission from Olsen KD. Tumors of the parapharyngeal space. Laryngoscope 1994;104(5 Pt 2 Suppl 63):4. Courtesy of the Mayo Clinic, Rochester, Minnesota.)

carotid artery, internal jugular vein, cranial nerves IX to XII, the cervical sympathetic chain, lymph nodes, and glomus bodies.

Second, a condensation of cervical fascia forms a band that extends from near the apex of the styloid process of the temporal bone to the angle and posterior border of the angle of the mandible (**Fig. 12.3**). This stylomandibular ligament and the posterior border of the mandible form the stylomandibular tunnel. The tunnel is a deep relation of the deep lobe of the parotid gland. Tumors of the deep lobe can extend into the parapharyngeal space through this tunnel giving rise to a dumbbell tumor.

■ Pathology

As mentioned above, parapharyngeal space tumors account for 0.5% of all head and neck masses. In a comprehensive review of the literature on parapharyngeal space tumors, Riffat et al identified approximately 70 different histologic subtypes of lesions.[3] Of these, 82% were benign and 18% malignant. The most common tumors were of salivary gland origin, accounting for 45% of all lesions. These arose in the prestyloid compartment. The vast majority (75%) were benign and 64% were pleomorphic adenomas. Adenoid cystic carcinoma and mucoepidermoid carcinoma were the most common reported malignant lesions.

Neurogenic lesions accounted for 41% of lesions in the parapharyngeal space. The majority of these lesions are benign and, of these, 52% were paragangliomas, 27% were schwannomas, and 9% were neurofibromas. Malignant lesions accounted for 5% of neurogenic lesions arising in the poststyloid space and the major subtype was malignant peripheral nerve sheath tumors.

A variety of miscellaneous lesions account for 12% of parapharyngeal space tumors. These include internal carotid artery aneurysms, branchial cleft cysts, hemangiomas, and meningiomas. Metastatic lesions account for 3% of lesions, and 2% of lesions are of lymphoid origin.

■ Clinical Presentation and Evaluation

These tumors are usually asymptomatic oropharyngeal masses, found on incidental examination for innocuous symptoms such

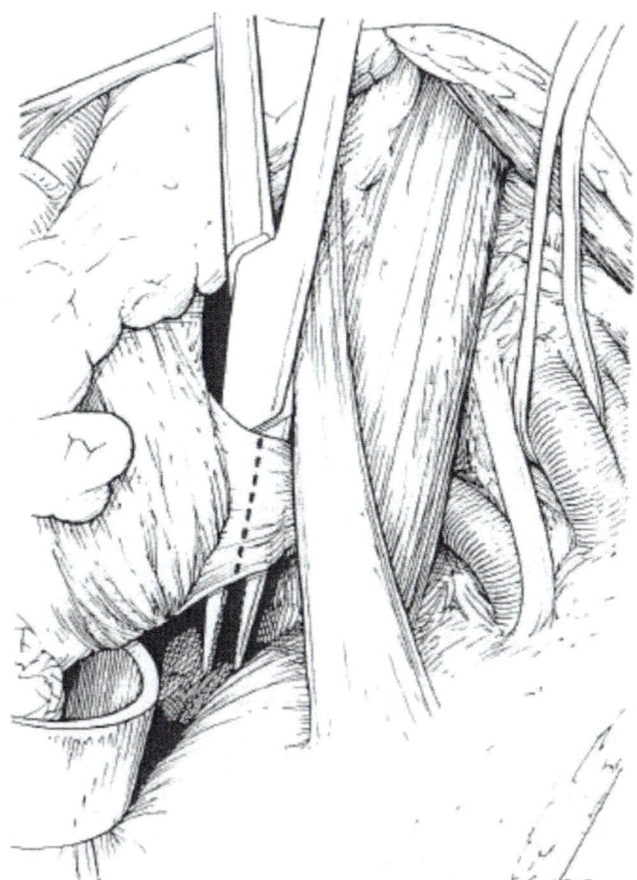

Fig. 12.3 Stylomandibular ligament of the left neck from styloid process to posterior border of mandible forming the stylomandibular tunnel. (Used with permission from Olsen KD. Tumors of the parapharyngeal space. Laryngoscope 1994;104(5 Pt 2 Suppl 63):21. Courtesy of the Mayo Clinic, Rochester, Minnesota.)

as sore throat. They need to be at least 3 cm before they become apparent and present as a neck mass. They may present with a simple nasal obstruction or snoring, or may present with hearing loss due to eustachian tube occlusion. Rarely, they may present with cranial nerve dysfunction, which may be due to pressure on or involvement of the hypoglossal, vagus, and glossopharyngeal nerves. They can also present with Horner syndrome.

Clinical evaluation requires assessment of the airway, speech, and swallowing; a full head and neck examination including cranial nerve examination; nasopharyngoscopy; and examination of the middle ear for effusion. Bimanual palpation and ballottement helps assess tumor mobility and size and appreciation of the displacement of the tonsil or the posterior pharyngeal wall provides clues to whether the lesion has its origins from the prestyloid or poststyloid compartment.[4]

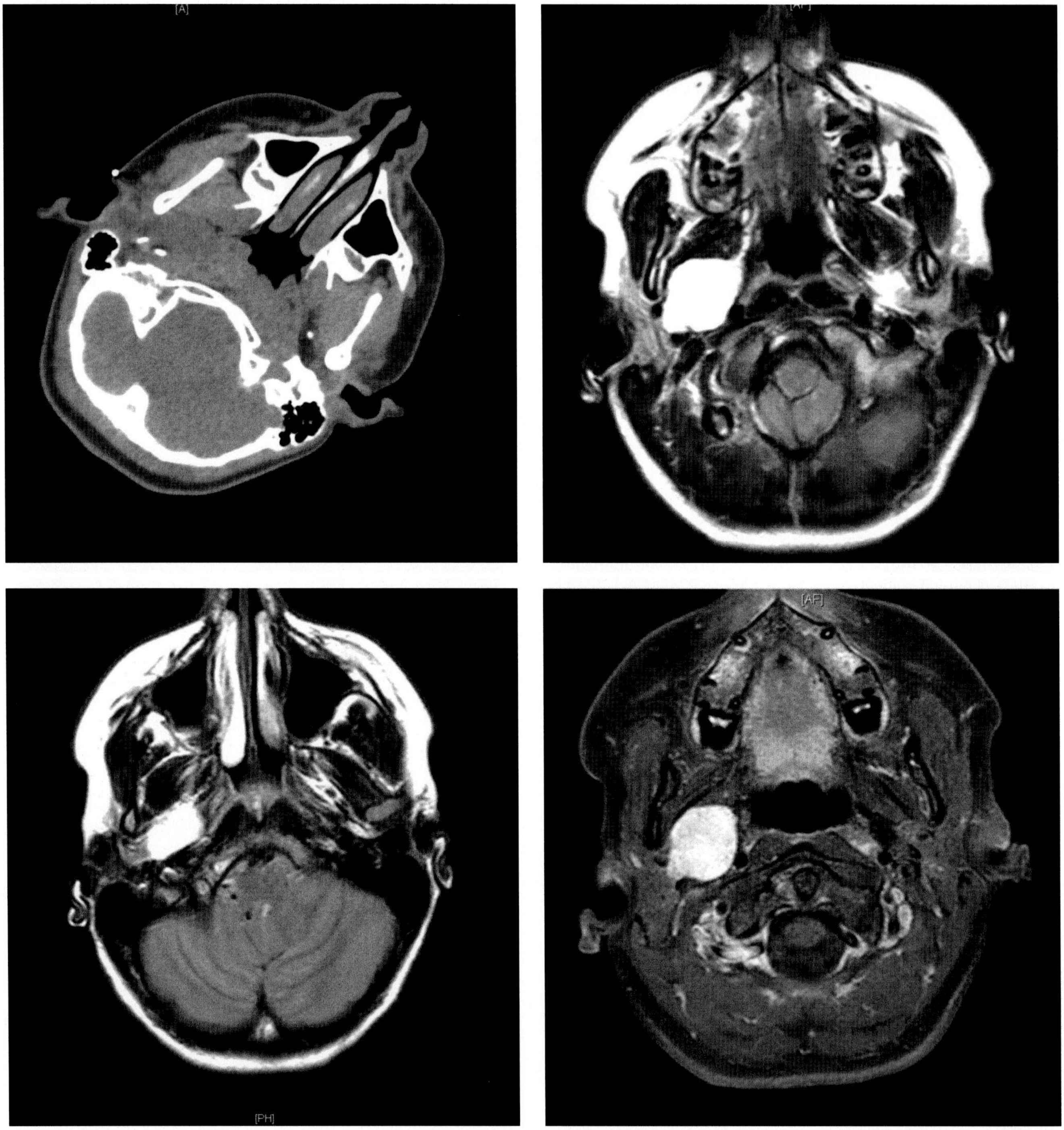

a b c d

Fig. 12.4 (a) Right parapharyngeal space (PPS) tumor on computed tomography showing PPS mass contiguous with deep lobe parotid. **(b)** Same right PPS tumor on magnetic resonance imaging (MRI) showing mass clearly arising from deep lobe of parotid. **(c)** Same right PPS tumor on MRI showing limited involvement of deep lobe of parotid. These lesions are suitable for a combined transcervical and transoral robotic surgery resection. **(d)** T1-weighted MRI with gadolinium and STIR sequence to suppress fat and demonstrate no fat plane in PPS between tumor and deep lobe of parotid.

Imaging

Accurate imaging of the parapharyngeal space is essential to planning surgical resection. Multiplanar imaging with fine slice CT and MRI provides the detail required. Further information regarding vascularity and relationship to the neurovascular structures can be gained from magnetic resonance angiography and carotid angiography.[5,6,7] Therapeutic interventions such as preoperative embolization or balloon occlusion studies can be performed at the same time.

The parapharyngeal space appears as a small triangular space on axial imaging with an image density or signal consistent with fat. Knowledge about the displacement patterns of fat and the internal carotid artery within the parapharyngeal space will aid in the localization of lesions.

The presence of a fat plane between the parotid and a lesion differentiates a truly parapharyngeal space lesion from an extension of a deep lobe parotid lesion through the stylomandibular tunnel into the parapharyngeal space (**Fig. 12.4**). A lesion arising in the prestyloid space may have a rim of parapharyngeal fat anteromedially, but displaces the parapharyngeal fat and internal carotid artery posterolaterally (**Fig. 12.5**), whereas a lesion in the poststyloid compartment will displace the parapharyngeal fat and internal carotid artery anteromedially. MRI with fat suppression sequences can help delineate this relationship clearly.

CT scans can show evidence of bony detail and erosion by these tumors and may also show calcification within tumors. MRI scans show soft tissue extension of these tumors including intracranial extension. MRI scan with gadolinium can also show involvement of nerves and perineural spread.

Some lesions have classic imaging characteristics like congenital cysts, which on CT are seen as low attenuation lesions with a thin uniformly smooth wall. On MRI, they appear as T1-weighted hypointense and T2-weighted hyperintense lesions with peripheral enhancement on postcontrast study. Schwannomas are fusiform, sharply circumscribed masses seen on CT as soft tissue density masses with few cystic areas within. They show uniform enhancement on postcontrast study. On MRI, they appear heterogeneously hyperintense on T2-weighted images and isointense to hypointense on T1-weighted images. There are no flow voids within them that help to differentiate them from paraganglioma. The flow voids in paraganglioma give them the characteristic "salt and pepper" appearance on MRI. Functioning paragangliomas may require further investigations including 24-hour urine screen for metanephrine.

Image guidance may be required to obtain a transcervical fine needle aspiration biopsy for lesions not obvious or accessible in the oropharynx by a transoral approach.[8]

Surgical Approaches

External transparotid, transcervical approaches to the parapharyngeal space have traditionally been considered the only safe access. The external approach was initially promoted in the 1950s mainly because of a poor understanding of the nature of these tumors and the surgical anatomic relationships. CT did not arrive until 1972 and was not in general use until 1979; the first MRI scanners arrived in the mid-1980s and were not in general use until the late 1990s. The improved imaging allowed consideration of approaches other than the traditional external approach.

In his treatise on parapharyngeal space surgery, Olsen provides a clear description of the variety of external approaches.[1] These include transcervical and in combination with a transcarotid approach with or without a mandibulotomy for tumors that extend into the intratemporal fossa. Other combinations including orbitozygomatic approaches as well as transmandibular

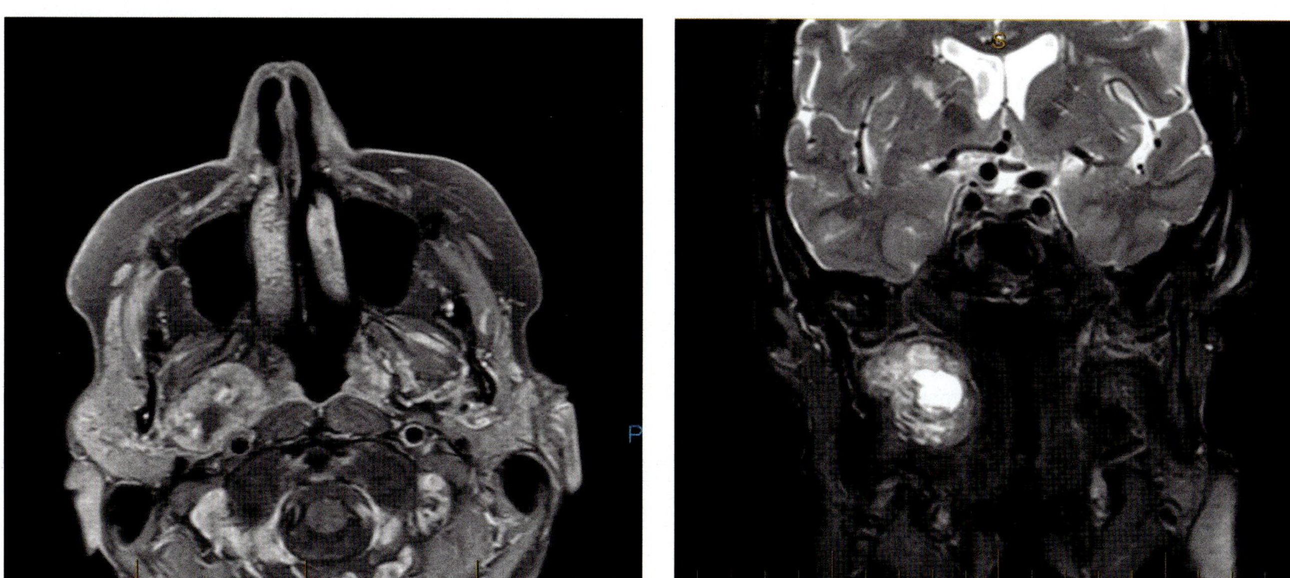

a b

Fig. 12.5 (a) Magnetic resonance imaging of right parapharyngeal space (PPS) tumor. Lesion of the right PPS with fat plane between tumor and deep lobe of parotid gland and rim of fat anteromedial to tumor. Lesion of the PPS in the prestyloid compartment displacing the carotid artery posteriorly. This variation is ideal for a transoral robotic surgical approach to resection. **(b)** Right PPS tumor displacing carotid artery laterally—favorable for transoral robotic surgery.

and transpalatal approaches have been described. These approaches all involve wide exposure and a significant disruption of the normal anatomy of the jaw and neck in order to facilitate safe resection of large or malignant neoplasms.

Transoral approaches have generally been discredited. This is predominantly related to the risk to adjacent neurovascular structures, the risk of tumors spilled during resection, the subsequent difficulty in dealing with recurrent tumor, and finally the risk of infection from contamination of oral commensals.

■ Transoral Robotic Surgery of the Parapharyngeal Space: The Paradigm Shift

Embarking on TORS of the parapharyngeal space requires addressing the concerns and criticisms of this approach. The first issue is the risk to vital neurovascular structures. The traditional transcervical approaches are mooted as safer. However, in practice these approaches provide clear visualization of the lower cervical component of parapharyngeal space tumors and their relationship to the neurovascular bundle in the neck. The superior component is often difficult if not impossible to visualize. A true inspection of the relationship of tumor to neurovascular bundle would require wide access techniques such as mandibular osteotomy and/or infratemporal fossa approaches. As most tumors are benign and of salivary gland origin the superior aspect of the dissection is often performed with blunt finger dissection and inferior traction of the tumor to displace it off the neurovascular bundle.

The da Vinci surgical robotic system has been used extensively in the treatment of benign and malignant tumors of the oropharynx and has had FDA approval for use in early oropharyngeal cancers since 2009. The use of TORS has expanded to involve lesions of the larynx, hypopharynx, nasopharynx, and skull base and, more recently, lesions in the parapharyngeal space. The transoral robotic approach does address some of the concerns previously leveraged against transoral approaches for parapharyngeal space lesions. The robot does provide better visual access to the oral cavity, oropharynx, and parapharyngeal space with excellent three-dimensional view with either a 0-degree scope or a 30-degree scope, which can be used to inspect the superior aspects of the parapharyngeal space up to the skull base as well as be rotated to inspect the inferior extent of tumors of the parapharyngeal space. It has overcome the line of sight limitations of the microscope and allows examination of the lateral aspects of the parapharyngeal space including the stylomandibular tunnel.

The second issue is the risk of tumor spillage. Undertaking a TORS approach requires meticulous study of the imaging and, at examination under anaesthesia, evaluation of the mobility of the tumor and its lateral, superior, and inferior relationships. The surgeon needs to understand the nature of the lesion, whether it is cystic, solid, or mixed, whether it is benign or malignant, the thickness of its capsule, and its relationship to the adjacent neurovascular structures.

The traditional support for external approach to the parapharyngeal space is based on a number of case series reports.[9,10,11,12] However, these are all retrospective, with a limited period of patient follow-up and with mixed pathologic type including vascular tumors. These papers still report recurrence of benign tumors and tumor spillage. In practice, it is not uncommon from the standard transcervical approach for lesions to have their capsule disrupted. Sometimes when tumors are displaced inferiorly by pulling down on the tumor, a fragment of tumor may split off from the main mass of tumor. Careful inspection of the parapharyngeal space cavity with a telescope and irrigation of small fragments is required.

In contrast there are few papers reporting the results of a transoral approach.[13,14,15,16] There have been case reports of neural sheath tumors, neurofibromas, branchial cleft cyst tumors, and benign mixed tumors being removed. Ducic et al reported transoral resection of a series of poststyloid salivary gland tumors that displaced the carotid artery anteriorly.[15] Since the introduction of CT scans and MRI and a better understanding of the cross-sectional anatomy of the parapharyngeal space, there has been renewed interest in transoral resection of parapharyngeal space tumors.

The advantages of the da Vinci robotic surgical system have also renewed interest in transoral resection of parapharyngeal space tumors. The first reports of transoral robotic resection of parapharyngeal space by O'Malley et al[17] described resection of a benign parapharyngeal space cyst without complications. The University of Pennsylvania's series reported 10 patients, one of whom was converted to an open transcervical approach due to difficulty in finger dissection and to avoid tumor spillage.[18,19] Dehiscence of the mucosal incision was observed in two patients; none of the patients had residual or recurrent neoplasms at a follow-up, on average, of 19.9 months. Their case series has reached 25 cases at the time of writing, with no recurrences and no patients requiring mandibulotomy or tracheostomy (personal communication). Several authors have reported their experience with TORS for parapharyngeal space tumor resection,[20,21,22,23,24,25,26,27,28] including a systematic review by Chan et al.[29]

Whereas the traditional transcervical approach allows you access to the bottom of the tumor and a blind finger dissection at the superior aspect of the tumor, a transoral approach allows access to all aspects of the tumor. O'Malley et al described combining the use of the robot to dissect the inferior and medial aspect of the tumor, with a blunt finger dissection to complete the superior and lateral dissection.[18] Patients in this institution are consented for a transoral robotic approach as well as for possible conversion to a transcervical approach with or without mandibulotomy if the transoral approach is not amenable to safe resection of tumor.

Cross-sectional imaging should distinguish vascular tumors, and if necessary, appropriate angiographic studies should be performed. The histological nature of tumors should be identified preoperatively by fine needle aspiration either by image control or by direct or transoral biopsy.

The transoral robotic technique has technical advantages, such as the three-dimensional high-resolution image with magnification, as well as the tremor filtration and motion scaling that allow delicate dissection. For tumors with a thin capsule or with a significant cystic component, however, consideration must be given to other methods to control the spillage of tumors. This may include blunt finger dissection particularly of the superior and lateral aspects of the tumor, or decompression of the tumor medially by a controlled perforation of the capsule and using either a microdebrider or coblator wand to evacuate the contents of the tumor within its cystic encasement before proceeding

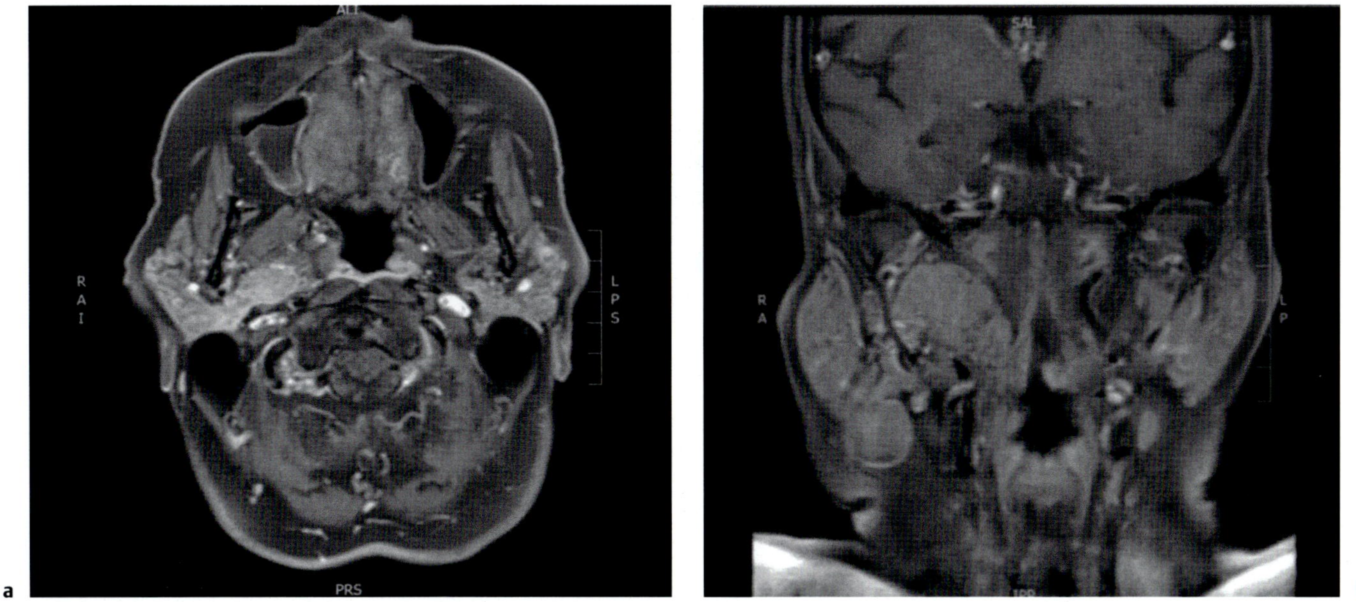

Fig. 12.6 (a) Axial magnetic resonance imaging (MRI) showing dumbbell tumor extensively involving the parotid gland with extension through the stylohyoid tunnel into the parapharyngeal space. Such tumors are not suitable for transoral robotic surgical resection. **(b)** Coronal MRI showing dumbbell tumor extensively involving the parotid gland with extension through the stylohyoid tunnel into the parapharyngeal space.

with lateral dissection. It is important that the lateral aspect of the tumor is dissected bluntly and carefully to ensure that tumor rupture is kept to a minimum. Usage of the robot allows careful inspection of the parapharyngeal space cavity after tumor removal to ensure that there is no residual tumor within the field.

Scaled movement and tremor filtration also allows for dedicated dissection around the tumor capsule ensuring resection with a margin.

Preoperative Assessment and Indication for Transoral Robotic Surgery

The use of TORS for parapharyngeal space resection does require accurate preoperative assessment. The focus of assessment is the relationship of the tumor to the carotid, tumor extent, tumor pathology, and the nature of the tumor in terms of thickness of capsule and whether the tumor is cystic or has cystic components. Fine needle aspiration biopsies done either by image control or by transoral biopsy are required as benign and low-grade malignancies are considered suitable for TORS.

The ideal indications for TORS parapharyngeal space resection are benign salivary gland tumors occurring in the prestyloid compartment, displacing the carotid artery posteriorly and laterally. These are the majority of parapharyngeal space tumors. Schwannomas and other benign neural tumors that are not deforming the carotid artery and not displacing the carotid artery medially are suitable for resection. Cystic lesions such as branchial cleft cysts are suitable for resection.

Relative indications include dumbbell tumors or tumors clearly arising in the parotid gland involving the deep lobe of the parotid gland. Such tumors with limited involvement of the deep lobe can be attacked by a combined transcervical and transoral approach as describe by Kim et al. An absolute contraindication is tumor that is adherent or involving the carotid artery. Other contraindications include dumbbell tumors arising clearly from the parotid gland with significant involvement of the parotid gland (**Fig. 12.6**), vascular tumors such as paragangliomas, tumors with bony involvement of the skull base, and malignant tumors.

Surgical Instrumentation

Surgery is performed under general anaesthesia with antibiotic prophylaxis at induction using cephazolin and metronidazole. The patient is intubated with an endotracheal tube. The patient is positioned with the neck extended using a bolster under the shoulder and appropriately draped and the eyes protected. The oral endotracheal tube can be left in the midline groove of the tongue and kept in position using the grooved tongue blade of the Boyle-Davis mouth gag. It can also be sutured to the contralateral side with an interdental suture and to the contralateral retromolar trigone to hold the tongue away from the tumor. The Boyle-Davis mouth gag is suspended using Draffin rods. The lips are protected using clear plastic photographic cheek retractors (**Figs. 12.7** and **12.8**).

The robot is docked in the standard fashion as is used for any transoral procedure. Our preference is to dock the robot at about 15 degrees to the operating table at approximately the junction of the forward one-third and the lower two-thirds of the table. The 0- and 30-degree scopes and the bipolar fenestrated forceps and spatula diathermy are our preferred robotic instruments.

The instruments that are used for intraoral exposure are Boyle-Davis retractors or the Crowe-Davis retractors, as used in standard tonsillectomy surgery. The assistant at the bedside will require instruments that can provide blunt retraction so

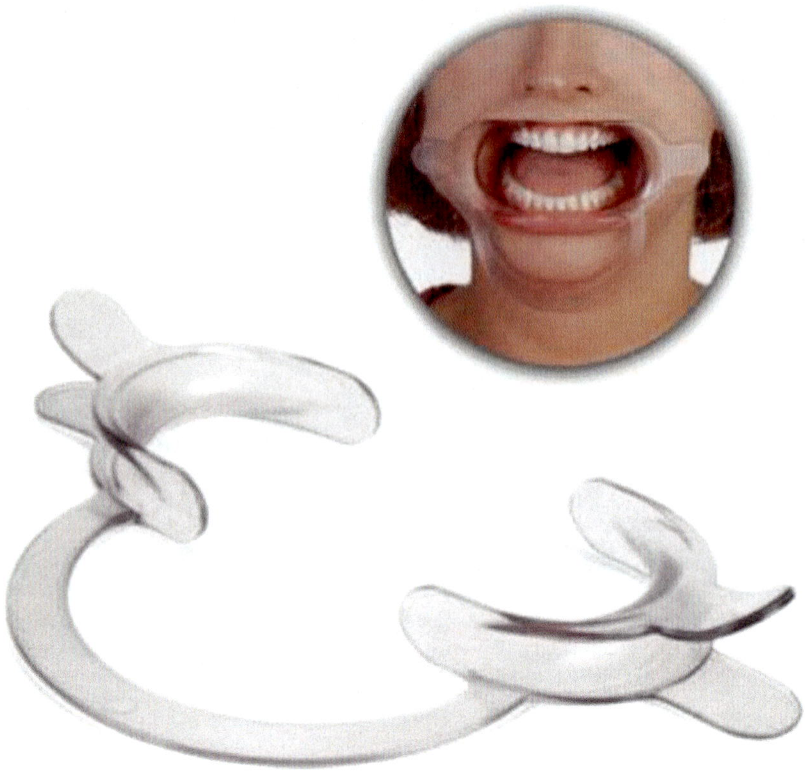

Fig. 12.7 Spandex cheek retractors to protect lips during transoral robotic surgery. (Courtesy of Almore International Inc., Beaverton, Oregon.)

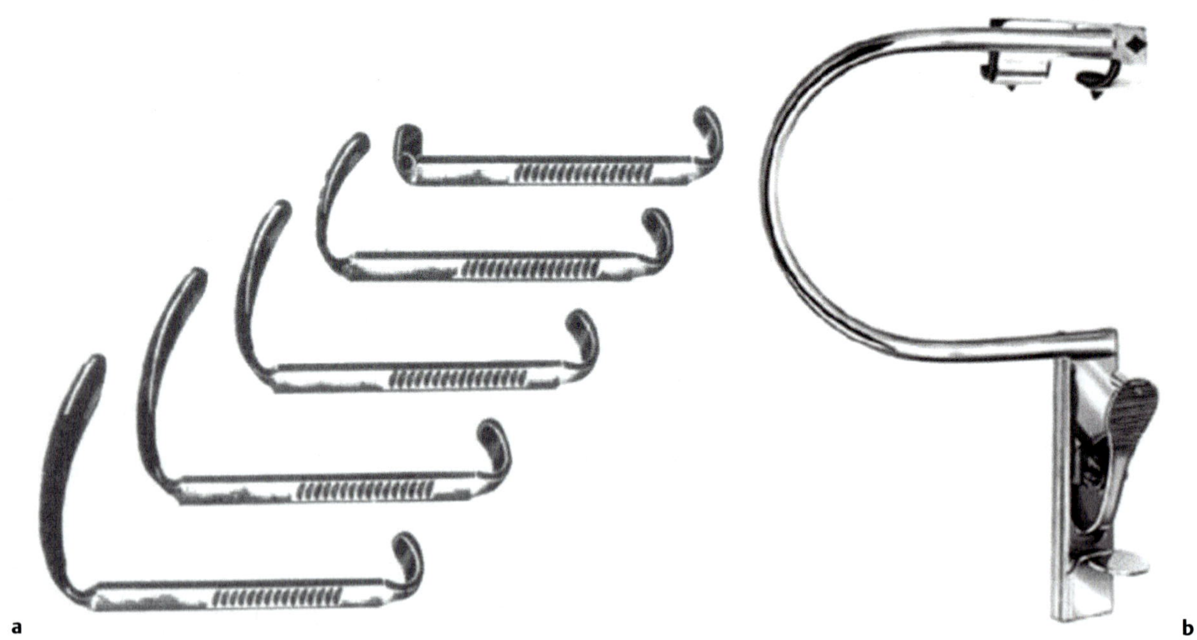

Fig. 12.8 (a,b) Crowe-Davis mouth gag.

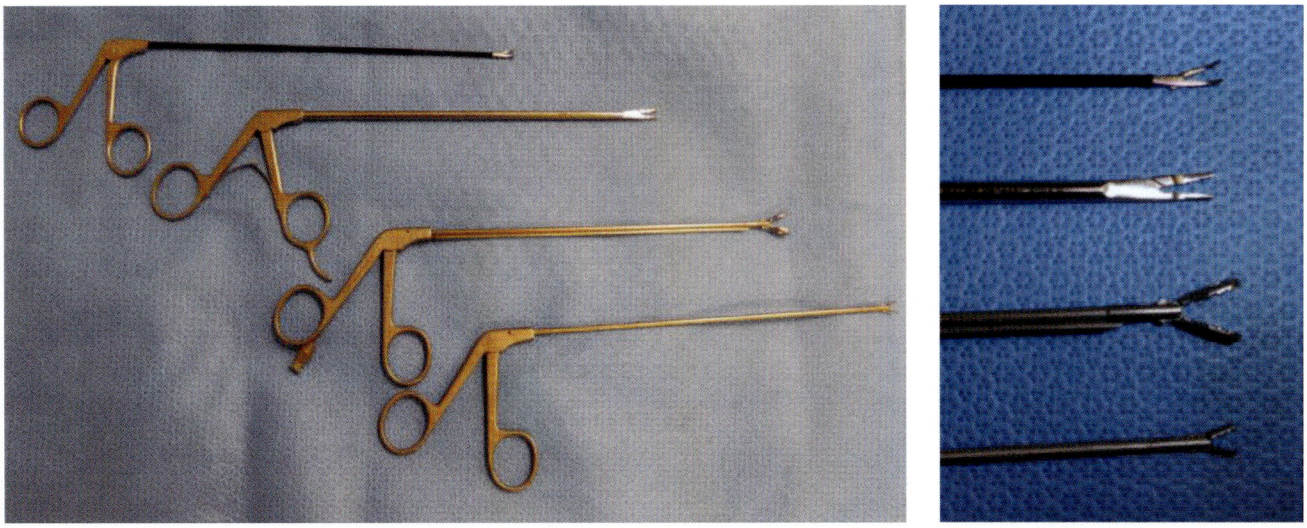

a b

Fig. 12.9 Microlaryngoscopy instruments (by Karl Storz GmbH, Tuttlingen, Germany) for use by assistant at bedside. **(a)** From above down, microlaryngoscopy insulated diathermy forceps, vascular clip applicator, large grasping forceps, and small grasping forceps. **(b)** Close-up of ends.

as not to traumatize the capsule of the tumor (**Figs. 12.9** and **12.10**). These could include malleable brain strips, dissecting peanut swabs mounted on a straight Negus clip, or the blunt end of a tonsil dissector. Two pediatric Yankauer suckers can also be used as a retractor and can provide suction to both evacuate any bleeding and provide the constant stream of warm air required to keep the telescope from fogging.

The assistant at the bedside is also provided with the Steiner LASER microlaryngoscopy range of instruments including the small and large toothed grasping forceps, the microlaryngoscopy forceps, the insulated diathermy forceps, and, essentially, the microlaryngoscopy vascular clip applicators.

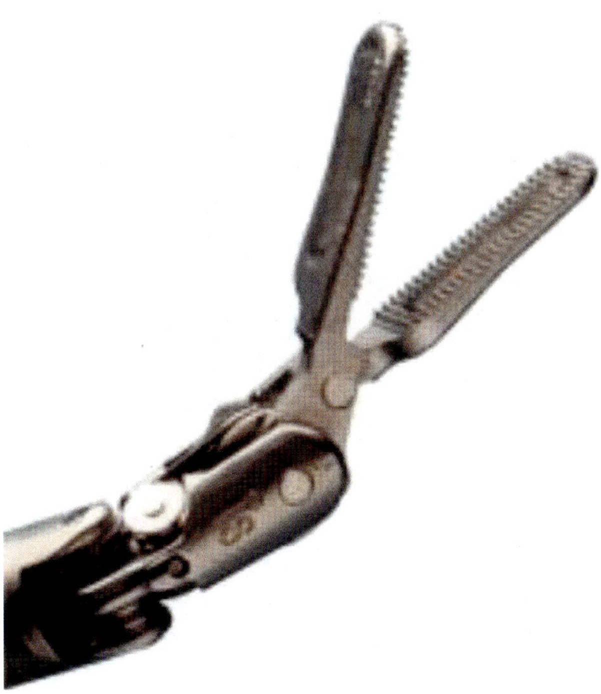

Fig. 12.10 Bipolar fenestrated EndoWrist (Intuitive Surgical, Inc.) robotic grasping forceps for gentle dissection, retraction, and hemostasis.

The Transoral Robotic Surgery Parapharyngeal Space Resection Step-by-Step

1. A straight incision is made over the crease in the oral mucosa made by the pterygomandibular raphe. Care is taken to make the incision superficial for large tumors and avoid cutting into the tumor (**Figs. 12.11** and **12.12**).
2. The pterygoid muscle is identified and palpated using the spatula of the robot diathermy instrument. It is used to bluntly dissect the constructor muscles medially and identify the tumor.
3. The superior aspect of the tumor is identified by extending the incision into the soft palate (**Fig. 12.13**). The incision is made close to the hamulus. The goal is to provide access to the superior aspect of the tumor and this can then be dissected by blunt dissection using the bipolar fenestrated diathermy forceps, which is flat. The usual Maryland forceps can be quite sharp and perforate the thin lining of the tumor, particularly the thin lining on cystic pleomorphic adenomas.
4. The thinned out constrictor and overlying pharyngeal mucosa is dissected from the medial surface of the tumor (**Fig. 12.14**).
5. This entire complex is gently displaced medially (using malleable brain strips, a peanut dissector, or the pediatric Yankauer sucker), exposing the tumor from its lateral wall. The medialized contents of the parapharyngeal space may expose rarely encountered arterial and venous branches, but if encountered, they can be clipped.
6. The bipolar fenestrated grasping forceps is used to pick up the medial edge of the medial pterygoid muscle, which can bulge medially. To separate the tumor from the muscle, the spatula tip cautery is used to transect the muscle. This has not been found to cause any long-term problems with trismus.

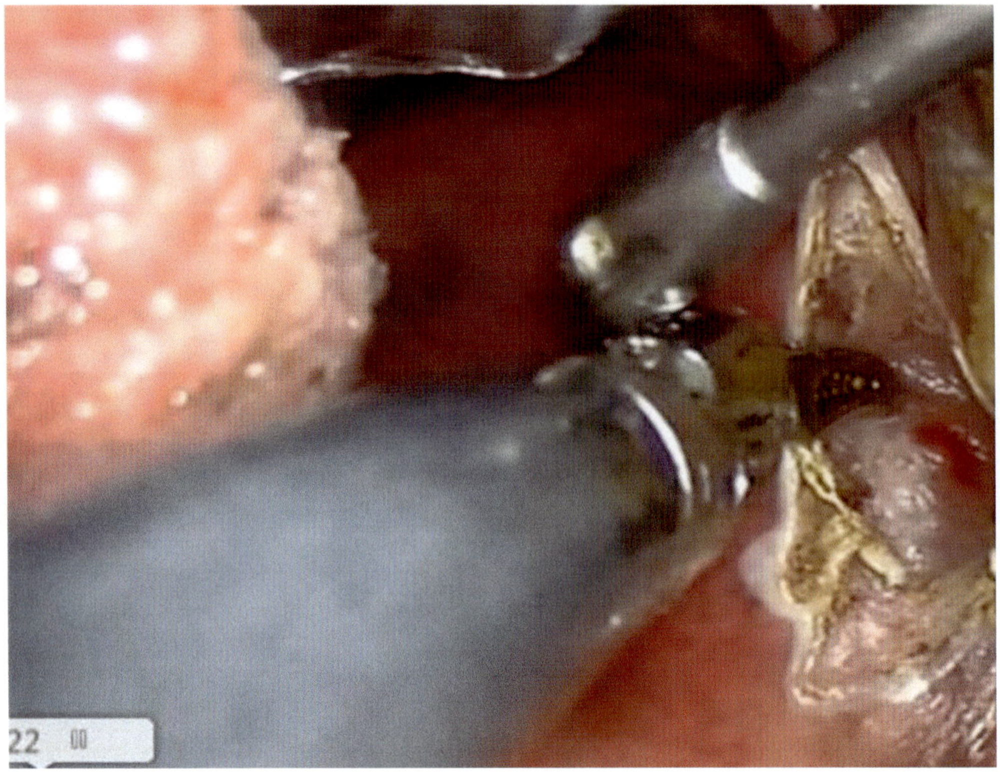

Fig. 12.11 Intraoral view of right parapharyngeal space pleomorphic adenoma. Top of picture is tongue base, tongue displaced to the right.

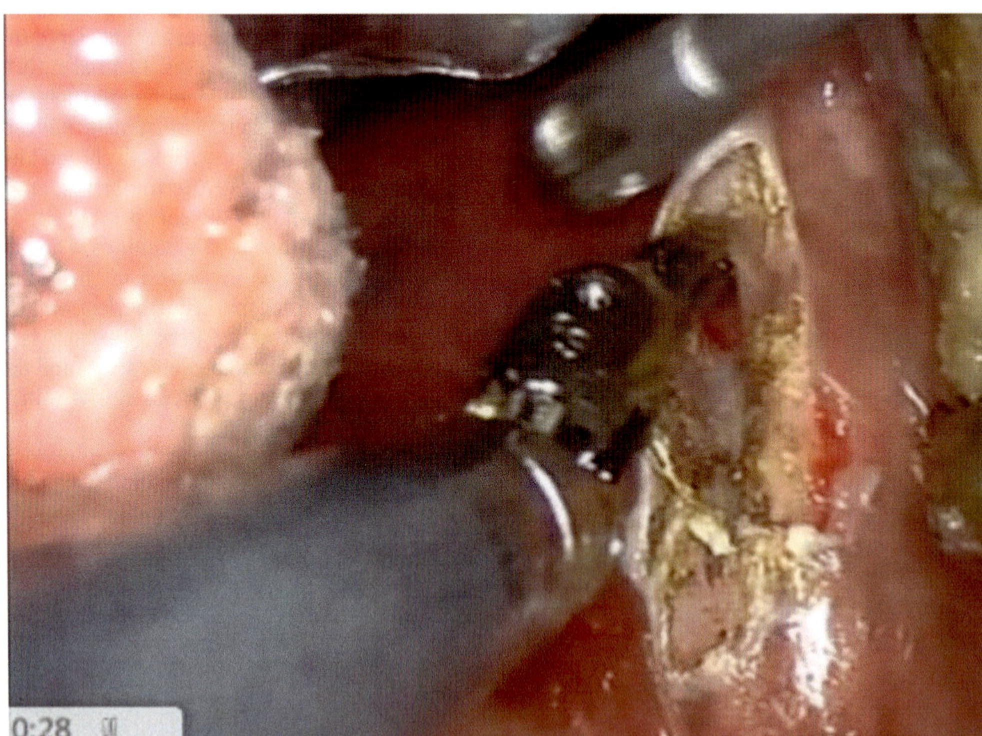

Fig. 12.12 Incision over pterygomandibular raphe.

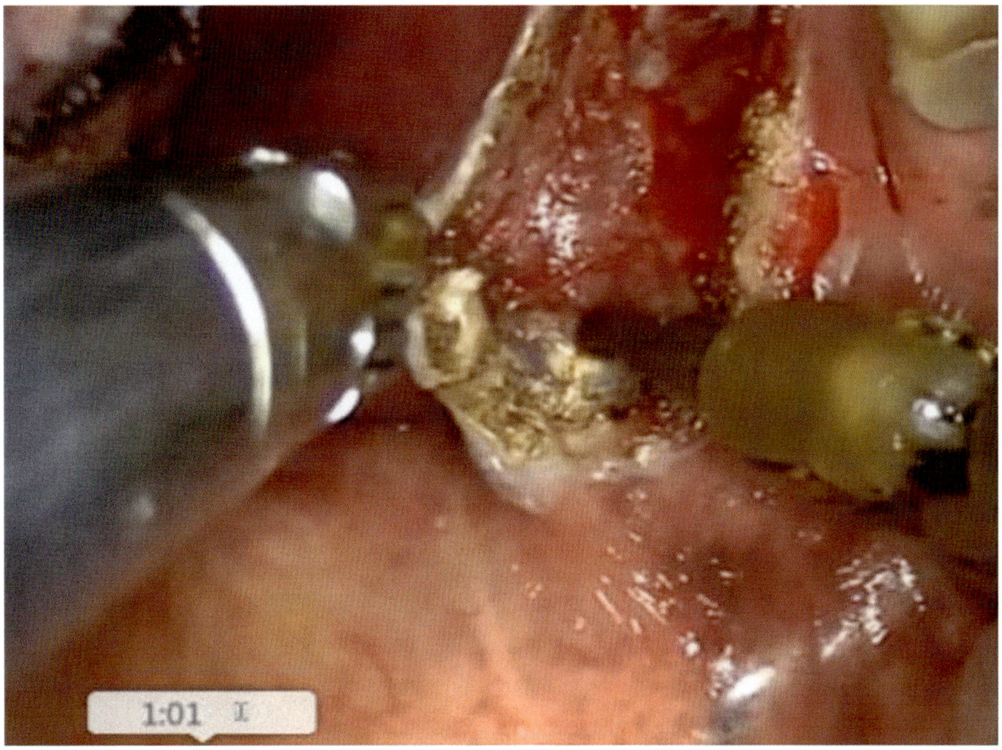

Fig. 12.13 Superior extension of incision into soft palate toward hamulus.

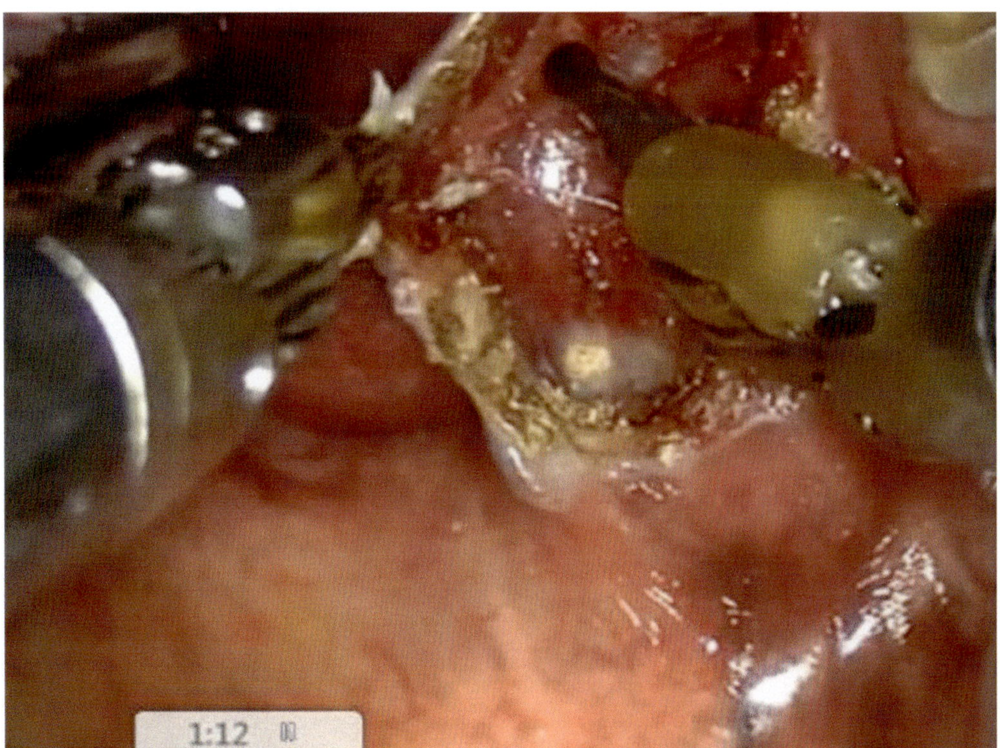

Fig. 12.14 Medial dissection lifting medial flap comprising pharyngeal mucosa and thinned out constrictor muscle.

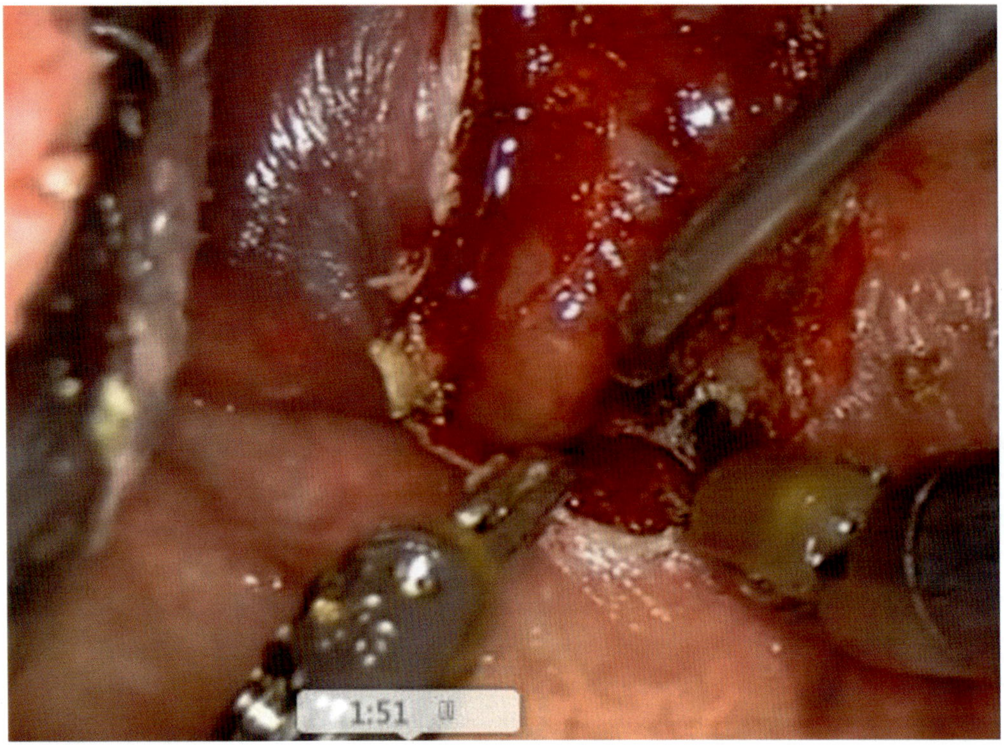

Fig. 12.15 Superior dissection peeling tumor from pterygoids using pediatric Yankauer sucker to gently retract tumor medially.

7. The blunt dissection of the posterior, superior, and lateral aspects of the tumor can be done very gently by using the bipolar fenestrated forceps (**Figs. 12.15** and **12.16**). The group from the University of Pennsylvania described the surgeon leaving the console, removing the robotic instruments and the mouth retractor, and using a finger to bluntly dissect the tumor. The blunt dissection is away from the tumor to avoid disrupting the capsule and sharp instrumentation is avoided lateral to the tumor to avoid tumor spillage laterally.

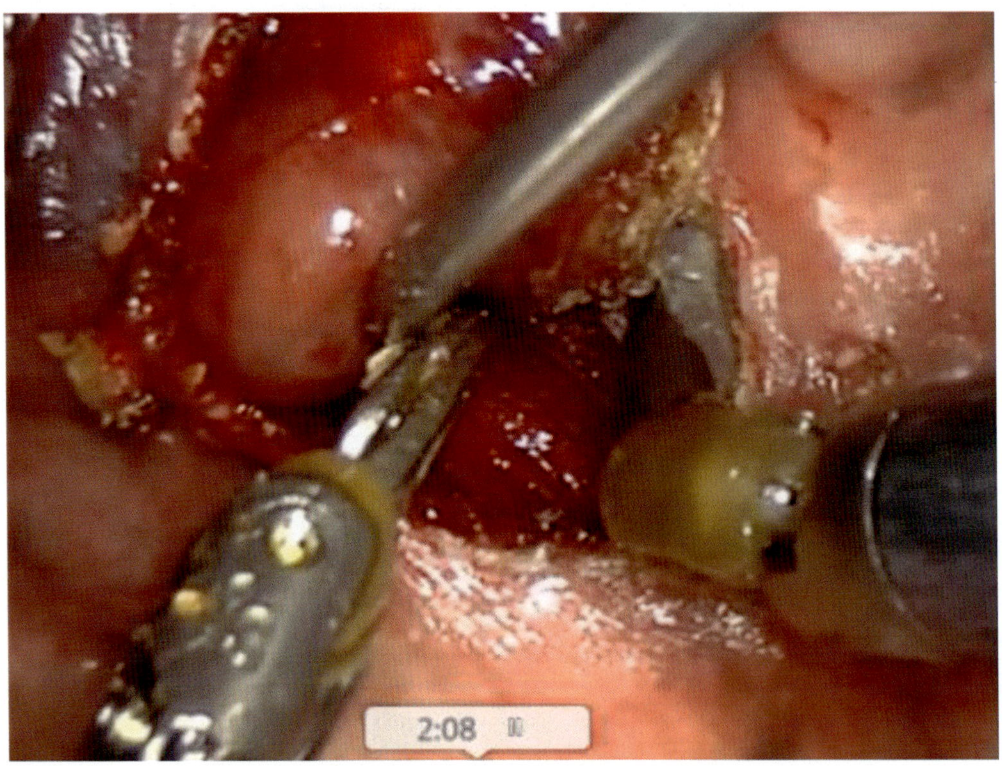

Fig. 12.16 Lateral dissection freeing tumor from palatoglossus and palatopharyngeus.

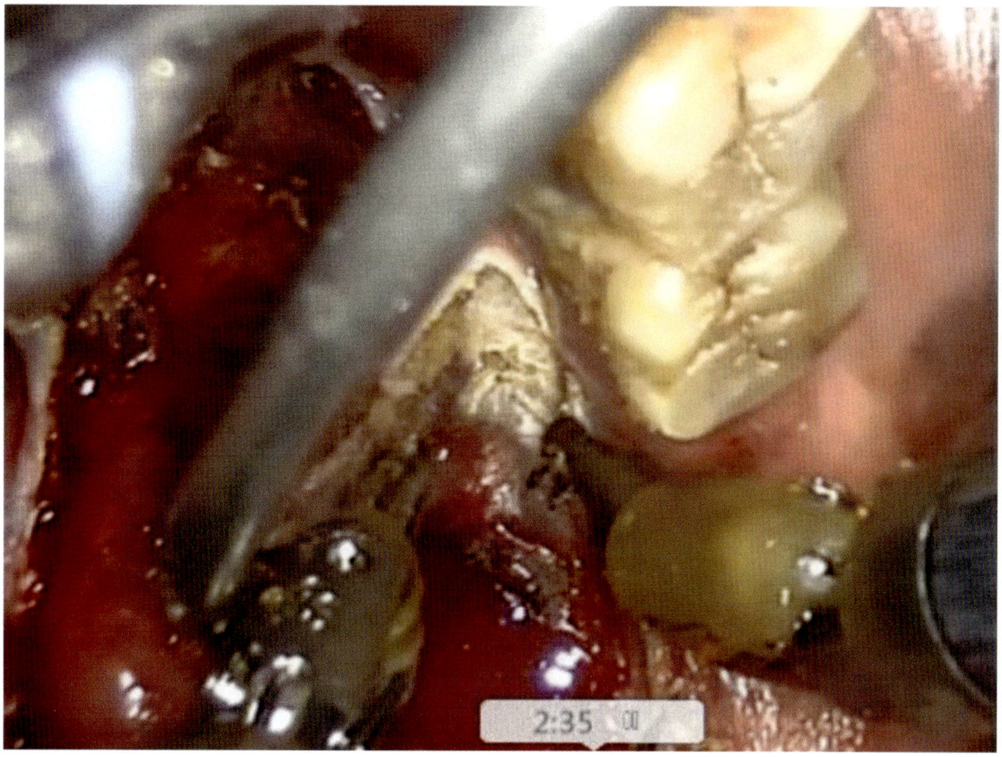

Fig. 12.17 Inferior dissection with extension of mucosal incision along anterior tonsillar pillar into floor of mouth.

To avoid tumor spillage and make dissection of the superior and lateral aspects easier, decompression of cystic lesions and controlled perforation and aspiration, microdebridement, or coblation of tumor contents has been described.

Another technique we have utilized is the infiltration of a 1:100,000 adrenaline in saline solution to "hydro-dissect" a plane of safety and to assist with dissection. We inject 30 mL in three 10-mL aliquots—each at the upper pole, lateral margin, and inferior pole of the tumor in a submucosal plane to hydro-dissect a surgical plane within the parapharyngeal space. This allows for easier dissection of the tumor and protects the capsule from rupture and tumor spillage.

8. The inferior dissection is performed by incising the mucosa of the anterior tonsillar pillar and extending this farther into the floor of the mouth than is usually done with TORS radical tonsillectomy (**Fig. 12.17**). The styloglossus muscle is usually displaced deep to the tumor and not encountered.
9. The mobilized tumor is gently peeled from its posterior, deep boundary (**Figs. 12.18** and **12.19**).
10. The tumor is removed, the wound is copiously irrigated with water, and bleeding is controlled with clips and bipolar cautery (**Fig. 12.20**).
11. The final step is assessment of the adequacy of resection by inspecting the tumor after removal to ensure that the shape matches the shape of the tumor on the scan and that the surface of the resected specimen is complete and intact (**Fig. 12.21**). Rents in the capsule are looked for and the tumor is oriented for the pathologist. The robot endoscope is introduced to inspect the cavity and all areas of the cavity are inspected using the 0- and 30-degree scopes to ensure that there is no residual tumor and that adequate hemostasis has been attained.
12. The mouth gag is relaxed, and if the soft tissues collapse and no visible cavity is present, our preference is to leave the wound open to drain and allow egress of blood and serous fluid out of the potential space. Others regularly close the wound with loose interrupted 3-0 Vicryl sutures and others have described using a drain.

■ Postoperative Care

All patients are managed in a high-dependency unit for airway observation and monitoring of potential oral bleeding that may embarrass the airway. Patients are usually extubated after surgery with no personal experience or reports of postoperative airway compromise and no patient requiring prolonged intubation or tracheostomy. Patients are kept nil by mouth overnight and allowed clear fluids on the first postoperative day, nourishing fluids on the second postoperative day, and a soft diet progressing to a normal diet from the third postoperative day. Subject to analgesic requirements patients are discharged on the second or third postoperative day.

■ Complications

The complications reported in surgery of the parapharyngeal space are related to vascular injury, lower cranial nerve injury, tumor spillage and recurrence, and first bite syndrome. Correct case selection and meticulous attention to preoperative imaging with respect to tumor relationship to vessels should prevent

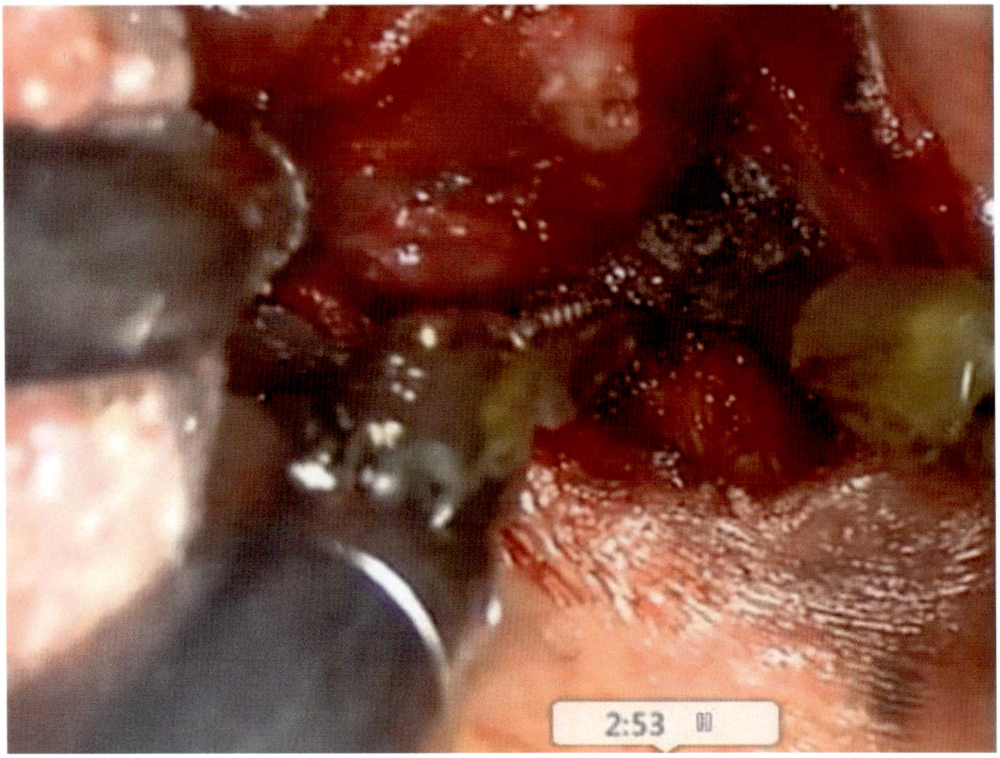

Fig. 12.18 Dissecting tumor from posterior and deep boundary.

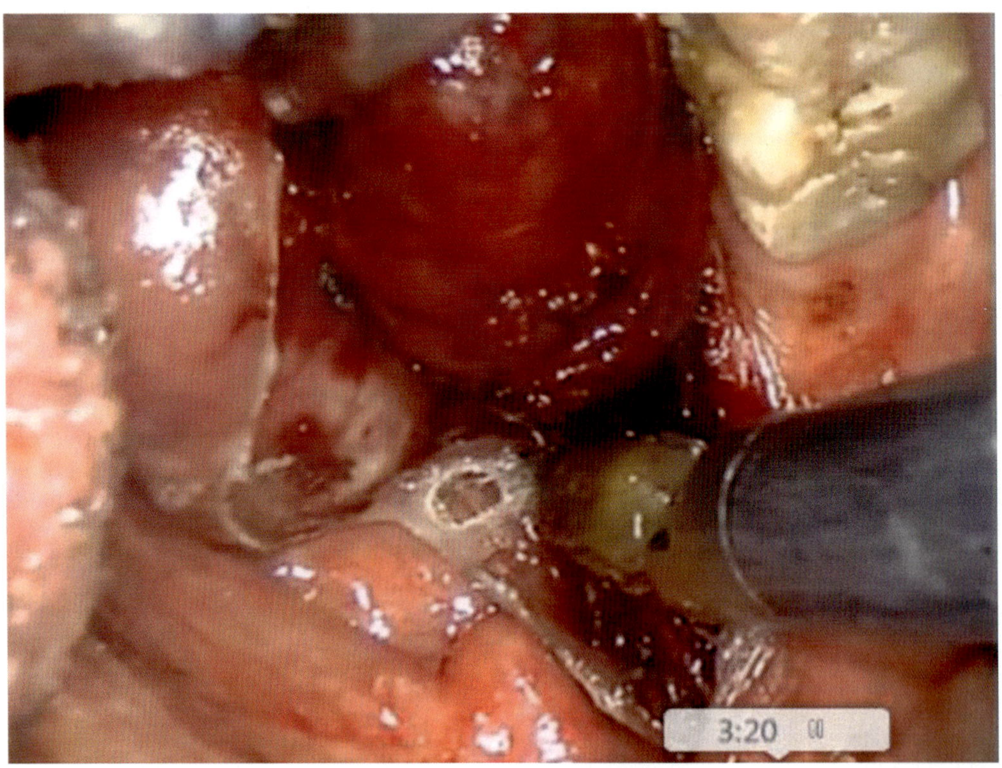

Fig. 12.19 Tumor mobilized.

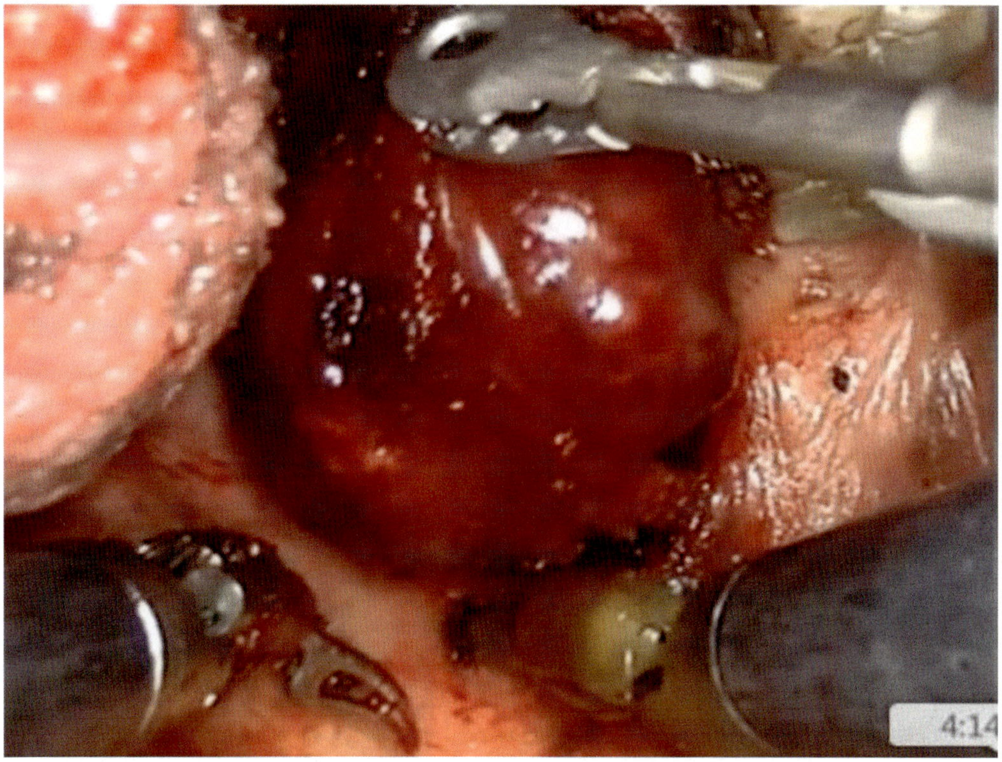

Fig. 12.20 Tumor being removed.

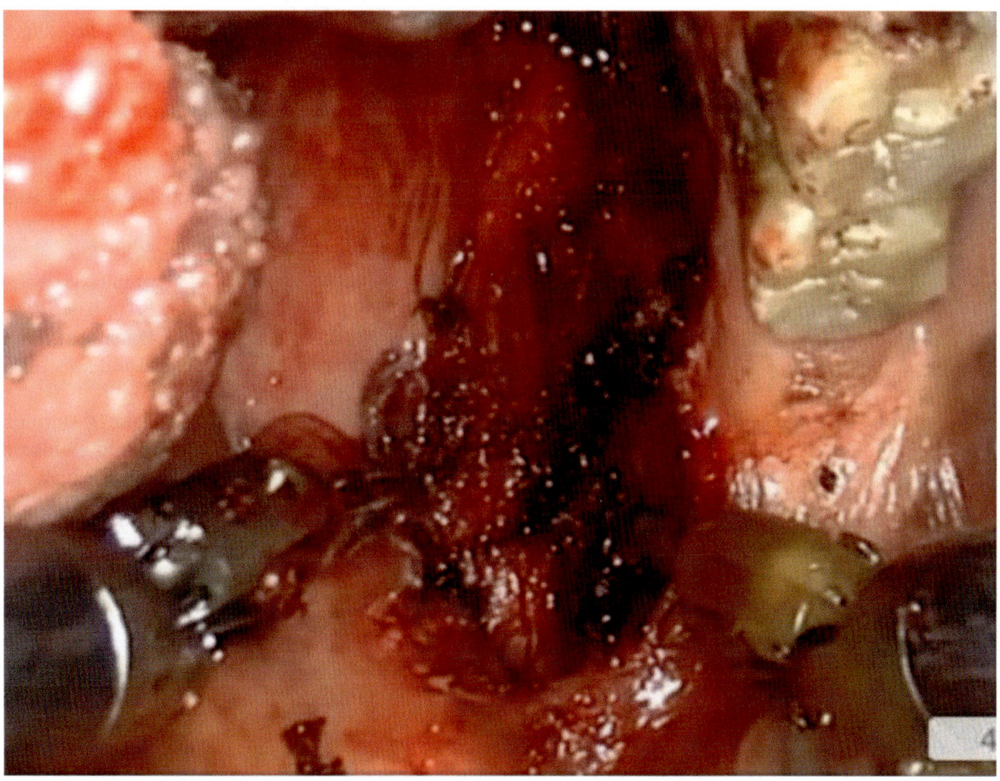

Fig. 12.21 Tumor bed being inspected; note how the potential space contracts after tumor removal.

risk of vascular injury in TORS for parapharyngeal space tumors. Similarly, because TORS avoids an external incision and avoids parotidectomy, there should be no risk to the facial nerve and its branches.

It is unclear if tumor spillage means definite recurrence. In the Mayo series reported by Hughes et al, tumor rupture was noted in 10 of the 68 cases, which is 15% of pleomorphic adenomas, but recurrence was only detected in 1 of those 10 ruptured cases.[10] In the Goodwin et al[14] and Ducic et al[15] reports, no tumor spillage was seen during transoral resection. Tumor spillage is not a common occurrence in carefully selected cases with thick capsules and no significant cystic components for TORS parapharyngeal space tumor resection and is no more common or worse than with transcervical blunt dissection. The important things are to avoid sharp dissection and to use blunt dissection particularly for the lateral, superior, and posterior aspects.

Bleeding can be avoided by meticulous hemostasis using hemoclips and the use of Tisseel or other tissue hemostatic agents.

Trismus may be present in the early postoperative period but is not a long-term complication, often resolving within 2 weeks of surgery.

The other complication reported in external approach surgery is first bite syndrome. As discussed by Chiu et al,[30] it has been postulated to be related to the loss of sympathetic supply to the parotid gland. This syndrome has not been seen in transoral resection and this is seen as a distinct advantage of transoral resection over external resection.

Future Directions and Conclusion

TORS for parapharyngeal space tumors is clearly advantageous for the true prestyloid benign salivary gland tumor, which is the most common tumor in this space. Its use in other tumors of this space is expanding with better understanding of tumor relationships to vital neurovascular structures through improved imaging. The advent of image guidance and real-time imaging may further enhance the cause of transoral surgery. Improvements in robotic instruments, particularly the imminent arrival of single port instruments, will improve access and precision of dissection. The introduction of haptic feedback may contribute to reducing the risk of capsular rupture and tumor spillage.

References

1. Olsen KD. Tumors of the parapharyngeal space. Laryngoscope 1994;104(5 Pt 2 Suppl 63):1–28
2. Bradley PJ, Bradley PT, Olsen KD. Update on the management of parapharyngeal tumors. Curr Opin Otolaryngol Head Neck Surg 2011;19(2):92–98
3. Riffat F, Dwivedi RC, Palme C, Fish B, Jani P. A systematic review of 1143 parapharyngeal space tumors reported over 20 years. Oral Oncol 2014;50(5):421–430
4. Eisele DW, Richmon JD. Contemporary evaluation and management of parapharyngeal space neoplasms. J Laryngol Otol 2013,127:550–555
5. Gupta A, Chazen L, Phillips D. Imaging evaluation of the parapharyngeal space. Otolaryngol Clin N Am 2012;45: 1223–1232
6 Wang C, Kandaria S, Fernandez-Miranda J, Duvvuri U. A description of arterial variants in the transoral approach to the parapharyngeal space. Clin Anat 2014;27(7):1016–1022
7. Arnason T, Hart R, Taylor SM, Trites JR, Nasser J, Bullock M. Diagnostic accuracy and safety of fine-needle aspiration biopsy of the parapharyngeal space. Diagn Cytopathol 2012;40(2): 118–123
8. Malone JP, Agrawl A, Schuller D. Safety and efficacy of transcervical resection of parapharyngeal space neoplasms. Ann Otol Rhinol Laryngol 2001;110(12):1093–1098
9. Hughes KV, Olsen KD, Maccaffrey TV. Parapharyngeal space neoplasms. Head Neck 1995;17(2):124–130
10. Carrau RL, Myers EN, Johnson JT. Management of tumors arising in the parapharyngeal space. Laryngoscope 1995;100: 583–589
11. Myatt HM, Remedios D. A transpalatal approach to the parapharyngeal space. J Laryngol Otol 1997;111:159–162
12. Goodwin WJ, Chandler JR Transoral excision of lateral parapharyngeal space tumors presenting intraorally. Laryngoscope 1988;98(3):266–269
13. Ducic Y, Oxford L, Pontius AT. Transoral approach to the superomedial parapharyngeal space. Otolaryngol Head Neck Surg 2006;134(3):466–470
14. Iseri M, Ozturk M, Kara A, Ucar S, Aydin O, Keskin G. Endoscope-assisted transoral approach to parapharyngeal space tumors. Head Neck Surg 2013;134(3):466–470
15. Varoquax A, Fakhry N, Gabriel S, et al. Retrostyloid parapharyngeal space tumors: a clinician and imaging perspective. Eur J Radiol 2013;82(5):773–782
16. Cassoni A, Terenzi V, Della Monaca M, et al. Parapharyngeal space benign tumors: our experience. J Craniomaxillofac Surg 2014;42(2):101–105
17. O'Malley Jr B, Weinstein GS. Robotic skull base surgery, preclinical investigations to human clinical application. Arch Otolaryngol Head Neck Surg 2007;133(12):1215–1219
18. O'Malley Jr B, Quon H, Leonhardt F, Chalian A, Weinstein G. Transoral robotic surgery for parapharyngeal space tumors. ORL J Otorhinolaryngol Relat Spec 2010;72(6):332–336
19. Rinaldi V, Pagani D, Torretta S, Pignataro L. Transoral robotic surgery in the management of head and neck tumors. Ecancermedicalscience 2013;7:359
20. Carrau RL, Prevedello DM, DeLara D, Durmus K, Ozer E. Combined transoral robotic surgery and endoscopic endonasal approach for the resection of extensive malignancies of the skull base. Head 2013;35(11):E351–358
21. Park YM, De Virgilio A, Kim WS, Chung HP, Kim S. Parapharyngeal space surgery via a transoral approach using robotic surgical system: transoral robotic surgery. J Laparoendos Adv Surg Tech A 2013;23(3):231–236
22. Arshad H, Durmus K, Oser E. Transoral robotic resection of selected parapharyngeal space tumors. Eur Arch Otorhinolaryngol 2013;270(5):1737–1740
23. Van Abel K, Moore EJ. The rise of transoral robotic surgery in the head and neck: emerging applications. Expert Rev Anticancer Ther 2012;12(3):373–380
24. Lee HS, Kim J, Lee HJ, Koh YW, Choi EC. Transoral robotic surgery for neurogenic tumors of the prestyloid pharyngeal space. Auris Nasus Larynx 2012;39(4):434–437

25. Tsang R, Mohr C. Lateral palatal flap approach to the nasopharynx and parapharyngeal space for transoral robotic surgery: a cadaveric study. J Robotic Surg 2013;7(2):119–123
26. Van Rompaey J, Suruliraj A, Carrau R, Panizza B, Solares A. Access to the parapharyngeal space: an anatomical study comparing the endoscopic and open approaches. Laryngoscope 2013;123(10):2378–2382
27. Beswick D, Vaezi A, Caicedo-Granados E, Duvvuri U. Minimally invasive surgery for parapharyngeal space tumor. Laryngoscope 2012;122(5):1072–1078
28. Betka J, Chovanec M, Klozar J, Taudy M, Plzak J, Kodetova D, Lisy J. Transoral and combined transoral-transcervical approach in the surgery of parapharyngeal tumors. Eur Arch Otorhinolaryngol 2010;267(5):765–772
29. Chan JYK, Tsang RK, Eisele DW, Richmon JD. Transoral robotic surgery of the parapharyngeal space: a case series and systematic review. Head and Neck 2015;37(2):293–298
30. Chiu AG, Cohen JI, Burningham AR, et al. First bite syndrome: a complication of surgery involving the parapharyngeal space. Head Neck 2002;24:996–999

13 Transaxillary Robotic Thyroidectomy

Jandee Lee and Woong Youn Chung

■ Introduction

In 2007, a century after Emil Theodor Kocher received the Nobel Prize in Medicine for his work on the thyroid gland, Dr. Chung's group in South Korea successfully performed the first robotic thyroidectomy using a gasless transaxillary approach.[1] The shift toward robotic thyroid surgery has reshaped the surgical approach for thyroid tumors in Asia and in Western countries. Its impact on South Korea, especially, has been remarkable and rapidly widespread.[2,3,4] With the promise of improved ergonomics and a shortened learning curve for the new robotic thyroid surgery technique, the field of head and neck surgery witnessed the revolution of the surgical management of thyroid cancer beyond conventional transaxillary endoscopic thyroid surgery.[5,6]

Remote access endoscopic surgery of the thyroid gland without neck scar has been reported to be a safe procedure resulting in excellent cosmetic satisfaction with postoperative scars.[7,8] Despite these benefits, transaxillary endoscopic thyroid procedures are difficult as they are performed in a deep and narrow neck space. Endoscopic instruments also have limitations, including two-dimensional visualization, reduced range of motion, and impaired eye–hand coordination. Robotic thyroid surgery can overcome limitations encountered with conventional transaxillary endoscopic techniques. The robotic system has reduced physiologic tremors of surgeons, enabling free dexterity of movement using articulated instruments, as well as enabling surgeons to control a three-dimensional (3D) camera.

A large number of studies describing surgery in selected low-risk thyroid cancer patients yielded good results, with low complication and conversion rates, and shorter hospital stay when compared with conventional open thyroidectomy.[9,10,11] As long-term survival data are limited, short-term measures of oncologic efficacy, including radioactive iodine-131 scan results, serum thyroglobulin (Tg) concentration after stimulation with thyroid-stimulating hormone (TSH), and the number of harvested cervical lymph nodes (LNs), have been used as indicators of surgical completeness and oncologic radicality. These measures confirmed the short-term oncologic efficacy and safety of robotic thyroidectomy and neck dissection.[2,3,4,5,12,13,14,15,16,17,18]

More recently, studies of robotic thyroidectomy have assessed quality-of-life (QoL) outcomes, since defining and improving QoL outcomes are necessary in assessing the efficacy of this procedure.[2,3,4,17,18,19,20,21,22,23,24,25,26,27,28,29,30,31] Patient satisfaction after neck surgery is highly associated with QoL outcomes such as cosmetic satisfaction, with poorer results causing significant long-term psychological distress. Recent prospective trials have found that patients undergoing open surgery have higher levels of dissatisfaction, especially with cosmetic outcomes, than do patients undergoing robotic surgery. Moreover, these studies showed that, compared with conventional open surgery, robotic thyroid surgery yielded favorable outcomes on functional assessments, including pain, neck stiffness, discomfort, sensory changes, voice changes, and swallowing difficulty.

This chapter provides an overview of robotic thyroid surgery and describes the latest advances in robotic thyroidectomy and radical neck dissection techniques. It also reviews three aspects of surgical outcomes after robotic thyroidectomy and radical neck dissection: (1) oncologic efficacy and safety; (2) patients' quality of life; and (3) surgeon's benefit.

■ Description of the Robotic System and Applied Anatomy

Robotic surgery has the potential to transform endoscopic surgery by providing, for the first time, instruments with distal ends that mimic the intricate movements of the human hand while at the same time providing the surgeon with a high-resolution, 3D view of the operative field. The surgeon sits at a console and manipulates master instruments on the console.[32] The console provides a magnified high-resolution, 3D binocular magnification of the operating field. The robot instruments offer 7 degrees of freedom, with high-precision movements that can be motion scaled to the surgeon's movements, and also have tremor-filtering systems.

Preparation for Robotic Thyroid Surgery

Patient evaluation consists of a physical examination and imaging modalities, including high-resolution ultrasonography (US) and neck computed tomography (CT). Preoperative diagnosis of thyroid nodules is based on the results of US-guided fine needle aspiration cytology (FNAC). Tumor characteristics assessed include size, location, presence of extrathyroid invasion, multiplicity, bilaterality, and presence of cervical lymph node metastasis. The inclusion and exclusion criteria for robotic thyroidectomy with or without radical neck dissection are described in **Table 13.1**.

The extent of thyroidectomy and radical neck dissection is based on revised American Thyroid Association (ATA)

Table 13.1 Indications and contraindications for robotic thyroidectomy with or without radical neck dissection

Indications	a) Benign thyroid nodule without substernal extension. b) Differentiated thyroid cancer without the following contraindications. * No absolute cut-off values in thyroid gland or thyroid nodule size or patient's body mass index
Contraindications	a) A history of previous head and neck surgery or irradiation. b) Uncontrolled thyrotoxicosis. c) Unrelated pathologic conditions of the neck or shoulder. d) Lesions located in the dorsal thyroid area, especially in the region adjacent to the tracheoesophageal groove (because of possible injury during surgery to the trachea, esophagus, or recurrent laryngeal nerve). e) Suspicious perinodal infiltration to adjacent structures such as the internal jugular vein or major nerves at lateral metastatic lymph nodes. f) Distant metastasis.

guidelines.[33] All patients with thyroid cancer undergo prophylactic central compartment neck dissection (CCND). Patients with lateral neck lymph nodes that are clinically palpable or appear suspicious on preoperative staging US and are assessed by FNAC also undergo total thyroidectomy with modified radical neck dissection (MRND). The preoperative presence of lateral lymph node metastasis is based on Tg concentrations in US-guided FNAC wash out fluid. In patients with N1b tumors, we follow the prescribed extent of MRND for PTC (levels IIA, III, IV, and Vb), whereas lymph nodes at levels IIB and VA are not routinely dissected. However, if palpation or preoperative imaging shows evidence of an enlarged or suspicious lymph node at level I, IIB, or VA, these compartments are included in en bloc dissection.[2,3,4]

Surgical Anatomy for Robotic Thyroid Surgery

In adapting a new surgical technique to the neck area, surgeons should familiarize themselves with the accurate neck anatomy and adjacent regional lymph node compartments. The biology of lymph node metastases is important in defining the extent of surgery, by correlating surgical and radiological landmarks. Because robotic surgery requires a lateral approach to the thyroid gland, complete understanding of neck anatomy is required to avoid injury to critical neck structures.

Our approach for remote access robotic thyroid surgery uses an incision in the axillary fold and proceeds to the neck via a dissection along the fascia of the pectoralis muscle. A directly visualized working space is created in the plane between the subcutaneous tissue and the pectoralis major muscle. The robotic working space consists of outer and inner spaces, and sufficient dissection is essential to maintain a proper working space. The ceiling of the outer space is formed by the subcutaneous and subplatysmal skin flaps, and its bottom by the clavicle, pectoralis major muscle, and soft tissues of the lateral neck. The borders of the inner working space consist of the sternal head of the sternocleidomastoid (SCM) and strap muscles, and the bottom by major vessels and the clavicular head of the SCM muscles (**Fig. 13.1**).[34]

■ Surgical Procedure

Patient Positioning

The patient is given general anesthesia and placed in the supine position, with mild extension of the neck with a small shoulder roll. The lesion-side arm is extended and raised to the target thyroid lobe superiorly (**Fig. 13.2a**).[1,9,10] A 5- to 6-cm vertical incision is marked in the anterior axillary fold along the lateral border of the pectoralis major muscle. It is recommend that the position of the skin incision be marked in the preoperative holding area with the patient sitting and with arms relaxed in a natural position to ensure adequate concealment of the incision. The arm also could then be secured in place with meticulous care to protect all pressure points and avoid undue stretching on the shoulder, elbow, or wrist joints.

Surgical Pearl: While positioning the patient, the arm on the lesion side should be raised superiorly but naturally within the range of shoulder motion to avoid brachial plexus injuries.[2,3,4,9] A modified patient position was developed in the United States especially for patients with a large body habitus. In this position, the lesion-side arm is extended to expose the patient's axillary area at the shoulder, the elbow is flexed to an angle of approximately 90 degrees, and the arm is padded and fixed to an arm board overlying the forehead (**Fig. 13.2b**).[10]

Surgical Pearl: Usually, the position of the skin incision has been marked in the preoperative holding area with the patient sitting with arms relaxed in a natural position to ensure adequate concealment of the incision.

A working space is generated under direct vision in the plane between the subcutaneous tissue of anterior chest and the pectoralis major muscle. The skin and subcutaneous fat are elevated medially to provide access to the midline from the thyroid notch to the sternal notch. A subplatysmal skin flap is made beyond the clavicle, until the bifurcation of the SCM muscles, between the sternal head and clavicular head, is exposed. After exposing the SCM, the dissection is approached through the avascular space of the two heads of the SCM muscles. Dissection is performed deep into the sternal head to expose and dissect the strap muscles off the thyroid gland.

Elevating the anterior portion of the SCM and underlying strap muscles from the carotid sheath structures and thyroid gland

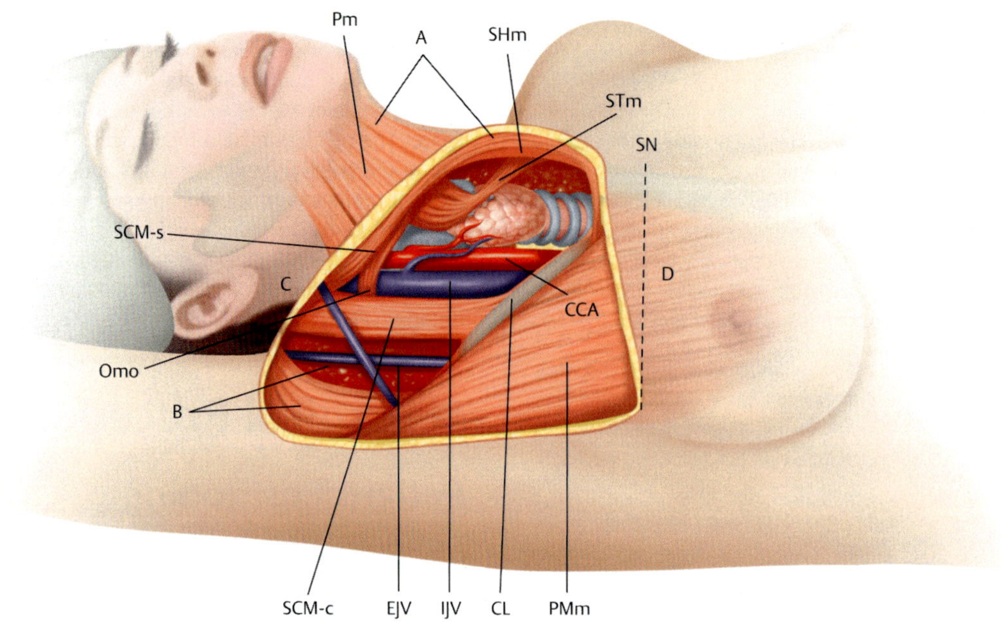

Fig. 13.1 An operation working space after the flap dissection and the external retractor setting. The outer space—(1) Ceiling: subcutaneous and subplatysmal skin flap (A). (2) Bottom: clavicle (CL), pectoralis major muscle (PMm), and soft tissues of the lateral neck (B) including the external jugular vein (EJV) and the anterior border of the trapezius muscle (Tm). (3) Superior border: subplatysmal skin flap of neck level V area (C). (4) Inferior border: sternal notch (SN) and an imaginary line from the sternal notch to the lower border of the axillary incision (D). The inner space—(1) Apex: sternal head of the SCM (SCM-s) and strap muscles (sternohyoid muscle [SHm], and sternothyroid [STm] muscle). (2) Bottom: common carotid artery (CCA), internal jugular vein (IJV), and clavicular head of the SCM muscles (SCM-c). (3) Superior border: omohyoid muscle (Omo) and the junction of the two SCM muscle branches. (4) Inferior border: strap muscles (STm, SHm) attached to the sternum.

provides access to the central compartment. Elevating the skin and subcutaneous fat over the pectoralis muscle, clavicle, and SCM muscle, as well as separating the anterior SCM muscle from the strap muscles to create a working space, requires the use of retractors and electrocautery devices of various lengths. After the omohyoid muscle is retracted superficially and posterolaterally, the strap muscles are elevated until the medial one-third portion of the contralateral lobe of the thyroid is exposed. To maintain a working space, an external retractor (Chung's retractor or comparable product) is placed under the strap muscles and elevated to expose the working field. The retractor is connected to continuous suction to achieve clear operating space.

> **Surgical Pearl**: After creating a working space, the incision entrance should be maintained to provide a height > 4 cm and the retractor blade should be > 1 cm from the anterior surface of the thyroid gland (**Fig. 13.3**). Particularly in obese patients, sufficient dissection is required to create a working space. Obese patients tend to have shorter and thicker necks, and the working space may easily collapse due to the excessive weight and tension from the patient's thick subcutaneous flap. Thus, robotic thyroid surgery requires considerably more time and effort in obese than in nonobese patients.[34]

Robot Docking Procedure

The da Vinci cart that carries the robotic arms is positioned on the side opposite the incision. After creation of working space, the patient cart should always be angled slightly contralateral to the location of the thyroid lesion, aligning the center column of the cart with the line of the retractor (approximately 60 to 85 degrees to the table). The camera arm is positioned with its setup joint toward the patient's head to ensure maximum clearance for the instrument arm. The camera arm should be positioned in the middle of the incision of the patient's axilla, such that the camera arm is in line with the camera cannula and center column of the patient cart. This "sweet spot" should be confirmed to maximize the range of motion for the instrument arms prior to docking. We align the blue arrow within the blue marker on the second joint or make a ~90-degree angle between the first and third joints on the camera arm. We also align the clutch button, the third joint of the camera arm, and the gray dot in da Vinci on the center column in a straight line. Once the camera arm is located correctly within its "sweet spot," the patient cart wheel is locked, the arms of the cart are extended over the patient, and the cannulas are placed within the incision site with the remote centers located just inside the skin edge.

A novel method of robotic thyroidectomy via a gasless transaxillary approach utilizes two skin incisions and uses three robotic arms (ProGrasp forceps, Maryland dissector, and Harmonic curved shears) and a single camera (Intuitive Surgical 30-degree endoscope); an axillary incision allows access of the camera and first and second robot arms and an anterior chest incision for the third robotic arm. In two-incision robotic thyroidectomy, the second skin incision, 0.6 to 0.8 cm long, is made on the medial side of the anterior chest wall to insert the third robot arm, 2 cm superiorly and 6 to 8 cm medially from the nipple. A ProGrasp forceps is inserted through this anterior chest wall incision (**Fig. 13.4a**).[1,14]

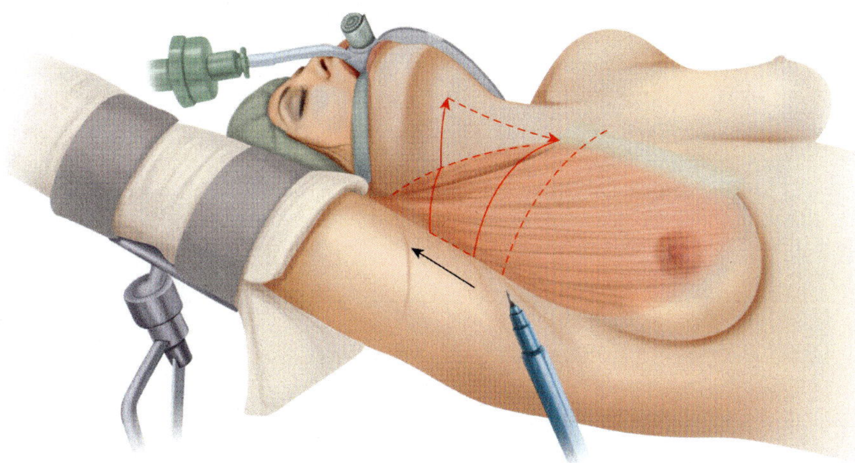

a

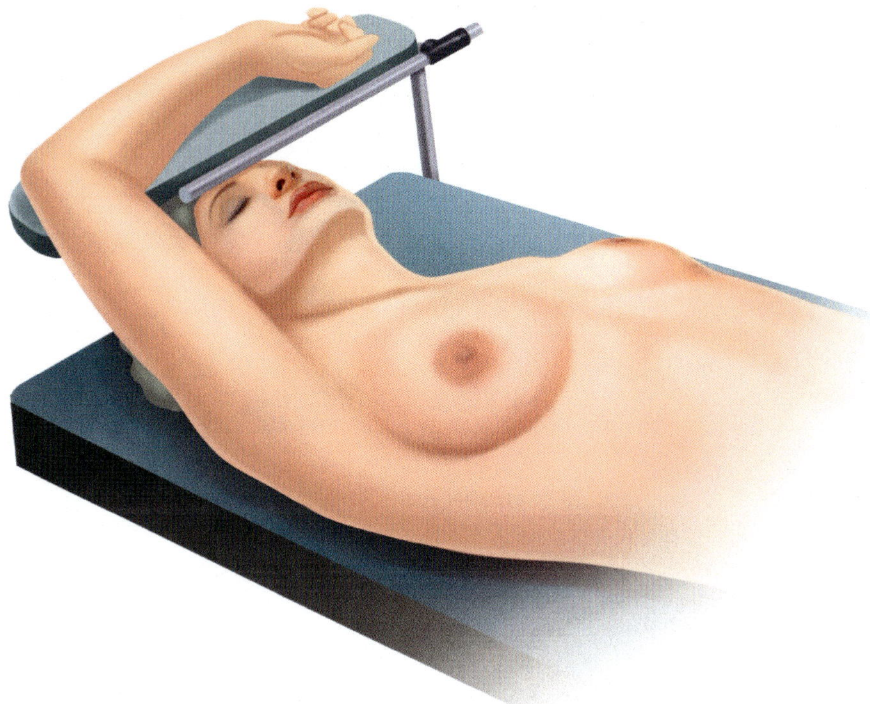

b

Fig. 13.2 Patient position during robotic thyroidectomy. **(a)** Standard patient position and skin incision line. The incision is made along the axillary skin crease on the lateral border of the pectoralis major muscle. This position is intended to expose the axillary fossa and to minimize the distance between the axilla and the anterior neck. **(b)** Modified arm position. The lesion-side arm was extended to expose the axillary area at the shoulder and flexed at the elbow at an approximately 90-degree angle to avoid brachial plexus injury.

After modification of this original docking method, we developed an advanced single-incision docking procedure, successfully.[35] In single-incision approach, four robotic arms are inserted through a single axillary incision. To make a conduit for robotic thyroidectomy via a single axillary incision, a dual-channel telescope is inserted in an upward direction and centered at the bottom of the incision (the external third joint should be placed in the lowest part, that is floor, of the incision entrance and the camera tip should be directed upward). Before the 8-mm cannula is positioned in the incision, the ProGrasp forceps is attached to the robot arm and the instrument should be fully inserted through the cannula. The tip of the ProGrasp forceps should then be positioned to the lesion side of the camera, beneath the anterior part of the skin incision parallel to the retractor blade. The 5-mm cannula for the Harmonic curved shears should be positioned at the edge of the incision (lesion side of the camera), and the 5-mm cannula of the Maryland dissector should be positioned on the opposite edge of the incision (opposite side of camera). Therefore, all three instruments and the camera are inserted through the axillary incision (**Fig. 13.4b**).[35]

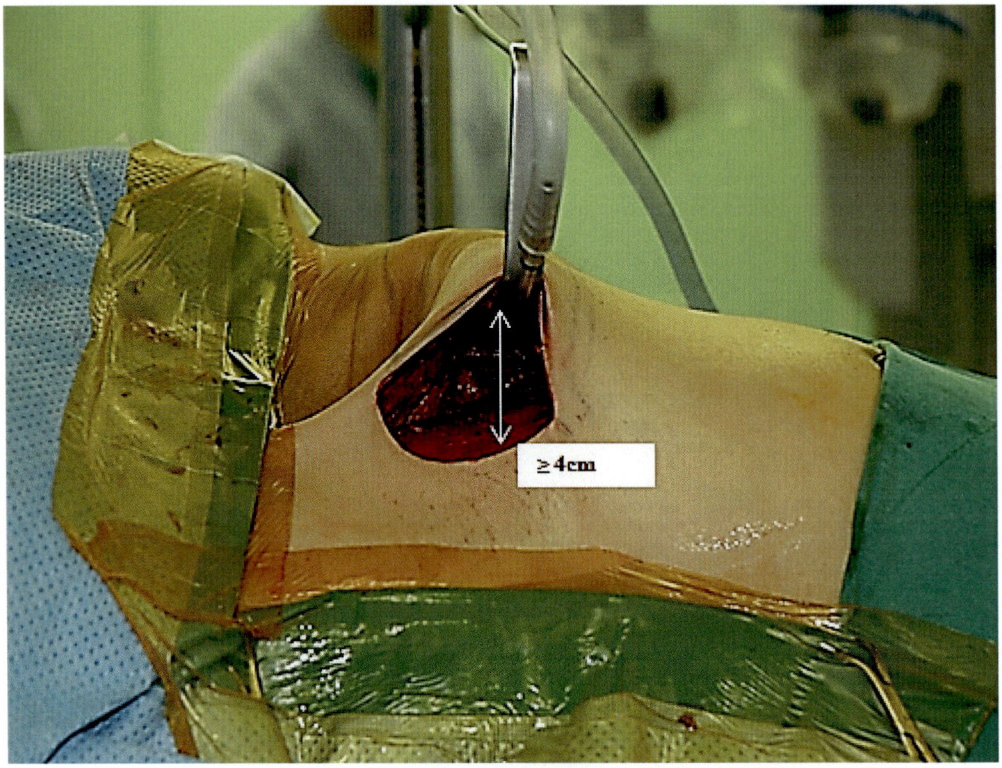

a

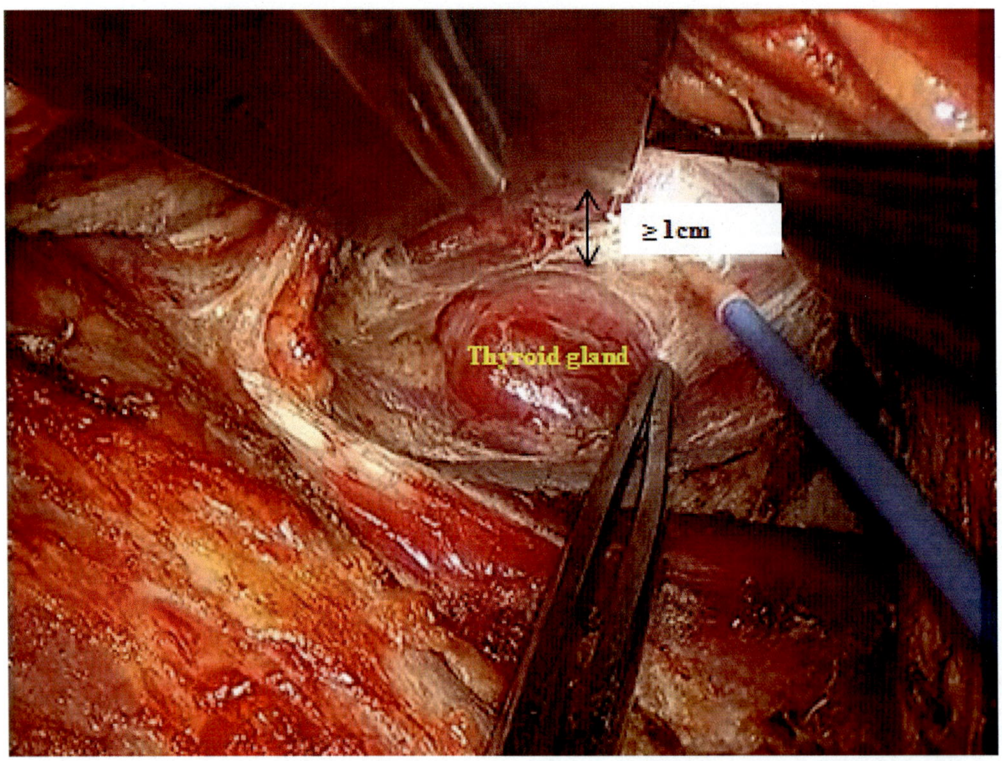

b

Fig. 13.3 To achieve an adequate working space after retractor blade positioning, **(a)** the axillary incision entrance should be maintained to provide a height of at least 4 cm, and **(b)** the retractor blade should be > 1 cm from the anterior surface of the thyroid gland to provide enough space for movement of the robotic instrument.

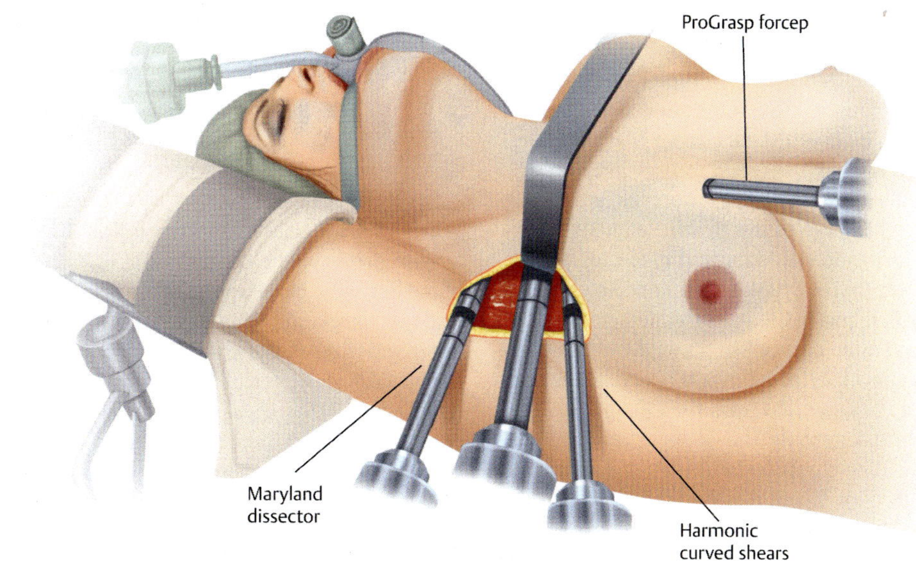

a

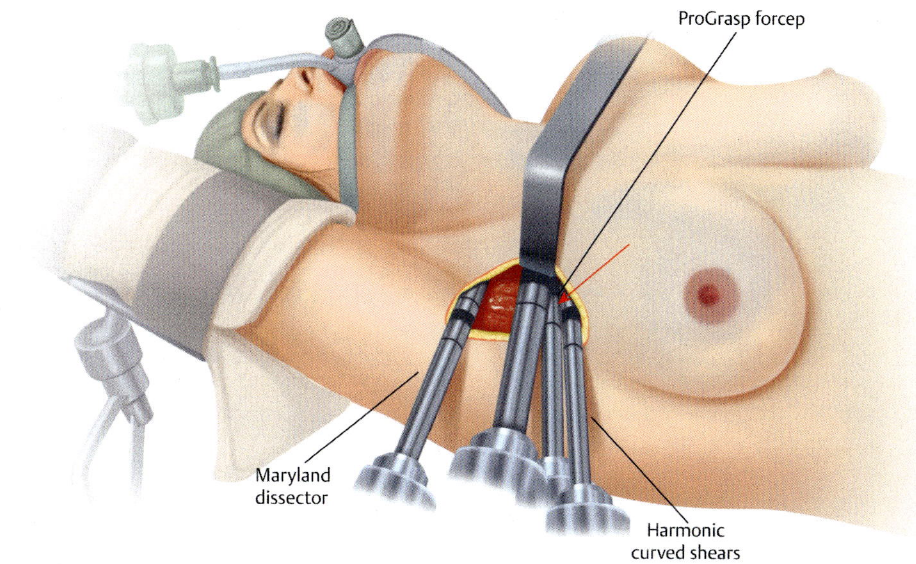

b

Fig. 13.4 (a) Schematic view of novel method of robotic thyroidectomy docking utilizing two skin incisions. A second 0.6–0.8 cm skin incision was created on the tumor side of the anterior chest wall to allow insertion of the fourth robotic arm (with ProGrasp forceps). **(b)** Schematic view of advanced method of robotic thyroidectomy docking with single skin incision. All four robotic instruments and the camera were inserted through the single axillary incision.

Surgical Pearl: During the docking stage, the angle and position of the da Vinci arm joints should be optimized to avoid collisions among robotic instruments and to provide free access to the thyroid bed. To make a conduit for robotic thyroidectomy via a single axillary incision, a 30-degree down dual channel telescope is inserted into the center of the incision in an upward direction, and ProGrasp forceps are placed caudal to the telescope and introduced beneath the anterior part of the skin incision parallel to the retractor blade. A Maryland dissector and Harmonic curved shears are placed on both lateral ends of the axillary incision, with the instruments positioned as far apart as possible. After the docking procedure, it is important to check for any external collisions and to adjust the positions of the arms as necessary to confirm full access to the target anatomy. We have described our robotic docking procedures in detail previously, and we have constructed a standard template for these procedures.[2,3,4,35]

Console Stage

After the docking procedure is complete, actual operation step is performed in the same manner as in conventional open thyroidectomy.

Surgical Pearl: During the console stage, the first assistant can provide additional contralateral traction during dissection, place sponges into the working space, provide suction, remove the specimen, and irrigate the incision. Therefore, both first assistants and beginning surgeons should be educated about neck anatomy and the entire robotic surgical procedure.

In robotic thyroidectomy, traction and counter-traction can be enhanced by the robot function of swapping arms between the ProGrasp forceps and the Maryland dissector.

Frequent swapping of the arms can be helpful to maximize the effect of traction and counter-traction, and to obtain optimal dissection planes. The thyroid gland is retracted using a ProGrasp forceps on the fourth robotic arm and dissection is performed using Harmonic curved shears and a Maryland dissector. This procedure allows the surgeon to use three robotic arms during thyroidectomy. The ProGrasp forceps is initially used to dissect the superior pole of the thyroid gland, retracting the thyroid downward, and the Maryland dissector is used to create traction on the thyroid tissue. The superior thyroid gland vessels are identified and individually ligated close to the thyroid gland using Harmonic curved shears to avoid injury to the external branch of the superior laryngeal nerve. The upper pole of the thyroid gland is separated from the cricopharyngeal and cricothyroid muscles, exposing the superior parathyroid gland and preserving it. The thyroid gland is then pulled in a superior and medial direction using the ProGrasp forceps, and the lateral side of the CCND is performed, from the common carotid artery (CCA) to the inferior thyroid artery superiorly and from the CCA to the substernal notch inferiorly. All dissections and ligations of vessels are performed using the Harmonic curved shears.

Surgical Pearl: During the console stage, all vessels are dissected and ligated using the Harmonic curved shears. These shears have been shown to be both useful and safe, providing an alternative to conventional methods of hemostasis. As hemostasis is achieved at low temperatures (range, 50–100°C) using Harmonic curved shears, energy and heat diffusion into the surrounding tissues is much lower than with other methods. Better hemostasis may be provided by controlling the superior, middle, and inferior thyroidal arteries and veins using a low-power level (70 μm vibration), whereas the other small vessels and surrounding connective tissues may be controlled using a higher power level (100 μm vibration) for easy cutting. Complete resection of the thyroid gland and cervical lymph nodes requires meticulous dissection around the major organs (recurrent/superior laryngeal nerve, trachea, esophagus, and major vessels), avoiding thermal or mechanical injury. Because the robot instruments have no tactile feedback, the thyroid gland should be meticulously detached from the trachea, especially in the Berry ligament area, to avoid direct or indirect thermal injury.

After exposing the CCA to the inferior thyroid artery, soft tissue and central compartment nodes are detached from the substernal notch until the anterior surface of the trachea is exposed. The inferior thyroid artery is divided close to the thyroid gland using the Harmonic curved shears, and the entire cervical course of the recurrent laryngeal nerve (RLN) is traced. In the Berry ligament area, the thyroid gland is meticulously detached from the trachea to avoid direct or indirect thermal injury to the RLN.

After resection of ipsilateral thyroid on isthmus portion, the contralateral lobe is drawn ventrally by the ProGrasp forceps and dissection is performed between the ventral aspect of the thyroid and the trachea using the Maryland forceps and Harmonic curved shears. Then, the contralateral superior pole is retracted inferomedially with the ProGrasp forceps and dissected using the Harmonic curved shears.

Surgical Pearl: During dissection of the contralateral lobe, the surgical table should be tilted to 10–15 degrees. Tilting the table could optimally expose the contralateral tracheoesophageal groove, especially in patients with a prominent trachea and a deeply located contralateral thyroid.

The inferior pole of the thyroid is also dissected subcapsularly to preserve the contralateral RLN and inferior parathyroid gland and its blood supply. After mobilization of the contralateral thyroid gland by dividing the superior and inferior pole, the posteromedial aspect of the contralateral lobe is only attached to the side of the cricoid cartilage by the posterior suspensory ligament of Berry. Because the contralateral RLN can be most consistently identified at the cricoid cartilage and is most vulnerable for injury in the vicinity of the ligament of Berry, special care should be taken to identify the contralateral RNL using the Maryland forceps. Once the contralateral RLN has been identified and preserved, the contralateral thyroid lobe can be removed from its tracheal attachments by dividing the ligament of Berry. The resected specimen is removed through an axillary skin incision. A 3-mm closed suction drain is inserted through a separate skin incision under the axillary skin incision. Wounds are closed cosmetically (**Fig. 13.5**). The axillary incision scar is completely covered when the arm is in its natural position (**Fig. 13.6**).

■ Operative Outcomes After Robotic Thyroid Surgery

Oncologic Effectiveness and Morbidity Rate

A large number of patients comparing robotic and conventional open thyroidectomy have been reported. **Table 13.2** summarizes comparisons of perioperative outcomes for robotic versus conventional open or endoscopic thyroid surgery, and shows that oncologic outcomes and morbidity rates were similar between robotic and conventional operative techniques.[5,12,13,14,15,17,18,19,20,21,22,23,24,25,26,27,28]

Recently, a study prospectively comparing the surgical completeness of robotic thyroidectomy with conventional open surgery in treating papillary thyroid cancer patients was published.[23] In this study, there were no significant differences in the number of harvested cervical lymph nodes and stimulated Tg levels acquired during 131-radioactive iodine (^{131}RAI) ablation scan between the open and robotic groups. In addition, the ablation success rate was similar between the two groups. Several studies also showed robotic thyroidectomy has similar oncologic outcomes as open surgery. However, its long-term outcomes cannot be compared with those of conventional operative technique, due to the recent development of robotic surgery.

Our recent study evaluating surgical complications after 3,000 cases of robotic thyroidectomy for thyroid cancer indicated the most common surgical complication was symptomatic hypocalcemia.[36] However, most cases of symptomatic hypocalcemia and

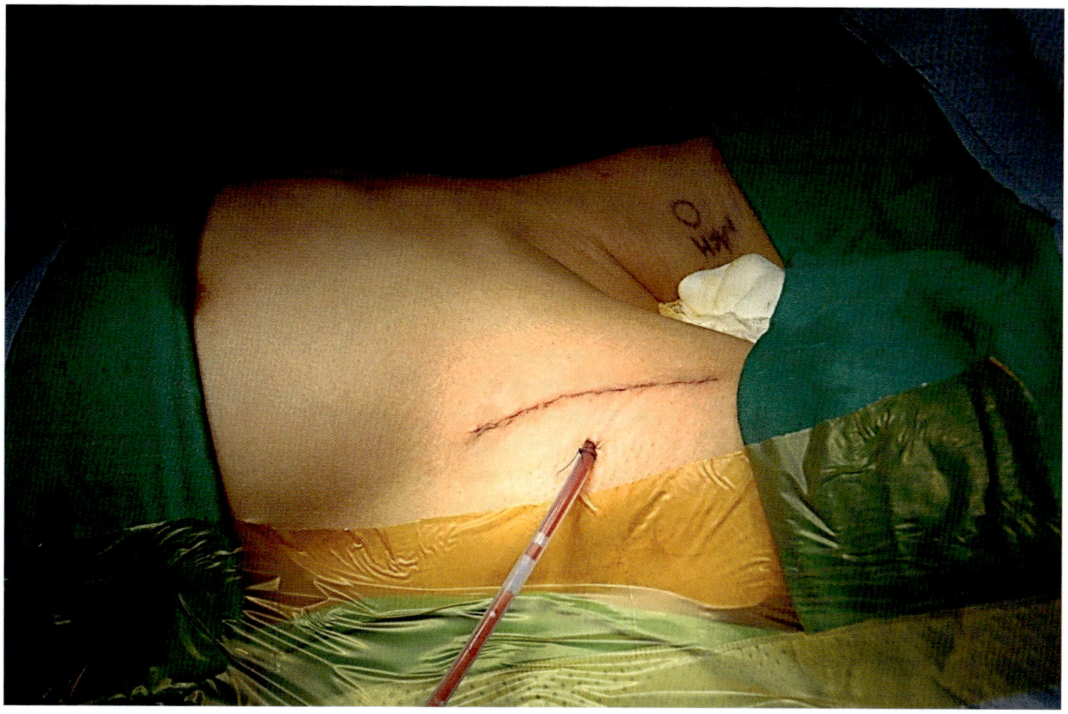

Fig. 13.5 Photograph of a postoperative scar. Immediate postoperative scar after transaxillary single-incision robotic thyroidectomy.

recurrent laryngeal nerve palsy were transient, and recovered spontaneously within 6 months. Other potential complications associated with robotic thyroid surgery, which were never seen in conventional open thyroidectomy, include brachial plexus injury, skin flap perforation, major vessel bleeding, and tracheal injury. These complications, however, can be minimized as surgeons overcome the surgical learning curve. Moreover, studies comparing robotic with conventional transaxillary endoscopic thyroidectomy have shown similar postoperative complication rates and these findings suggest that robotic thyroidectomy is feasible and safe, and can overcome some of the technical limitations associated with conventional transaxillary endoscopic procedures (**Table 13.2**).[5,12,13,14,15,17,18,19,20,21,22,23,24,25,26,27,28]

Until now, there have been no randomized controlled trials comparing oncologic outcomes and complication rates of conventional open and robotic thyroid surgery techniques. Nevertheless, the considerable evidence from nonrandomized comparative studies suggests that robotic and open surgery result in similar surgical completeness and extent of radical neck dissection, as well as similar surgical morbidity rates.

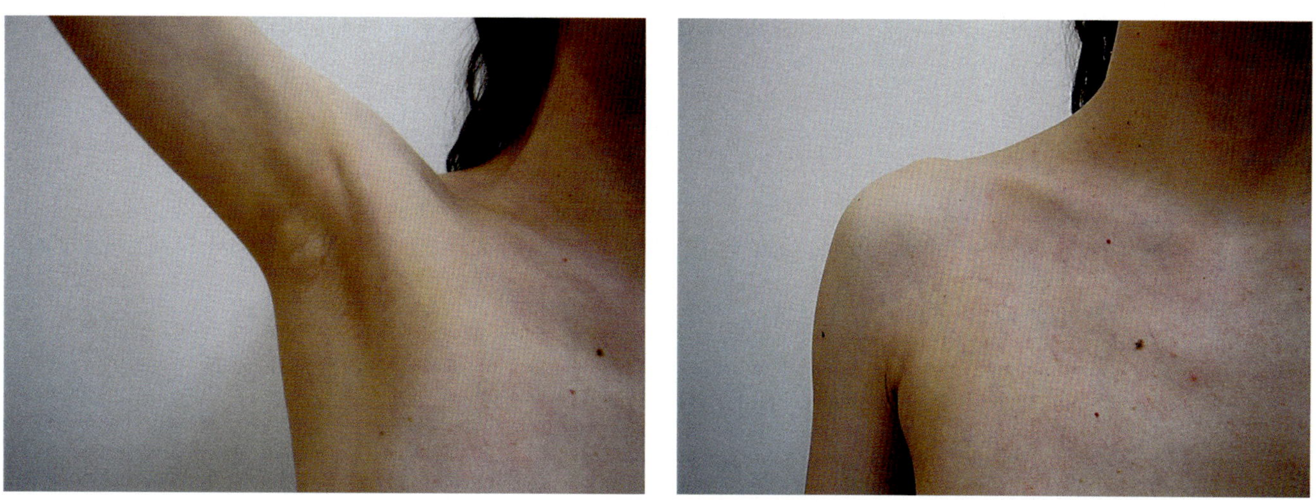

a b

Fig. 13.6 Photographs of a postoperative axillary scar after robotic thyroidectomy. **(a)** Operative scar 3 months after single-incision robotic thyroidectomy. **(b)** Concealment of an axillary scar by her arm in the natural position.

Table 13.2 Comparative studies for oncologic outcomes, complication rates, and other perioperative parameters between robotic (RT) versus conventional open (OT) (or endoscopic [ET]) thyroidectomy

Author	Cases (number)	Oncologic outcomes (measured by number of harvested cervical LN, stimulated Tg level, ^{131}RAI scan, and US)	Complication rates	Operation Time	Other perioperative outcomes (including hospital stay, estimated blood loss, and amount of drainage, etc.)
Lee et al (2010)[17]	OT (43) vs. RT (41)	No difference (number of harvested LN)	No difference	RT>OT	No difference
Tae et al (2011)[18]	OT (163) vs. RT (41)	Number of harvested cervical LN; OT>RT	No difference	RT>OT	No difference
Landary et al (2011)[15]	OT (25) vs. RT (25)		Brachial plexus injury; RT>OT	RT>OT	Estimated blood loss; RT>OT
Tae et al (2012)[19]	OT (226) vs. RT (75)	No difference (stimulated Tg level, ^{131}RAI scan, neck US) Number of harvested LN; OT>RT	Transient hypoparathyroidism; OT>RT	RT>OT	No difference
Lee et al (2012)[13]	OT (266) vs. RT (192)	No difference (stimulated Tg level, ^{131}RAI scan, neck US) Number of harvested LN; OT>RT	No difference	RT>OT	No difference
Ryu et al (2013)[22]	OT (45) vs. RT(45)	No difference (number of harvested LN)	No difference	RT>OT	No difference
Yi et al (2013)[20]	OT (423) vs. RT (98)	No difference (stimulated Tg level, ^{131}RAI scan, number of harvested LN)	Transient hypoparathyroidism; RT>OT	RT>OT	Hospital stay; RT>OT
Aliyev et al (2013)[21]	OT (30) vs. RT (16)	No difference (stimulated Tg level, ^{123}I uptake, number of harvested LN)	No difference	RT>OT	No difference
Lee et al (2014)[23]	OT (51) vs. RT (43)	No difference (stimulated Tg level, ^{123}I uptake, number of harvested LN, ^{131}RAI uptake ratio)	No difference		

Lee et al (2013)[24]	O-MRND (66) vs. R-MRND (62)	No difference (stimulated Tg level, ^{131}RAI scan, number of harvested LN)	No difference	R-MRND>O-MRND	No difference
Lee et al (2011)[12]	ET (96) vs. RT (163)	Number of harvested cervical LN; RT>ET	No difference	ET>RT	No difference
Lang et al (2011)[25]	ET (39) vs. RT (7)		No difference	RT>ET	No difference
Lee et al (2011)[14]	ET (570) vs. RT (580)	Number of harvested LN; RT>ET No difference (stimulated Tg level, ^{123}I uptake, neck US)	Transient hypoparathyroidism; RT>ET	ET>RT	No difference
Yoo et al (2012)[26]	ET (165) vs. RT (46)	No difference (stimulated Tg level)	No difference	RT>ET	No difference
Lee et al (2012)[5]	ET (843) vs. RT (1769)	Number of harvested LN; RT>ET	No difference	ET>RT	No difference
Tae et al (2013)[27]	ET (105) vs. RT (113)	No difference (stimulated Tg level, ^{131}RAI scan, number of harvested LN)	No difference	ET>RT	No difference
Cabot et al (2012)[28]	OT (30), ET (30), vs. RT (30)		No difference	ET>RT>OT	No difference

Abbreviations: LN, lymph nodes; Tg, thyroglobulin; ^{131}RAI, 131-radioactive iodine; US. ultrasonography; R-MRND, robotic modified radical neck dissection; O-MRND, open modified radical neck dissection.

Quality-of-Life Outcomes for Patients After Robotic Thyroid Surgery

Recently, the paradigm for assessing the surgical quality includes the evaluation of the operative benefits on patient perception and satisfaction with robotic thyroid surgery. These studies have analyzed QoL outcomes after this technique, such as pain, discomfort, sensory changes, voice and swallowing recovery, and cosmetic satisfaction. **Table 13.3** summarizes the QoL categories in studies comparing robotic and conventional open (or endoscopic) thyroid surgery techniques.[17,18,19,21,22,24,25,29,30,31] All of these studies comparing patient satisfaction and regret after open or robotic surgery have found higher levels of dissatisfaction and regret, especially with cosmetic outcomes, in patients undergoing open surgery (**Figs. 13.6** and **13.7**).

Several prospective and retrospective clinical trials comparing the degree of pain and sensory changes after robotic surgery or conventional open surgery found that postoperative discomfort in the neck was significantly more frequent in the open than in the robotic surgery group. These findings suggest that robotic thyroidectomy may offer advantages for patients with thyroid cancer by reducing postoperative neck discomfort and sensory changes. Studies of postoperative voice and swallowing changes using subjective and objective validated parameters showed that short-term voice and swallowing outcomes were superior or at least similar after robotic than after conventional open thyroidectomy.[17,24,30,31]

Although these prospective controlled trials have fully addressed QoL outcomes using objective and subjective measures after robotic and conventional open thyroidectomy, the follow-up period was insufficient to determine any long-term effects on patients' QoL. Moreover, as patients were not randomized, it would certainly be premature to claim that robotic surgery is definitely superior to the conventional approach. Further analyses of robotic thyroidectomy, including long-term follow-up and randomized controlled trials, are needed.

■ Benefits for Surgeons of Robotic Thyroid Surgery

Any new surgical procedure is subject to a surgical learning curve. Robotic thyroid surgery can overcome some of the limitations imposed by conventional transaxillary endoscopic instrumentation, including counterintuitive hand movements, two-dimensional visualization, limited degrees of instrument motion within the body, and ergonomic difficulties and tremor amplification. Therefore, robotic thyroidectomy was associated with a shorter operation time than conventional transaxillary endoscopic thyroidectomy. Several studies evaluating surgical learning curves have found that learning curves were significantly shorter for the robotic technique compared to conventional transaxillary endoscopic thyroidectomy. In these studies, the operation time required by a robot- naïve surgeon to perform robotic thyroidectomy plateaued after 35 to 50 operations.[5,11,12] Evaluation of learning curves by two pioneering surgeons from South Korea and the United States showed that the console times for robotic thyroidectomy reached a steady state after about 40 to 45 operations.[9,16]

A Korean multicenter study also represented surgical learning curves for robotic thyroidectomy by analyzing several perioperative parameters, including operation time, complication rate, intraoperative blood loss, length of hospital stay, number of harvested lymph nodes, and serum thyroglobulin concentration.[11] This study showed that operation times and complication rates stabilized in all robot-naïve surgeons after completing 50 total and 40 subtotal robotic thyroidectomies with CCND. In addition, robot-naïve surgeons achieved postoperative outcomes similar to those of experienced surgeons once the learning curve was overcome.

A prospective survey-based study of 2,014 patients with thyroid cancer who underwent robotic thyroidectomy evaluated surgeons' ergonomic considerations for each thyroidectomy procedure, using a questionnaire comparing the type and magnitude of musculoskeletal stress during open, transaxillary endoscopic, and robotic thyroidectomy.[6] In this study, although the operation time for robotic surgery performed by robot-naïve surgeons was longer than for conventional open surgery, surgeons had better ergonomic outcomes after robotic surgery than after conventional operative technique.

However, these studies have assessed the learning curves for robotic thyroidectomy by surgeons with prior experience in performing transaxillary endoscopic thyroidectomy. Although prior experience in transaxillary endoscopic surgical techniques could improve the learning curves for robotic thyroidectomy, little is known about the robotic thyroidectomy learning curves for beginning surgeons with no prior experience with endoscopic surgery. Further studies evaluating surgical learning curves for robotic thyroidectomy by beginning surgeons without transaxillary endoscopic surgery experience are required. Moreover, the ergonomic outcomes reported by several surgeons examined were rather varied, and may be influenced by subjective measures. Additional studies using objective measures are needed to determine the magnitude of the muscle forces used during each procedure.

■ Future Directions and Conclusion

The robotic approach is the new frontier of thyroid cancer surgery, with several advantages over conventional open and endoscopic techniques. Studies to date have shown that the short-term oncologic effectiveness of robotic thyroidectomy, assessed by measuring serum Tg level after TSH stimulation with ^{131}RAI scanning, as well as its morbidity rate and safety, compare favorably with those of conventional open thyroidectomy. Recent assessments of QoL outcomes have also found that patients undergoing robotic thyroid surgery experience lower levels of dissatisfaction and regret than patients undergoing conventional open thyroid surgery, largely due to differences in cosmetic outcomes. Prospective trials evaluating functional parameters, including pain, neck discomfort, and sensory changes in the neck, have favored robotic over conventional open thyroid surgery. Similarly, objective and subjective evaluations of

Table 13.3 Comparative studies for quality of life outcomes following robotic versus conventional open (or endoscopic) thyroidectomy

Author (year)	Study design	Cases (number of patients)	QoL measures	QoL outcomes
Cosmetic satisfaction				
Lee et al (2010)[17]	Prospective	OT (43) vs. RT (41)	Verbal response scale	RT much better than OT
Tae et al (2011)[18]	Prospective	OT (163) vs. RT (41)	Verbal response scale	RT much better than OT
Tae et al (2012)[19]	Retrospective	OT (226) vs. RT (75)	Verbal response scale	RT much better than OT
Tae et al (2013)[27]	Retrospective	ET (105) vs. RT (113)	Verbal response scale	RT similar to ET
Lee et al (2013)[24]	Prospective	O-MRND (66) vs. R-MRND (62)	Verbal response scale	R-MRND much better than O-MRND
Jackson et al (2013)[29]	Meta-analysis	OT (794), ET (965), vs. RT (1122)	Verbal response scale	RT much better than OT
Pain				
Lee et al (2010)[17]	Prospective	OT (43) vs. RT (41)	Postoperative analgesic use, pain score	RT similar to OT
Tae et al (2011)[18]	Prospective	OT (163) vs. RT (41)	Pain score	RT similar to OT
Lang et al (2011)[25]	Retrospective	ET (39) vs. RT (7)	Pain score	RT similar to ET
Tae et al (2012)[19]	Retrospective	OT (226) vs. RT (75)	Pain score	RT similar to OT
Aliyev et al (2013)[21]	Prospective	OT (30) vs. RT (16)	Postoperative analgesic use, pain score	RT similar to or worse than OT
Tae et al (2013)[27]	Retrospective	ET (105) vs. RT (113)	Pain score	RT similar to ET
Ryu et al (2012)[22]	Prospective	OT (45) vs. RT (45)	Postoperative analgesic use, pain score	RT better than or similar to OT
Lee et al (2013)[24]	Prospective	O-MRND (66) vs. R-MRND (62)	Pain score	R-MRND much better than O-MRND
Jackson et al (2013)[29]	Meta-analysis	OT (794), ET (965), vs. RT (1122)	Pain score	RT similar to or better than OT
Sensory changes				
Lee et al (2010)[17]	Prospective, single surgeon	OT (43) vs. RT (41)	Sensory score	RT better than OT
Tae et al (2012)[19]	Retrospective, single surgeon	OT (226) vs. RT (75)	Sensory score	RT similar to OT
Lee et al (2013)[24]	Prospective, single surgeon	O-MRND (66) vs. R-MRND (62)	Sensory score	RT better than OT

(continued)

Table 13.3 Comparative studies for quality of life outcomes following robotic versus conventional open (or endoscopic) thyroidectomy *(continued)*

Author (year)	Study design	Cases (number of patients)	QoL measures	QoL outcomes
Voice and swallowing disability				
Lee et al (2010)[17]	Prospective	OT (43) vs. RT (41)	Subjective score	Voice: RT similar to OT Swallowing: RT better than OT
Lee et al (2013)[24]	Prospective	O-MRND (66) vs. R-MRND (62)	Subjective score	Voice: R-MRND similar to O-MRND Swallowing: R-MRND better than O-MRND
Tae et al (2012)[30]	Prospective	OT (61) vs. RT (50)	Subjective score and objective parameters	Voice: RT better than OT Swallowing: RT similar to OT
Lee et al (2012)[31]	Prospective	OT (46) vs. RT (42)	Subjective score and objective parameters	Voice: RT similar to OT
Movement disability				
Lee et al (2013)[24]	Prospective, single surgeon	O-MRND (66) vs. R-MRND (62)	Subjective score and objective parameters	R-MRND similar to O-MRND

Abbreviations: ET, endoscopic thyroidectomy; O-MRND, open modified radical neck dissection; OT, open thyroidectomy; QoL, quality of life; R-MRND, robotic modified radical neck dissection; RT, robotic thyroidectomy.

voice and swallowing discomfort were improved in patients undergoing robotic thyroidectomy. Thus, use of a robot results in overall increases in cosmetic satisfaction and decreases in several measures of postoperative discomfort compared with the conventional open thyroid technique. Moreover, for surgeons, the use of a robot offers a shorter operation time and a shorter learning curve compared with conventional transaxillary endoscopic thyroidectomy, and causes less musculoskeletal discomfort than open or endoscopic thyroidectomy. **Table 13.4** summarizes the advantages and disadvantages of robotic compared with conventional open (or endoscopic) thyroid surgery.

The main drawbacks of robotic thyroid surgery in its present form are its longer operation times and higher surgical costs than conventional open thyroid surgery. Another drawback for the current robot surgical system is the lack of tactile feedback and limited instrumentation. The final current limitation of robotic surgery is the need to train teams, including attending surgeons, surgical assistant(s), and nurses, to become proficient in this technique (**Table 13.4**). However, as more robotic thyroid surgery procedures are being performed and as technological advances are making robotic systems even more useful, robotic surgery may become more feasible and cost-effective. Technicians and surgeons are also trying to advance the current robotic system to overcome current disadvantages.

Robotic MRND for thyroid cancer patients with lateral neck node metastasis (N1b) is increasingly being performed by robot

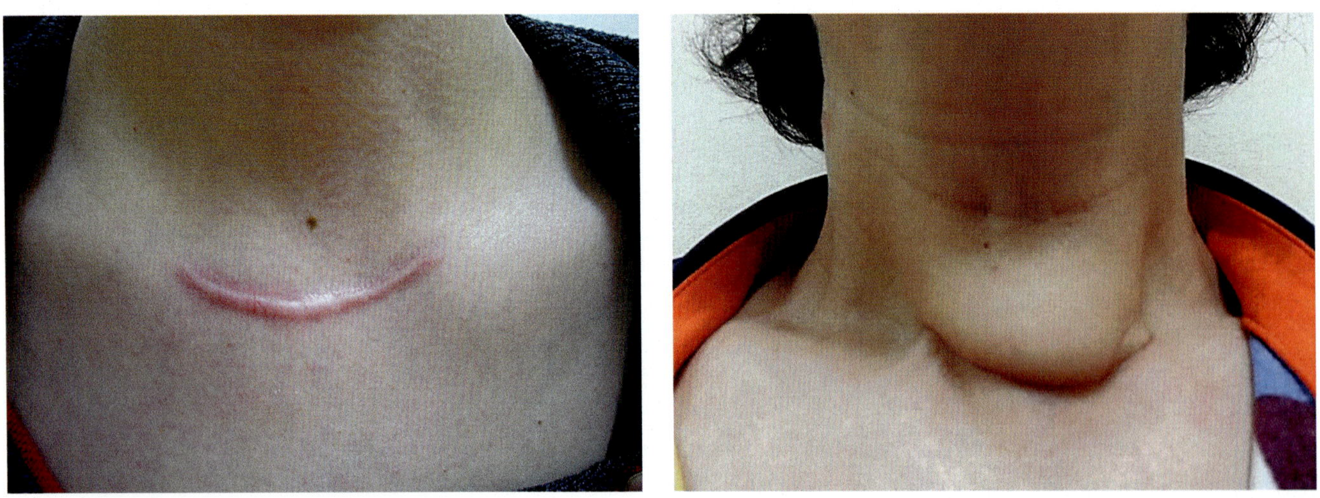

a b

Fig. 13.7 Photographs of a postoperative anterior neck scar after conventional open surgery. **(a)** Hypertrophic scar 6 months after open thyroidectomy. **(b)** Wrinkled scar with a conventional collar incision 6 weeks after open thyroidectomy.

Table 13.4 Summary of merits and demerits of robotic compared with conventional open or endoscopic thyroidectomy

	Robotic thyroidectomy (RT)	versus	Open thyroidectomy (OT)	Robotic thyroidectomy (RT)	versus	Endoscopic thyroidectomy (ET)
Oncologic efficacy	RT	similar to	OT	RT	better than	ET
Safety	RT	similar to	OT	RT	similar to or better than	ET
Cosmetic satisfaction	RT	much better than	OT	RT	similar to	ET
Patient's functional outcomes (pan, sensory changes, voice and swallowing disability)	RT	better than	OT	RT	no available data	ET
Operation time	RT	worse than	OT	RT	better than	ET
Surgical learning curve	RT	no available data	OT	RT	better than	ET
Surgeon's ergonomic consideration	RT	better than	OT	RT	much better than	ET
Surgical cost	RT	worse than	OT	RT	worse than	ET
Tactile feedback	RT	worse than	OT	RT	worse than	ET
Bulky character of operative theater	RT	worse than	OT	RT	worse than	ET
Demand to train all operative team members	RT	worse than	OT	RT	worse than	ET

surgeons, but the ultimate impact of such techniques remains unclear. Our previous studies have shown robot techniques have yielded favorable postoperative outcomes, including oncologic efficacy and safety, comparable to conventional operative techniques, without additional complications.[37,38] Considering recent evidence indicating that robotic thyroidectomy is as safe and oncologically effective as conventional open thyroidectomy, as determined by postoperative ^{131}RAI scans, serum Tg concentrations, and number of retrieved cervical lymph nodes, we found that robotic thyroid surgery was both well tolerated and feasible in thyroid cancer patients. In addition, robotic thyroidectomy with MRND was found to enhance QoL outcomes relative to conventional open thyroidectomy with MRND. Among the QoL benefits of robotic MRND, excellent cosmetic results and reductions in neck sensory changes, voice, and swallowing discomfort after surgery have already been published.[24]

References

1. Kang SW, Jeong JJ, Yun JS, et al. Robot-assisted endoscopic surgery for thyroid cancer: experience with the first 100 patients. Surg Endosc 2009;23:2399–2406
2. Lee J, Chung WY. Current status of robotic thyroidectomy and neck dissection using gasless transaxillary approach. Curr Opin Oncol 2012;24:7–15
3. Lee J, Chung WY. Robotic thyroidectomy and neck dissection: past, present and future. Cancer J 2013;19:151–161
4. Lee J, Chung WY. Robotic surgery for thyroid disease. Eur Thyroid J 2013;2:93–101
5. Lee J, Yun JH, Choi UJ, et al. Robotic versus endoscopic thyroidectomy for thyroid cancers: a multi-institutional analysis of early postoperative outcomes and surgical learning curves. J Oncol 2012;2012:734541
6. Lee J, Kang SW, Jung JJ, et al. Multicenter study of robotic thyroidectomy: short-term postoperative outcomes and surgeon ergonomic considerations. Ann Surg Oncol 2011;18: 2538–2547
7. Ikeda Y, Takami H, Sasaki Y, Takayama J, Niimi M, Kan S. Clinical benefits in endoscopic thyroidectomy by the axillary approach. J Am Coll Surg 2003;196:189–195
8. Ikeda Y, Takami H, Sasaki Y, Takayama J, Kurihara H. Are there significant benefits of minimally invasive endoscopic thyroidectomy? World J Surg 2004;28:1075--1078
9. Kang SW, Lee SC, Lee SH, et al. Robotic thyroid surgery using a gasless, transaxillary approach and the da Vinci S system: the operative outcomes of 338 consecutive patients. Surgery 2009;146:1048–1055

10. Kuppersmith RB, Holsinger FC. Robotic thyroid surgery: an initial experience with North American patients. Laryngoscope 2011;121:521–526
11. Lee J, Yun JH, Nam KH, et al. The learning curve for robotic thyroidectomy: a multicenter study. Ann Surg Oncol 2011;18: 226–232
12. Lee J, Lee JH, Nah KY, Soh EY, Chung WY. Comparison of endoscopic and robotic thyroidectomy. Ann Surg Oncol 2011;18:1439–1446
13. Lee S, Ryu HR, Park JH, et al. Early surgical outcomes comparison between robotic and conventional open thyroid surgery for papillary thyroid microcarcinoma. Surgery 2012;151:724–730
14. Lee S, Ryu HR, Park JH, et al. Excellence in robotic thyroid surgery; a comparative study of robot-assisted versus conventional endoscopic thyroidectomy in papillary thyroid microcarcinoma patients. Ann Surg 2011;253:1060–1066
15. Landry CS, Grubbs EG, Morris GS, et al. Robot assisted transaxillary surgery (RATS) for the removal of thyroid and parathyroid glands. Surgery 2011;149:549–555
16. Kandil EH, Noureldine SI, Yao L, Slakey DP. Robotic transaxillary thyroidectomy: an examination of the first one hundred cases. J Am Coll Surg 2012;214:558–564
17. Lee J, Nah KY, Kim RM, Ahn YH, Soh EY, Chung WY. Differences in postoperative outcomes, function, and cosmesis: open versus robotic thyroidectomy. Surg Endosc 2010;24:186–194
18. Tae K, Ji YB, Jeong JH, Lee SH, Jeong MA, Park CW. Robotic thyroidectomy by a gasless unilateral axillo-breast or axillary approach: our early experiences. Surg Endosc 2011;25:221–228
19. Tae K, Ji YB, Cho SH, et al. Early surgical outcomes of robotic thyroidectomy by a gasless unilateral axillo-breast or axillary approach for papillary thyroid carcinoma: 2 years' experience. Head Neck 2012;34:617–625
20. Yi O, Yoon JH, Lee YM, et al. Technical and oncologic safety of robotic thyroid surgery. Ann Surg Oncol 2013;20:1927–1933
21. Aliyev S, Taskin HE, Agcaoglu O, et al. Robotic transaxillary total thyroidectomy through a single axillary incision. Surgery 2013; 153:705–710
22. Ryu HR, Lee J, Park JH, et al. A comparison of postoperative pain after conventional open thyroidectomy and transaxillary single-incision robotic thyroidectomy: a prospective study. Ann Surg Oncol 2013;20(7):2279–2284
23. Lee S, Lee CR, Lee SC, et al. Surgical completeness of robotic thyroidectomy: a prospective comparison with conventional open thyroidectomy in papillary thyroid carcinoma patients. Surg Endosc 2014;28(4):1068–1075
24. Lee J, Kwon IS, Bae EH, Chung WY. Comparative analysis of oncological outcomes and quality of life after robotic versus conventional open thyroidectomy with modified radical neck dissection in patients with papillary thyroid carcinoma and lateral neck node metastases. J Clin Endocrinol Metab 2013;98(7):2701–2708
25. Lang BH, Chow MP. A comparison of surgical outcomes between endoscopic and robotically assisted thyroidectomy: the authors' initial experience. Surg Endosc 2011;25:1617–1623
26. Yoo H, Chae BJ, Park HS, et al. Comparison of surgical outcomes between endoscopic and robotic thyroidectomy. J Surg Oncol 2012;105:705–708
27. Tae K, Ji YB, Jeong JH, Kim KR, Choi WH, Ahn YH. Comparative study of robotic versus endoscopic thyroidectomy by a gasless unilateral axillo-breast or axillary approach. Head Neck 2013; 35:477–484
28. Cabot JC, Lee CR, Brunaud L, et al. Robotic and endoscopic transaxillary thyroidectomies may be cost prohibitive when compared to standard cervical thyroidectomy: a cost analysis. Surgery 2012;152:1016–1024
29. Jackson NR, Yao L, Tufano RP, et al. Safety of robotic thyroidectomy approaches: meta-analysis and systemic review. Head Neck 2014;36(1):137–143
30. Tae K, Kim KY, Yun BR, et al. Functional voice and swallowing outcomes after robotic thyroidectomy by a gasless unilateral axillo-breast approach: comparison with open thyroidectomy. Surg Endosc 2012;26:1871–18771
31. Lee J, Na KY, Kim RM, et al. Postoperative functional voice changes after conventional open or robotic thyroidectomy: a prospective trial. Ann Surg Oncol 2012;19:2963–2970
32. Veronesi G. Robotic surgery for the treatment of early-stage lung cancer. Curr Opin Oncol 2013;25:107–114
33. American Thyroid Association (ATA) Guidelines Taskforce on Thyroid Nodules and Differentiated Thyroid Cancer, Cooper DS, Doherty GM, et al. Revised American Thyroid Association management guidelines for patients with thyroid nodules and differentiated thyroid cancer. Thyroid 2009;19:1167–1214
34. Lee S, Park S, Lee CR, et al. The impact of body habitus on the surgical outcomes of transaxillary single-incision robotic thyroidectomy in papillary thyroid carcinoma patients. Surg Endosc 2013;27:2407–2414
35. Ryu HR, Kang SW, Lee SH, et al. Feasibility and safety of a new robotic thyroidectomy through a gasless, transaxillary single-incision approach. J Am Coll Surg 2010;211:e13–19
36. Ban EJ, Yoo JY, Kim WW, et al. Surgical complications after robotic thyroidectomy for thyroid carcinoma: a single center experience with 3,000 patients. Surg Endosc 2014;28(9):2555–2563
37. Kang SW, Lee SH, Ryu HR, et al. Initial experience with robot-assisted modified radical neck dissection for the management of thyroid carcinoma with lateral neck node metastasis. Surgery 2010;148:1214–1221
38. Kang SW, Lee SH, Park JH, et al. A comparative study of the surgical outcomes of robotic and conventional open modified radical neck dissection for papillary thyroid carcinoma with lateral neck node metastasis. Surg Endosc 2012;26:3251–3257

14 Robotic Neck Dissection

Hyung Kwon Byeon and Yoon Woo Koh

Clinical Background

Since the advent of robotics in the field of surgery, transoral robotic surgery (TORS) has been perceived and adopted by many surgeons worldwide as a promising surgical modality in resecting primary tumors of the head and neck area. Under strict and appropriate clinical indications, this so-called minimally invasive surgery is being regarded as an alternative surgical method to the conventional radical open surgical approach methods. There is a general consensus that from TORS, a patient's postoperative morbidity has been dramatically reduced.[1,2] However, regarding the management of the neck, not much has changed in terms of the surgical method of neck dissection. If a decision is made that the neck must be surgically treated, then a conventional neck dissection utilizing a transcervical incision is still the mainstay of neck surgery. So the patient is still left with a grossly noticeable neck scar even though he or she may have received the minimally invasive TORS. Not only will the patient be displeased in aesthetic aspects with the neck scar, but the patient will be now more prone to specific postoperative complications such as cervical lymphedema, cervical fibrotic band formation, or incisional wound dehiscence. Therefore, it can be considered that this is not really a minimally invasive head and neck surgery.

Consequently, the authors have been actively engaged in the investigation of minimally invasive surgical methods of neck dissection. Robotic neck dissection was first reported by Kang et al from Korea,[3] who presented their technique of robotic selective neck dissection including levels IIA, III, IV, and VB in thyroid papillary carcinoma with lateral neck node metastasis. They have utilized the same transaxillary (TA) port in performing the total thyroidectomy; however, from this approach, the upper cervical level I and posterior cervical levels IIB and VA were difficult to access because of the limited axis of view and restriction of instrumentation. Comprehensive neck dissection is commonly required in the neck management of head and neck carcinoma with positive cervical metastasis, so we have developed an alternative route—a novel retroauricular (RA) approach that could provide easier access to the superior and posterior cervical levels. Though this is not a minimally invasive surgery in the strict sense but is more of a remote access surgery, the authors strongly believe that many of the postoperative clinical problems stated above can be solved from this surgical approach of neck dissection, and therefore it can be said that this can be viewed as a minimally invasive surgery in the broad sense. Since 2010, the authors have developed and actively performed robotic neck dissection for patients with head and neck cancer with cN+ necks as well as cN0 necks.[4,5,6,7,8,9,10,11,12,13,14,15]

The Advantages and Disadvantages of Various Surgical Methods of Neck Dissection

The conventional open type of neck dissection utilizing a transcervical incision offers the surgeon the best surgical view since direct approach is possible. So far, if there is an overt, extensive extracapsular invasion of the metastatic node, then the best surgical option would be open neck dissection. Although there are currently many types of neck dissection that have been refined from the classic radical neck dissection to preserve vital structures and certain neck levels so that significant surgical morbidities can be minimized, the resulting scar on the neck following the operation is still unavoidable. Despite the efforts to minimize scarring, some patients may still suffer from disfiguring hypertrophic scar or keloid formation, which can adversely affect the patient's quality of life. Fibrotic band formation on the surgically treated neck can develop, and sometimes if there is a trifurcation incisional wound on the neck, skin dehiscence may develop from skin margin necrosis, which may lead to drastic secondary complications such as carotid artery exposure. Lymphedema is also one of the frequent complaints that the patient can have after conventional neck dissection. The long transverse incision in the neck can disrupt normal lymphatic drainage from the head to the neck area and, consequently, this disruption will result in facial or neck edema.

The authors have personal surgical experiences of robotic neck dissections via a transaxillary-retroauricular (TARA) approach that have been performed in our initial period of robotic neck dissection.[15,16,17,18] We have realized that though it can be cosmetically superior for the patient since the surgical wounds are hidden in areas not normally visible, the surgical access gained from the TA port only is restricted, especially in areas of level I, IIB, and VA. Therefore, aid from an extra remote access port, the RA port, was considered vital to complete the neck dissection.

Through the accumulation of our surgical experiences of robotic neck dissections, we have realized that the surgical procedure can be confidently performed through the RA port alone. All levels of the ipsilateral neck could be reached with the RA approach, and by eliminating the TA approach, the area of dissection is greatly reduced. In addition, the area of dissection required is much less for the RA approach than the TA approach, as has been investigated by Terris et al.[19,20] Another strong advantage for the RA approach is that the surgical anatomy will be much more familiar for the head and neck surgeon and, unlike the TA approach, any chances of intraoperative complications due to the surgical procedures related to the obstructing clavicle will be completely eliminated. However, this cosmetically excellent procedure has some drawbacks. First, the overall operation time to complete the required neck dissection is longer than conventional methods, mainly due to additional skin flap elevation and working space creation. Second, this specific surgical technique requires a considerable level of technical proficiency so it is not an easy procedure for an inexperienced surgeon especially in the area of endoscopic surgery.[21] Finally, the total medical cost from robotic surgery is more expensive than with conventional neck dissection.

■ Indications and Contraindications

Indications for RA robotic neck dissection are as follows:

1. Biopsy-proven head and neck cancer requiring elective neck dissection (cN0) or therapeutic neck dissection (cN+)
2. No previous treatment for head and neck cancer
3. cN0 neck or cN+ neck with minimal extracapsular spread of metastatic node on preoperative imaging studies

Contraindications for this procedure are as follows:

1. Patients expressing refusal of the procedure
2. Chemoradiation for primary definitive treatment due to refusal of surgery
3. Salvage neck surgery
4. Inoperable state due to distant metastasis
5. Unresectable metastatic cervical nodes with overt extracapsular spread
6. Advanced nodal stage more than N2
7. Patients who require cervical skin incision for removal of advanced primary cancers
8. Patients who require free flap reconstruction. The authors have recently started to conduct simultaneous robotic neck dissection and free flap reconstruction via the same RA approach and with success, so the necessity for free flap reconstruction would be a relative contraindication.[22]
9. Past history of neck surgery of any kind
10. A patient with a short, obese neck. The length and circumference of the patient's neck are important determinants of good exposure for robotic neck dissection. A patient who has a slender, long neck provides the best exposure for working space creation, although the procedure was equally feasible in patients with shorter, more obese necks. Therefore, the somatometry of the patient is not considered an absolute contraindication.

■ Special Equipment

1. Retractors for skin flap elevation
   - Skin hook
   - Army-Navy retractor
   - Right-angle breast retractor
   - Self-retaining retractor (Sangdosa Inc.)
2. Instruments for dissection under direct vision
   - Monopolar cautery tips with variable length (spatula tip is preferred)
   - Harmonic curved shears (Harmonic Ace 23E; Johnson & Johnson Medical)
   - DeBakey forceps or Russian forceps
   - Yankauer suction
3. Robotic instruments (da Vinci Robotic System, Intuitive Surgical, Inc.)
   - 12-mm, 30-degree face-down endoscope
   - 5-mm Maryland forceps
   - 5-mm Harmonic curved shears
   - 8-mm ProGrasp forceps
4. Vessel ligation system
   - Hem-o-lok Ligation System (Teleflex Inc.)

■ Surgical Procedure

Generally, the procedure of robotic neck dissection can be divided into two main parts: gross dissection under direct vision, and robotic dissection. Most of the procedure can be conducted under direct vision and the robot merely aids the procedure in dissecting the areas difficult to access under the naked eye. So strictly speaking the correct terminology for this procedure is robot-assisted neck dissection, or RAND, rather than robotic neck dissection, as in this chapter's title. The procedure of robotic neck dissection has a distinct difference whether levels IV and V are included in the procedure or not. Therefore, the relevant surgical procedure is discussed and illustrated according to two distinct types of neck dissection as follows. For all types of RAND, the patient is positioned supine with the head rotated to the contralateral side of the dissection. The neck is generally relaxed in its natural position. There is no need for neck extension with a shoulder roll.

Selective Neck Dissection (Levels I–III)

Skin Incision Design

An RA or modified facelift (MFL) incision is adopted with consideration of the type and extent of surgery. The RA incision is placed at the RA sulcus where it is curved to the occipital direction at midpoint level to angulate smoothly downward 0.5 cm inside and along the hairline (**Fig. 14.1a**). The MFL incision is the same incision for conducting conventional parotidectomy. It is similar to the RA incision except that it has an additional preauricular limb. When neck dissection is performed via the MFL incision, dissection can be much easier since the working space created from skin flap elevation would be larger.

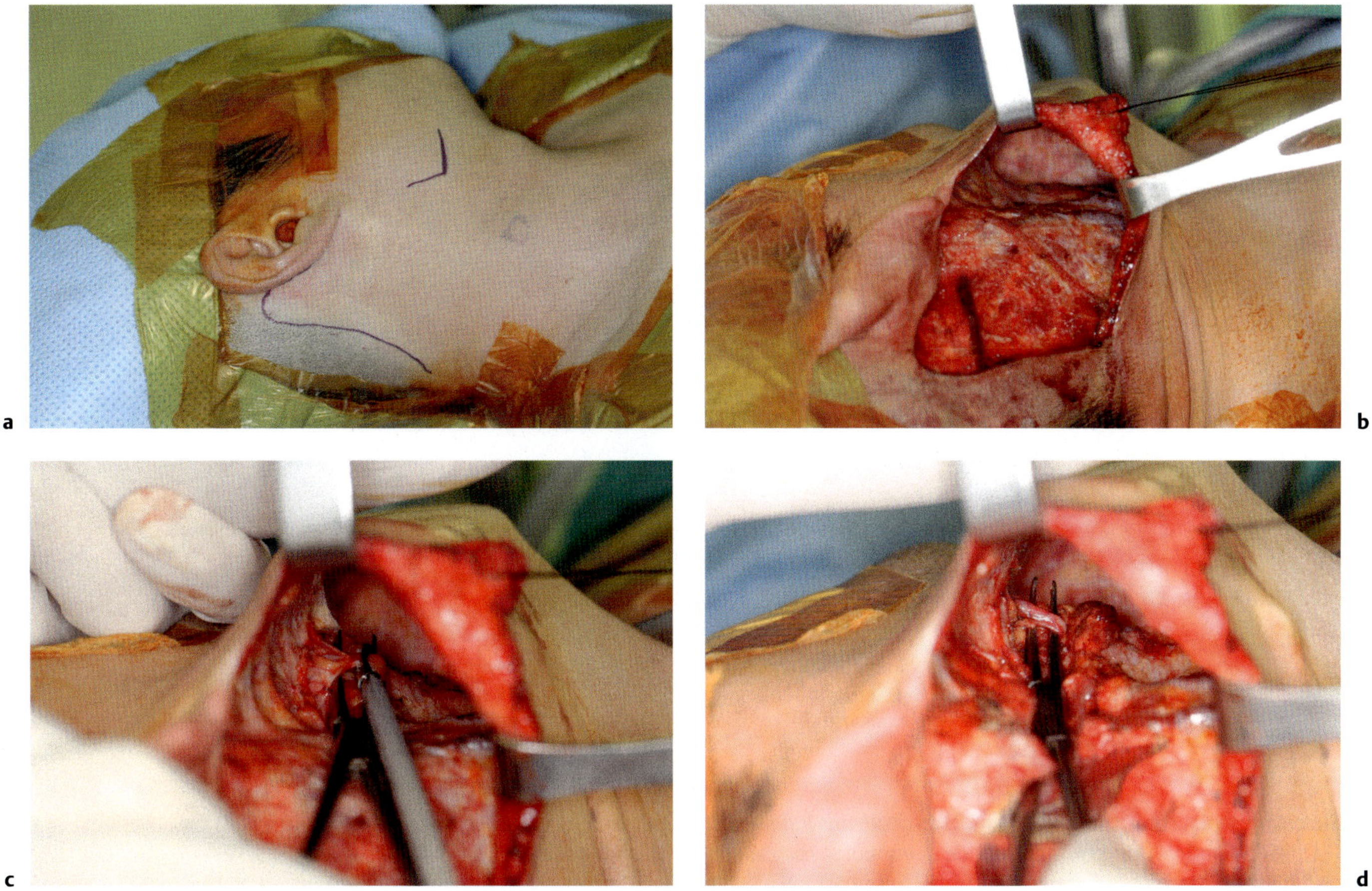

Fig. 14.1 Skin incision and upper neck dissection using the conventional techniques. **(a)** Position of the patient and design of the retroauricular skin incision. **(b)** The greater auricular nerve and external jugular vein are preserved superficial to the sternocleidomastoid muscle. **(c)** Distal facial vein and marginal mandibular branch of the facial nerve. The perivascular lymph nodes should be dissected after preserving the mandibular branch. **(d)** The distal facial artery located deep to the mandibular branch; may be a good landmark.

Working Space Creation

After skin incision, subplatysmal skin flap is elevated just above the sternocleidomastoid (SCM) muscle using a monopolar electrocautery under direct vision. The greater auricular nerve and external jugular vein can be identified located superficial to the SCM muscle (**Fig. 14.1b**). The skin flap is elevated until the anterior extent reaches the midline of the anterior neck, the superior extent the inferior border of the mandible, and the inferior extent the level of omohyoid muscle. Skin flap elevation below the mandible should be performed carefully to minimize injury to the nearby marginal branch of the facial nerve. Normally two assistant surgeons are required to comfortably lift up the skin flap with an Army–Navy retractor or a right-angle breast retractor. After obtaining a sufficient amount of working space, a self-retaining retractor (Sangdosa) is applied through the space and is secured (**Fig. 14.1b**).

Upper Neck Dissection Under Direct Vision

Before robotic dissection procedure, neck dissection under direct vision is performed using conventional technique. First, the marginal branch of the facial nerve is identified referring to the distal portion of facial artery and facial vein as landmarks, which are located along the inferior border of mandible (**Fig. 14.1c,d**). The perifacial lymph nodes surrounding the marginal nerve and the nearby lymphoadipose tissue are cautiously dissected with preservation of the facial nerve. Next the parotid tail is divided from its surrounding tissue and the dissection is further directed anteriorly, along the inferior border of the submandibular gland (SMG), revealing the posterior belly of the digastric muscle underneath. The anterior border of SCM muscle is opened and followed inferiorly until the level of the omohyoid muscle. Dissecting the area between the inferior border of digastric muscle and the anterior border of SCM enables the visualization of the internal jugular vein contour. The transverse process of atlas can be palpated at this region, which is a reliable landmark to localize the spinal accessory nerve.

The spinal accessory nerve is identified and skeletonized and level IIB is dissected (**Fig. 14.2**). The specimen is directed anteriorly toward the carotid sheath and lymphoadipose tissues of levels IIA and III are sequentially dissected.

Robot-Assisted Neck Dissection Technique

The robotic arms are docked through the RA port. Three robotic arms are used: a 30-degree dual-channel endoscope (Intuitive

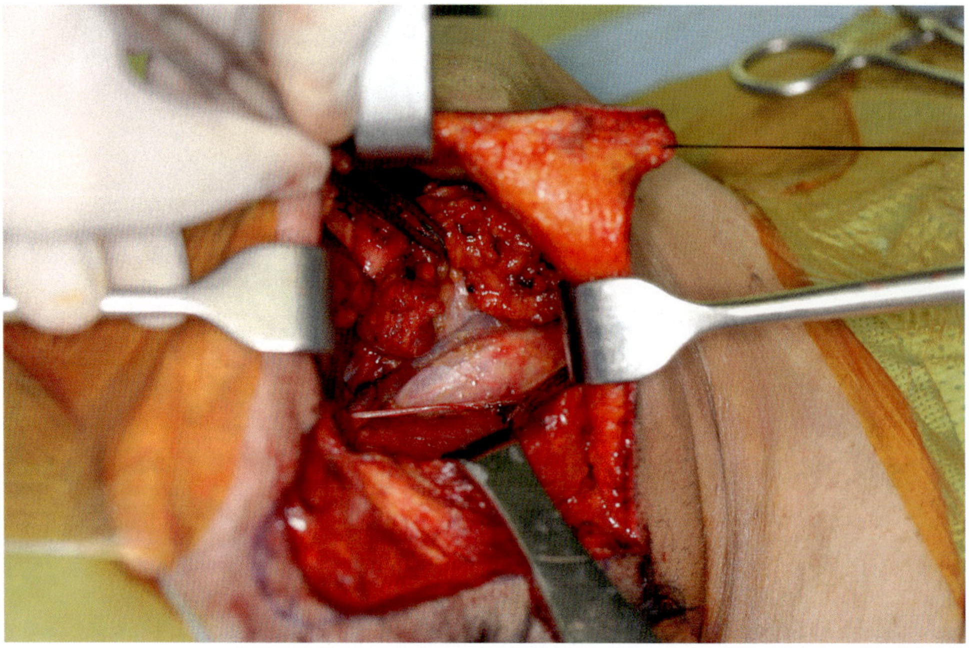

Fig. 14.2 Identifying the spinal accessory nerve and level IIB dissection. The lymphofatty tissues are dissected from the medial border of the sternocleidomastoid muscle and the specimen is directed anteriorly toward the carotid sheath, and lymphoadipose tissues of levels IIB and IIA are sequentially dissected.

Surgical) is placed at the center, and Harmonic curved shears (Intuitive Surgical) or a 5-mm spatula monopolar coagulator and a 5-mm Maryland dissector (Intuitive Surgical) are placed at either side of the central arm (**Fig. 14.3**). Additional aid from a fourth arm such as a ProGrasp forceps is not applicable with this approach; however, its role can be substituted by an endoscopic alligator forceps, which are held by a patient-side assistant surgeon.

The robotic dissection is commenced at the remaining undissected anterior portion of level I. The dissection of level I is performed in a lateral to medial manner. Confirming the posterior belly of the digastric muscle, the proximal facial artery

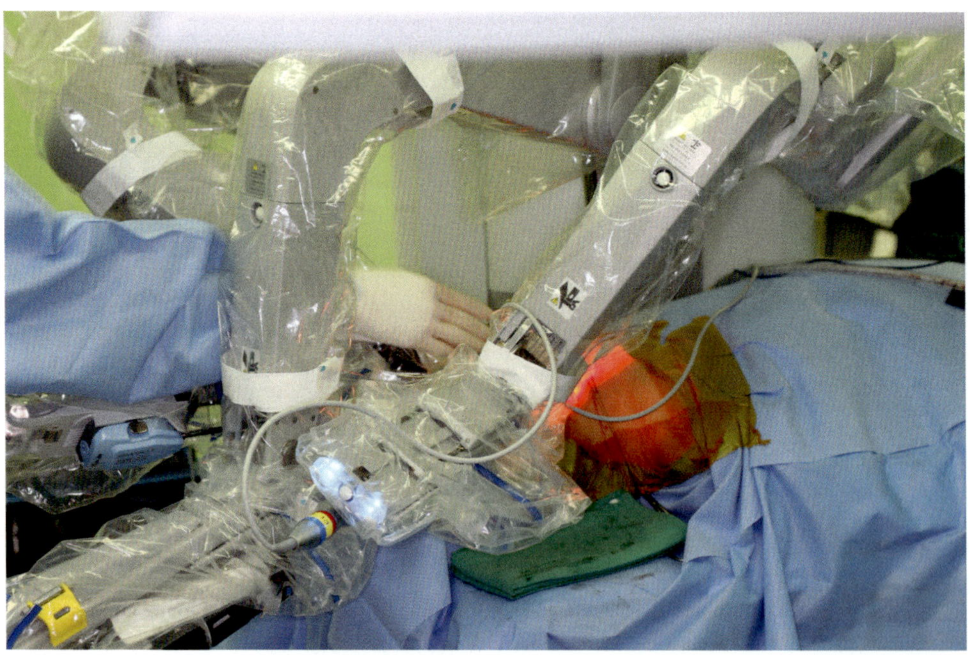

Fig. 14.3 Docking of the robotic arms. A face-down 30-degree endoscope is used for visualization of the surgical field, and two robotic instrument arms, equipped at either side of the endoscopic arm with 5-mm Maryland forceps and 5-mm Harmonic curved shears, respectively, are utilized throughout the operation.

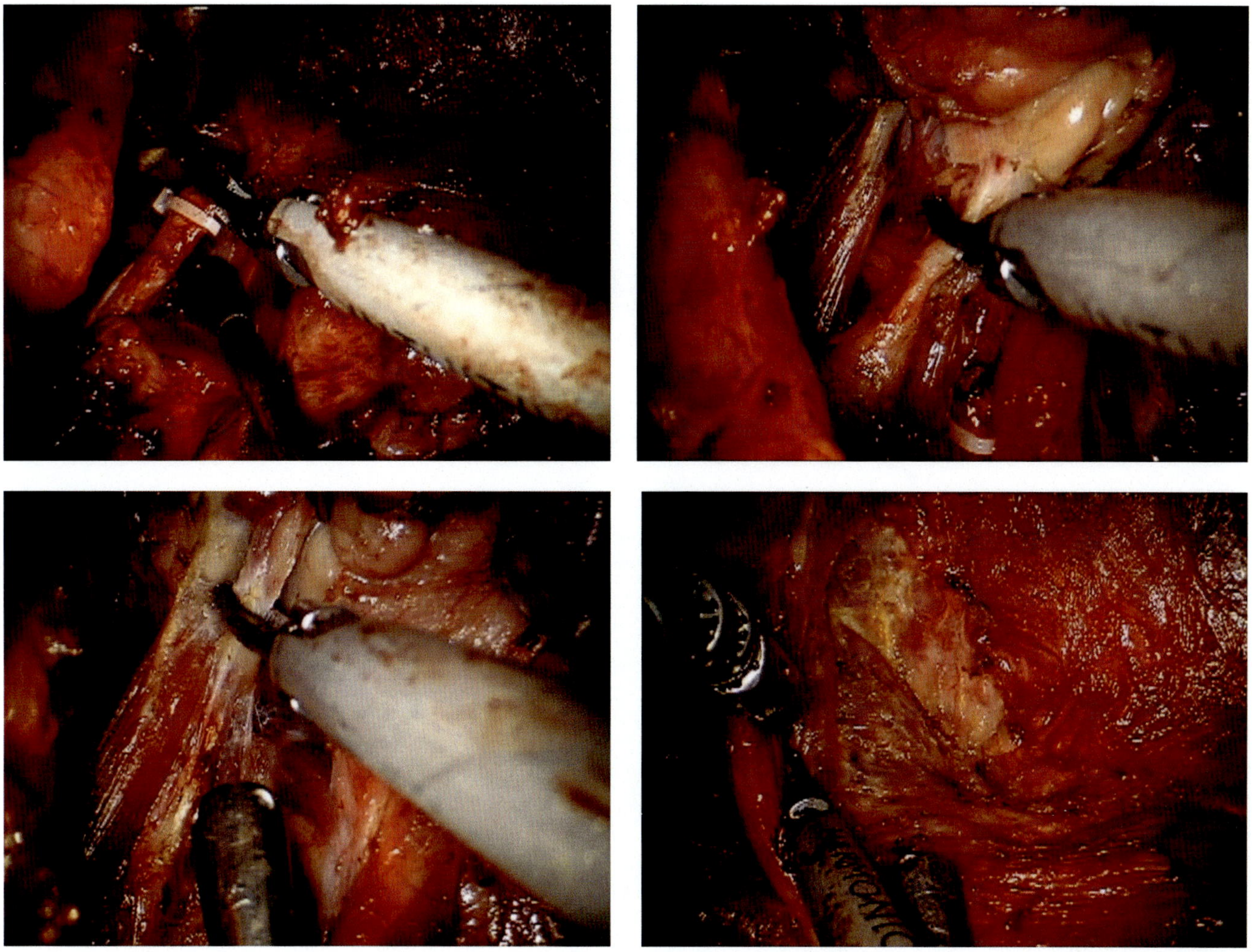

a b c d

Fig. 14.4 Dissection of level I. **(a)** Ligation of proximal facial artery. **(b)** Lingual nerve and submandibular ganglion. **(c)** Wharton's duct: The duct is ligated deep to the mylohyoid muscle. **(d)** Level IA dissection. Fibroadipose tissues of level IA between the posterior belly of digastric muscle are removed.

is identified at the posterior border of the SMG, which is then sealed with Harmonic curved shears or double ligated with the Hem-o-lok Ligation System (Teleflex Inc.) by the assistant (**Fig. 14.4a**). Handling the fibroadipose tissue with the Maryland forceps, level I tissue containing the SMG is dissected away from its surrounding tissue. During the dissection of SMG, the marginal mandibular branch of facial nerve, lingual nerve, and hypoglossal nerve should be clearly identified and safely preserved.

The mylohyoid muscle is revealed at the anterior border of the SMG, where the SMG ganglion (**Fig. 14.4b**) and the Wharton's duct (**Fig. 14.4c**) are visualized by retracting the specimen posteriorly. Each are consequently sealed off with Harmonic curved shears. The submental artery can be brought into view during this step and can also be ligated with Harmonics. Using the same instrument, fibrofatty tissues of level IA between the two anterior bellies of digastric muscle on each side are dissected and detached (**Fig. 14.4d**).

Following the completion of level I dissection, the previously dissected tissues of levels II and III are reflected medially using the Maryland dissector (**Fig. 14.5a**) and dissected from the carotid sheath using Harmonic curved shears (**Fig. 14.5b**). Dissection is then conducted inferiorly to the superior belly of the omohyoid muscle and medially to the lateral border of the strap muscles. The superior thyroid artery and ansa cervicalis can be easily identified (**Fig. 14.5c**). After completion of the dissection the specimen is delivered through the RA port (**Fig. 14.5d**).

Modified Radical Neck Dissection (Levels I–V or II–V)

Just as in the conventional modified radical neck dissection, the SCM muscle, spinal accessory nerve (SAN), or the internal jugular vein (IJV) can be resected where indicated; however, the authors believe that resecting any of these vital structures fails to correspond to the notion of minimally invasive surgery of functional and aesthetic superiority so we make all efforts to preserve all structures including SCM muscle, SAN, and IJV in all cases. Robot-assisted modified radical neck dissection should therefore be performed under strict indications where there are no gross, extensive invasions of the metastatic node.

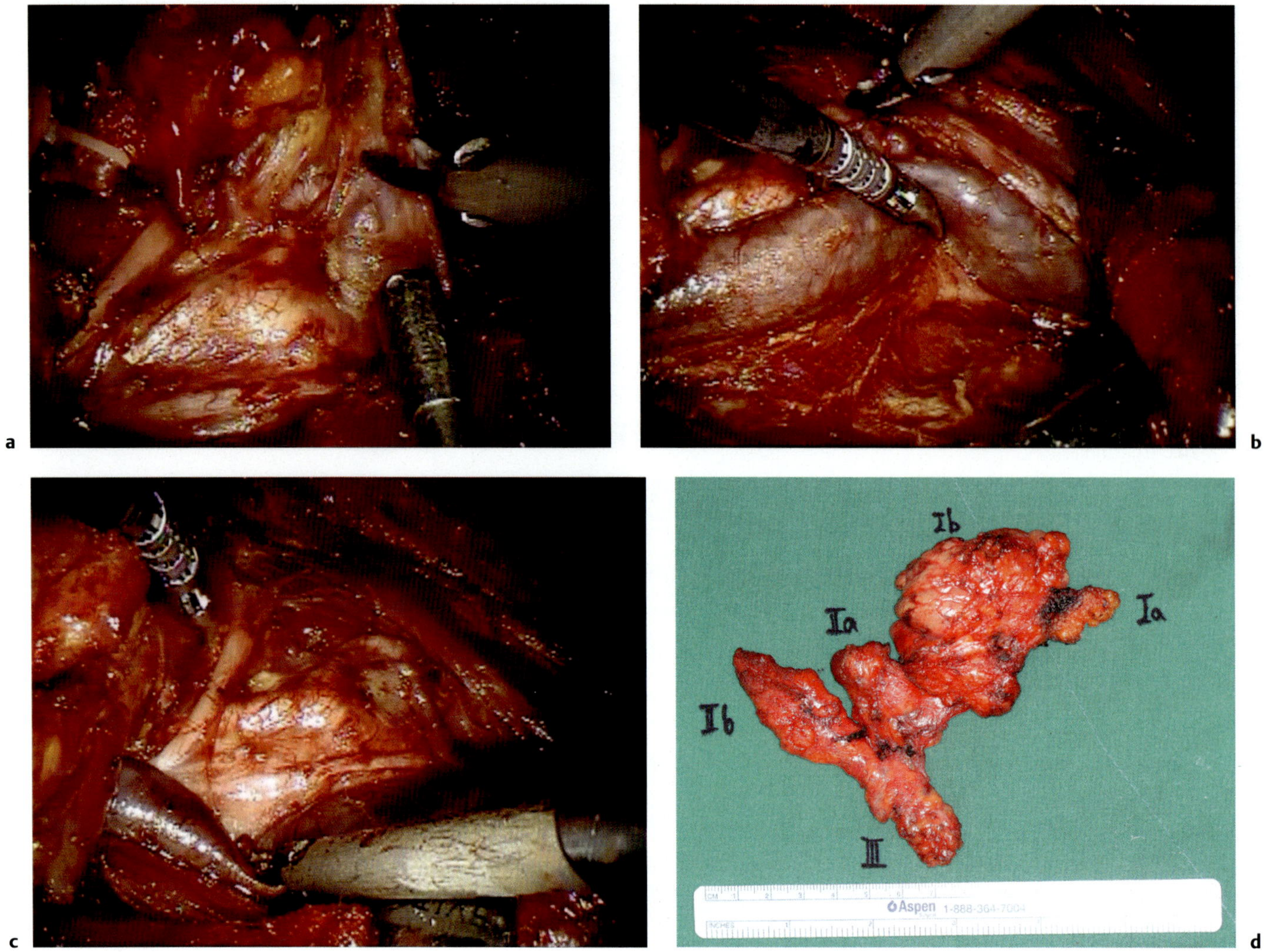

Fig. 14.5 Dissection of levels II and III. **(a)** Superior thyroid artery, carotid bifurcation, and hypoglossal nerve can be easily visualized through the magnified view provided by the endoscopic camera. **(b)** Level III dissection to the omohyoid muscle. Dissection is then conducted inferiorly to the superior belly of the omohyoid muscle and medially to the lateral border of the strap muscles. **(c)** Completion of selective neck dissection level I–III. Superior thyroid artery, hypoglossal nerve, and ansa hypoglossi can be easily visualized through the magnified view provided by the endoscopic camera. **(d)** Surgical specimen.

Skin Incision and Flap Elevation

If level I dissection is omitted, there is no need to elevate the skin flap as high up as the inferior border of the mandible; however, the working space must cover as far below so that the clavicle is reached for levels IV and V to be accessible. Also, the skin–subplatysmal flap should be raised more laterally with reference to the posterior border of the SCM so that the lymph nodes of level V are sufficiently addressed. This procedure could be greatly facilitated if the operator is positioned above the patient's head and faced caudally.

Upper Neck Dissection Under Direct Vision

Great efforts should be made to preserve the SCM muscle, SAN, and IJV at all times whenever robot-assisted modified radical neck dissection is performed. For the comprehensive neck dissection, the marginal branch of the facial nerve is identified first as described above for the selective neck dissection of levels I–III. When performing the neck dissection of levels II–V, the initial dissection is made along the inferior border of the SMG and the tail of parotid gland, where the posterior belly of the digastric muscle is identified underneath these structures. Following along the posterior belly of the digastric muscle and retracting it superiorly enables the visualization of the IJV. The SAN is then identified near the IJV after palpating and checking the location of the transverse process of the atlas. Next the fascia of the anterior border of SCM is opened and the muscle is followed down at the medial border and is continued inferiorly as far below as possible. The entire course of the SAN is skeletonized from its exit near the skull base to its entry at the trapezius muscle. The operator then opens up the fascia along the posterior border of the SCM muscle, where it is then lifted upward using an Army–Navy retractor so that the fibrofatty tissue inside and under the

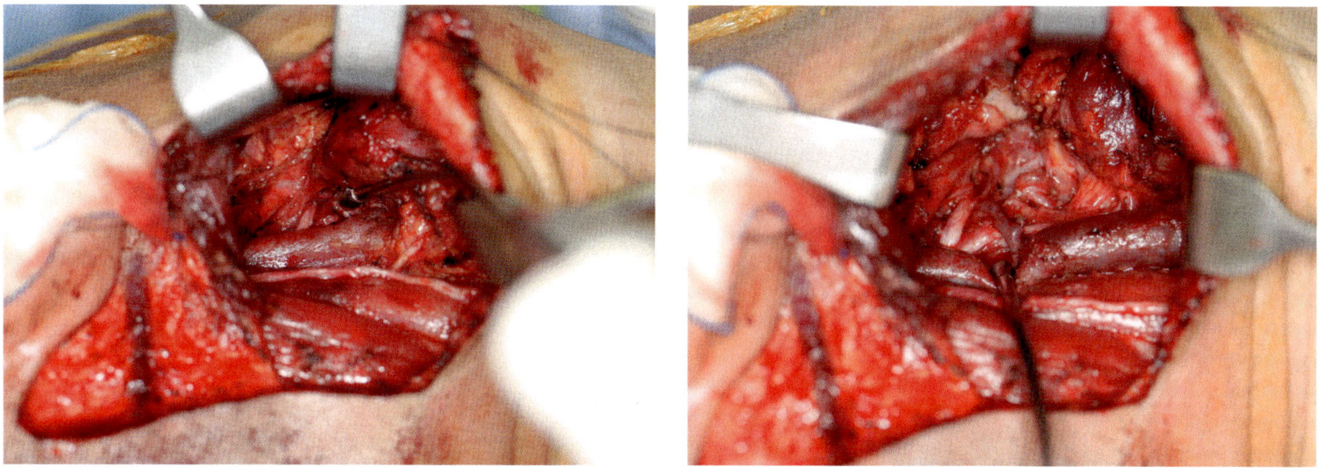

a b

Fig. 14.6 The surgical view of modified radical neck dissection. **(a)** Levels IIB, VA, IIA, and upper III dissections of the right side neck under direct vision. With the upward retraction of the skeletonized sternocleidomastoid muscle, the spinal accessory nerve is identified near the transverse process of the atlas and traced to the insertion to the trapezius muscle. **(b)** Hypoglossal nerve and ansa hypoglossi are identified during levels IIA and III dissection.

SCM muscle is dissected. The fibroadipose tissue is collectively dissected off the SCM muscle during this procedure, and during this step care must be taken not to damage the SAN near its entry to the trapezius muscle (**Fig. 14.6a**).

The SCM muscle is maintained in its retracted position using the self-retaining retractor so that levels IIB, VA, and the lateral aspect to the carotid sheath of IIA and upper III are dissected under direct vision. A considerable portion of the upper neck can be accomplished under direct vision including also the levels IIA and III medial to the carotid sheath. The hypoglossal nerve is identified and preserved near the carotid bifurcation area and the superior thyroid and lingual artery are identified and preserved (**Fig. 14.6b**). The final step of this procedure is primarily removing the dissected specimen so that a clear surgical view is obtained for robotic dissection. While separating the specimen for removal, care should be taken not to violate or transect any lymph nodes nearby. Making sure the SCM muscle is secured in its elevated status, the robotic arms are now introduced.

Robot-Assisted Neck Dissection Technique (Video 14.1)

If level I dissection is included in the operation, the surgery from the robot console is initiated at level I. When docking the robotic arms the axis should be parallel to the inferior border of the mandible. The specific procedures for level I dissection are identical as described above for selective neck dissection (I–III). The specimen obtained from the procedure is removed before moving on to levels IV and V dissection. For the dissection of levels IV and V, the robotic arms must be realigned so that they are addressed toward level IV and V (cephalocaudal direction). The previously dissected portion of level III is dissected from the robotic console in a superior to inferior manner, to continue down to levels IV and VB. The lymphofatty tissue is carefully dissected from the IJV using Harmonic curved shears. Any branches of the IJV can be identified during carotid sheath dissection and controlled in advance with Harmonic curved shears or Hem-o-lok Ligation System to minimize unnecessary bleeding at the operating field. Dissection of level V is conducted in a posterior to anterior manner and generally this procedure is fairly manageable since the working space is already secured after elevation of skin flap and SCM muscle. The fibrofatty tissue of level VB is dissected in a lateral to medial direction and the omohyoid muscle, which is encountered during this process, is cut using Harmonic curved shears. The transverse cervical artery and vein are identified and preserved during the process of level VB and IV dissection (**Fig. 14.7a**).

Just like the conventional procedure, the level of dissection done must be above the facial carpet so that structures like the phrenic nerve or the brachial plexus are safely preserved. The specimen is then retracted superiorly and medially to move on to the following level IV dissection. The lymphoadipose tissue around the carotid sheath at level IV is carefully dissected using Harmonic curved shears (**Fig. 14.7b**). The vagus nerve, carotid artery, and IJV are all identified and preserved by carefully opening up the carotid sheath. When conducting the inferior part of level IV dissection, the lymphatic or thoracic duct should be anticipated around the IJV (**Fig. 14.7c**). Hemoclips or the Hem-o-lok Ligation System should be used to control the lymphatic or thoracic duct not only when there is an evident injury but also when it is undisturbed to prevent any future incidence of chyle leakage (**Fig. 14.7d**). Surgical management of postoperative chylous fistula would often be difficult since the relevant area is reached distally from the RA port.

After completion of the neck dissection, the specimen is delivered through the RA incision port (**Fig. 14.8**).

■ Pearls and Pitfalls

- The key point of this surgical technique is acquiring a sufficient amount of working space. Reflecting our personal

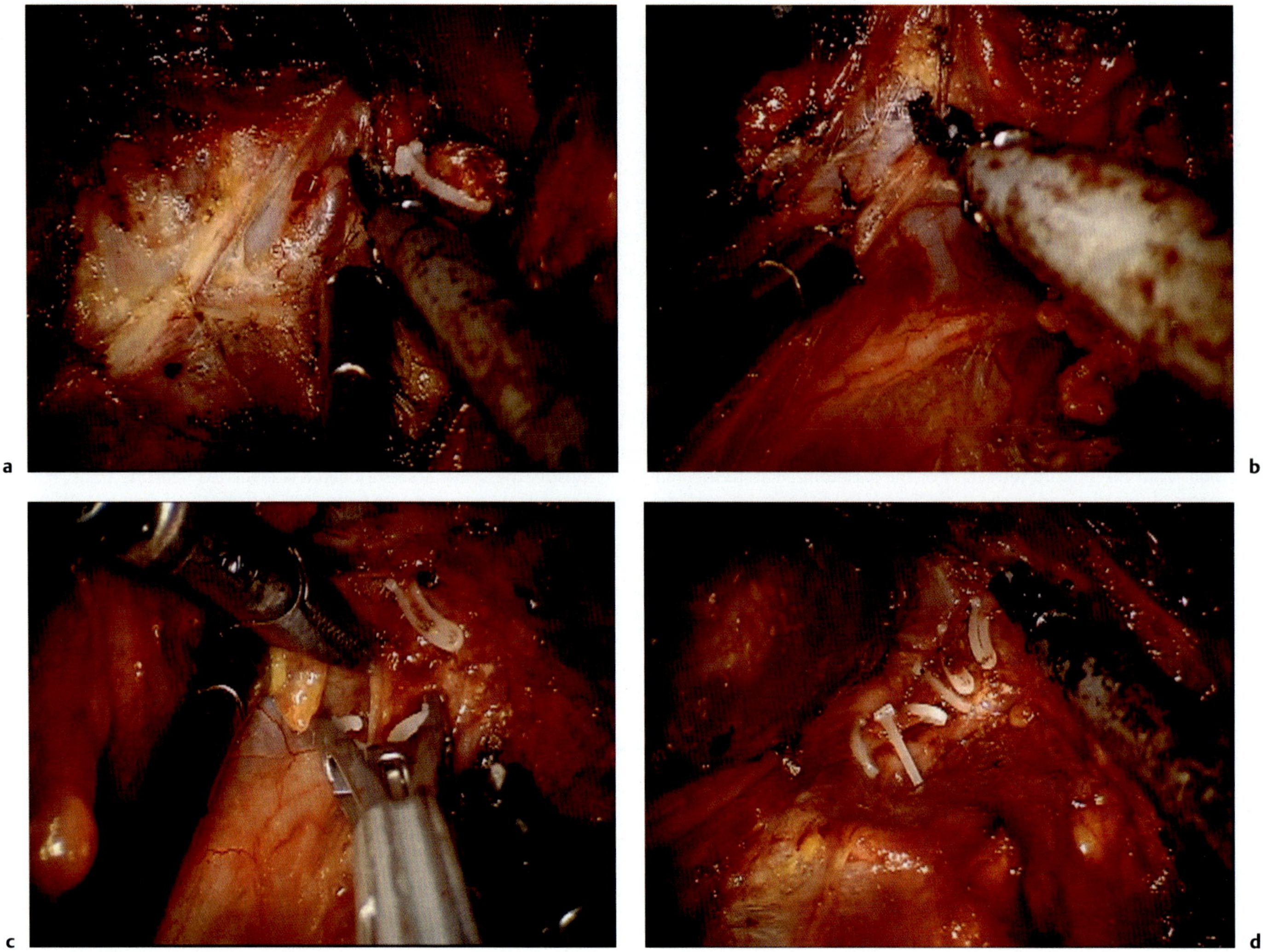

Fig. 14.7 The surgical view of modified radical neck dissection of the right side neck. **(a)** Level VB dissection. The cervical plexus and the transverse cervical artery are identified and the external jugular vein is ligated. **(b)** Carotid sheath dissection in levels III and IV. The fibrofatty tissues near the carotid space are dissected with preservation of the vagus nerve using Harmonic curved shears. **(c)** Identification of the lymphatic duct. The lymphatic duct is sealed with Hem-o-lok to prevent a chyle leakage. **(d)** The surgical view of level IV and V area. The transverse cervical artery and the vagus nerve are well preserved. The omohyoid muscle is securely ligated.

surgical experience, the height of the skin flap raised after securing the self-retaining retractor should be at least 4 cm. If that height is not obtained, it is advised that the RA incision be extended to an MFL incision or the hairline incision portion be extended more caudally.

- Identification of the greater auricular nerve and the external jugular vein may aid in finding the correct subplatysmal plane when performing skin flap elevation. Keeping the correct surgical plane after identifying the platysma muscle is mandatory before proceeding with elevation of the skin flap to the mandible. Elevation of the skin flap without identification of the platysma muscle may lead to thinning of the skin flap, which could result in postoperative skin depression or even perforation of the skin.
- Digital palpation and identification of the distal facial artery just below the mandible provides an anatomical landmark to identify the marginal branch of the facial nerve.
- A patient-side assistant should be well trained to provide a good surgical view during the robotic dissection. The equipment that the assistant can use during the operation are the Army–Navy retractor, Yankauer suction, and endoscopic alligator forceps. Sometimes, robotic arms alone are not enough to provide adequate surgical view and instrumentation.
- For a beginner to this procedure, an MFL incision may be more convenient to acquire an adequate working space at first. Identifying the marginal branch of the facial nerve would be easier also with this incision.
- Since robot-assisted dissection of level I may be somewhat more complex, including the risk of marginal branch injury and dissection or ligation of the facial artery, submandibular ganglion, and Wharton's duct, a beginner may initially attempt performing a selective neck dissection of level II or, III for cN0 oropharyngeal or hypopharyngeal cancer treated with transoral approach or transoral robotic surgery.

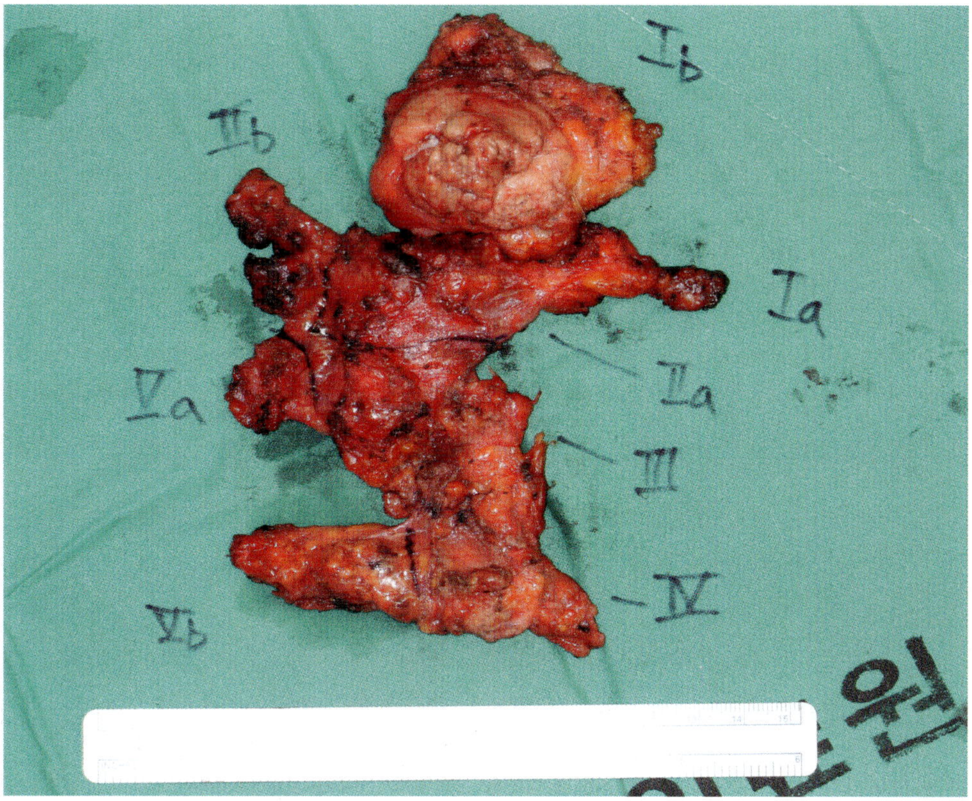

Fig. 14.8 The surgical specimen can be separately removed with level-by-level strategy.

- The authors recommend beginners to conduct endoscopic or robot-assisted submandibular gland excision via RA approach primarily before practicing RAND. The experience will help them especially in aspects of level I dissection.[23,24]
- Damage to the RA hair follicles during hairline skin incision and flap elevation may cause loss of hair and the scar to be more visible postoperatively.
- Thermal injury to the marginal branch of the facial nerve during skin flap elevation may lead to functional deficit in the movement of the lower lip.

■ Complications

Possible complications of this surgical procedure include:

- Nerve injury (marginal branch of facial, greater auricular, hypoglossal, lingual, spinal accessory, vagus nerves)
- Necrosis or discoloration of the skin flap
- Hair loss
- Hematoma
- Infection
- Keloid/scar formation

These are similar to possible complications of a conventional neck dissection. Mouth corner deviation from injury of the marginal branch of the facial nerve can result during the dissection of the area or from the traction made by the external retractors. In addition, the operator should be especially careful when changing instruments during dissection under direct vision or robotic dissection so as not to cause unnecessary trauma to the nerve.

When performing RAND, the surgical field is relatively narrow so the risk of any complications due to major neurovascular structure injury would be greater. Therefore a comprehensive knowledge of the local anatomy and a sufficient level of surgical experience are prerequisites to minimize such complications.

In terms of complications relating to the specific skin incision of RAND, skin ischemia or necrosis can occur at the RA skin flap in some cases. These specific complications can be prevented by limiting the upper end of the flap to the level of the external auditory meatus and avoiding an acute angle of the skin curvature. Hair loss can occur at the skin incision within the hairline in some cases. This can be prevented by beveling the incision at this portion within the hairline.

■ Review of Available Data

The authors have previously reported the surgical techniques of RAND via RA incision on both clinically node negative and positive necks, which were proven to be not only feasible but also satisfactory in terms of cosmesis, since the resulting scar is hidden by the auricle and hair (**Fig. 14.9, Tables 14.1** and **14.2**).

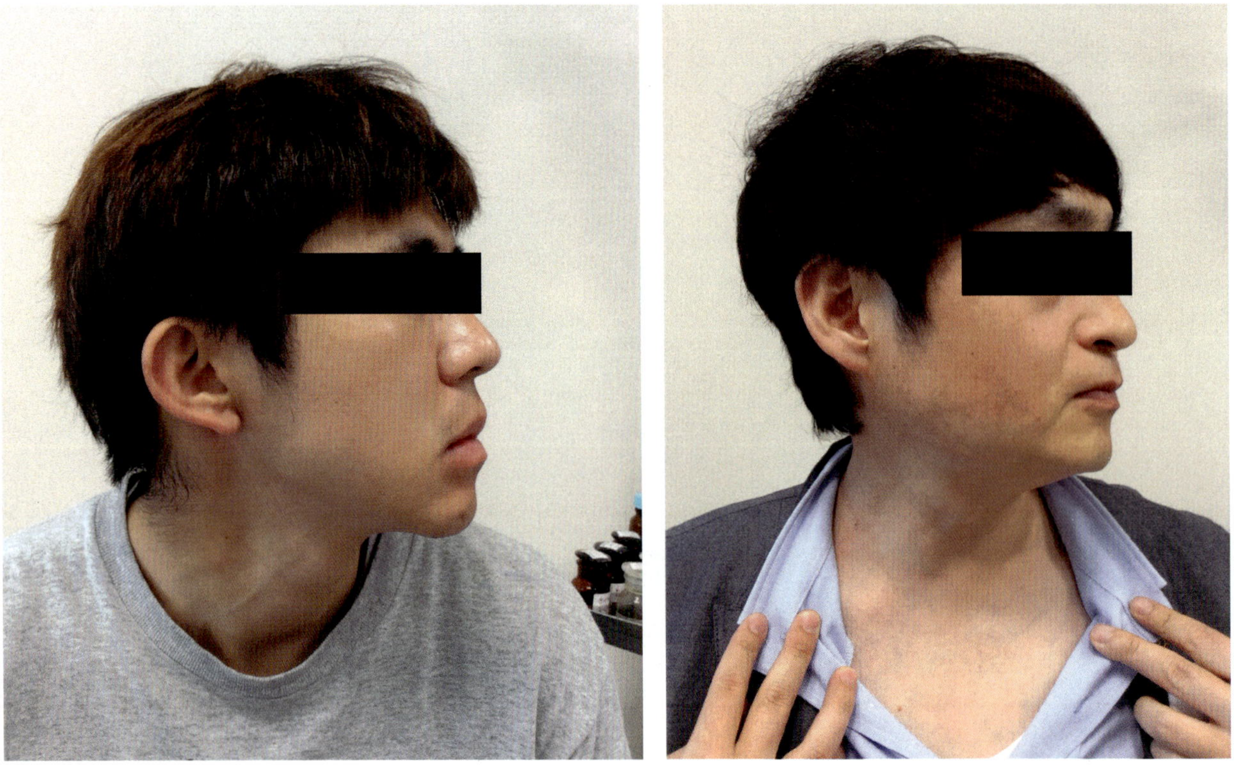

a b

Fig. 14.9 Postoperative photographs. **(a)** Photograph after robot-assisted supraomohyoid neck dissection level I–III of the right side. **(b)** Photograph after robot-assisted modified radical neck dissection of the right side. Postoperative scar is hidden by the auricle and hair without any significant lymphedema or fibrotic change of the dissected area.

Table 14.1 Postoperative outcome of robot-assisted and conventional supraomohyoid neck dissection

Variables	RAND (n = 10)	CND (n = 16)	p value
Operation time (min)	157 ± 18	78 ± 6	0.001
Amount of drainage (mL)	258 ± 40	240 ± 38	0.286
Duration of drainage (d)	5.6 ± 0.8	5.3 ± 1.6	0.241
Hospital stay (d)	9.1 ± 1.6	10.8 ± 5.1	0.897
Retrieved lymph nodes	22 ± 4	20 ± 4	0.310
Satisfaction of scar	4.0 ± 0.7	2.2 ± 0.8	0.001
Complications			
Numbness of earlobe	6	4	0.109
Temporary mouth corner deviation	2	2	0.625
Shoulder syndrome			
Shoulder droop	0	0	
Shoulder pain score	2.25	2.29	0.872
Shoulder motion score	2.75	2.84	0.412
Adjuvant therapy			
CCRT	1	2	
RT	2	2	
Median follow-up (months)	6	6	

Abbreviations: CCRT, concurrent chemoradiotherapy; CND, conventional neck dissection; RAND, robot-assisted neck dissection; RT, radiotherapy.
Source: Data from Lee HS, Kim WS, Hong HJ, et al. Robot-assisted Supraomohyoid neck dissection via a modified face-lift or retroauricular approach in early-stage cN0 squamous cell carcinoma of the oral cavity: a comparative study with conventional technique. Ann Surg Oncol 2012;19:3871–3878.

Table 14.2 Operative parameters of therapeutic robot-assisted and conventional neck dissection

Characteristics	RAND (n = 20)	CND (n = 33)	p value
Operation time (min)	186 ± 37	150 ± 23	0.000
Estimated blood loss during neck dissection (mL)	259 ± 76	239 ± 71	0.354
Amount of drainage (mL)	894 ± 424	794 ± 306	0.327
Duration of drainage (d)	9.7 ± 4.0	8.2 ± 2.0	0.145
Hospital stay (d)	17.0 ± 8.1	15.5 ± 7.8	0.522
Free flap reconstruction	3	8	0.503
SCM muscle sacrifice	6	10	1.000
Internal jugular vein ligation	3	7	0.725
Intentional SAN sacrifice	2	3	1.000
Conversion to conventional ND	0	-	
Perioperative complications			
Seroma	4	5	0.715
Hematoma	2	1	0.549
Chyle leakage	2	4	1.000
Skin flap necrosis/dehiscence	0	1	1.000
Orocervical fistula[a]	0	2	0.521
Lingual nerve injury	0	0	
Hypoglossal nerve injury	0	0	
Phrenic nerve palsy	0	0	
SAN injury[b]	0	1	1.000
Vagus nerve injury	0	0	
Sympathetic trunk injury	1	0	
Temporary mouth corner deviation	4	3	0.405
Satisfaction of scar	3.6 ± 1.1	2.8 ± 1.1	0.023
Adjuvant therapy			
CCRT	13	21	
RT	6	9	
Median follow-up (mo)	8.0	9.3	0.456
Nodal recurrence	0	2	0.521

[a]Orocervical fistula in cases of oropharynx cancer.
[b]Unexpected SAN injury or resection.
Abbreviations: CCRT, concurrent chemoradiotherapy; CND, conventional neck dissection; RAND, robot-assisted neck dissection; RT, radiotherapy; SAN, spinal accessory nerve; SCM, sternocleidomastoid muscle.
Source: Data from Kim WS, Byeon HK, Park YM, et al. Therapeutic robot-assisted neck dissection via a retroauricular or modified facelift approach in head and neck cancer: A comparative study with conventional transcervical neck dissection. Head Neck 2015;37(2):249–254

The perioperative surgical outcomes of RAND were comparable to the conventional type of neck dissection (CND). The average operation times with RAND, however, were generally longer than with CND because of the additional time created for skin flap elevation, working space establishment, and robotic arms docking. The mean operation times for each of the types of RAND and the relative time with respect to the corresponding type of CND are shown in **Table 14.3**. The complication rates and oncologic outcomes of RAND were comparable to CND (**Tables 14.1** and **14.2**). The average yield of lymph nodes according to each type of RAND is depicted in **Table 14.4**. The mean numbers of retrieved lymph nodes according to each sublevel in the RAND group were not significantly different from those in the CND group.

Table 14.3 Operating times according to type of operation

Type of RAND	No.	Mean (SD) console time (minutes)	Mean (SD) total operation time (minutes)	Percentage of CND time[a]
Selective (levels I,II,III)	3	56 (1)	123 (4.4)	137
Selective (levels II,III / II,III,IV)	14	83.2 (67.3)	134.3 (82.4)	149
Selective (levels I-V / II-V)	25	113.0 (68.0)	190.2 (75.1)	127

[a]The crude mean times for conventional selective neck dissection I, II, III; II, III, IV; and I–V in our institution are 90 minutes, 90 minutes, and 150 minutes, respectively. The mean total time consumed for each type of RAND is expressed as a percentage of the mean duration of CND.
Abbreviations: CND, conventional neck dissection; RAND, robot-assisted neck dissection; SD, standard deviation.
Source: Data from Byeon HK, Holsinger FC, Kim DH, et al. Feasibility of robot-assisted neck dissection followed by transoral robotic surgery. Br J Oral Maxillofac Surg 2015;53:68–73.

■ Future Directions and Conclusion

The current robotic application to the neck dissection has enabled the procedure from a remote access port, thereby allowing excellent aesthetic outcomes. However, in terms of the specific operative procedure, the relatively restricted working space can sometimes hinder the operation, for both the console surgeon and the patient-side assistant surgeon since there is scarcely any extra free space once all three robotic arms have been docked. Considering this one limitation of RAND, there is still much room for development of robotic surgery. In the near future, if a single-arm, multi-instrumentation robotic system becomes available commercially for application, it would open up another era of head and neck surgery. RAND would be easier to practice, and even more, the same operation with a smaller incision would be possible. The application of a flexible endoscopic arm will also be beneficial.[25,26]

The central concept of this novel technique of neck dissection is not the application of the robotic system but the adoption of a remote access port that will demonstrate comparable oncologic control and be functionally and aesthetically superior. By shifting the conventional transcervical incision posteriorly behind the ear and the hairline, this technique will be expected to show universal application in the field of head and neck surgery. Already the authors are actively performing various head and neck surgeries via RA approach such as submandibular gland resection, thyroidectomy, free flap reconstruction, and even excision of hypopharyngeal tumors via lateral pharyngotomy.[5,23,24] Further investigation and evaluation of its surgical outcomes need to be conducted to verify its feasibility and oncologic safety.

Table 14.4 Yield of lymph nodes according to type of robot-assisted neck dissection

Type of RAND	No.	Mean (SD) no. of lymph nodes invaded	Mean (SD) no. of lymph nodes retrieved
Selective (levels I, II, III)	3	1.3 (0.6)	24.3 (6.0)
Selective (levels II, III/II, III, IV)	14	0.4 (1.1)	14.1 (7.5)
Selective (levels I–V/II–V)	25	3.0 (2.9)	37.9 (16.7)

Abbreviations: RAND, robot-assisted neck dissection; SD, standard deviation.
Source: Data from Byeon HK, Holsinger FC, Kim DH, et al. Feasibility of robot-assisted neck dissection followed by transoral robotic surgery. Br J Oral Maxillofac Surg 2015;53:68–73.

References

1. Richmon JD, Feng AL, Yang W, Starmer H, Quon H, Gourin CG. Feasibility of rapid discharge after transoral robotic surgery of the oropharynx. Laryngoscope 2014;124:2518–2525
2. Kelly K, Johnson-Obaseki S, Lumingu J, Corsten M. Oncologic, functional and surgical outcomes of primary transoral robotic surgery for early squamous cell cancer of the oropharynx: a systematic review. Oral Oncol 2014;50:696–703
3. Kang SW, Lee SH, Ryu HR, et al. Initial experience with robot-assisted modified radical neck dissection for the management of thyroid carcinoma with lateral neck node metastasis. Surgery 2010;148:1214–1221
4. Byeon HK, Holsinger FC, Kim DH, et al. Feasibility of robot-assisted neck dissection followed by transoral robotic surgery. Br J Oral Maxillofac Surg 2015;53:68–73
5. Byeon HK, Holsinger FC, Tufano RP, et al. Robotic total thyroidectomy with modified radical neck dissection via unilateral retroauricular approach. Ann Surg Oncol 2014;21:3872–3875
6. Koh YW, Choi EC. Robotic approaches to the neck. Otolaryngol Clin North Am 2014;47:433–454
7. Kim WS, Byeon HK, Park YM, et al. Therapeutic robot-assisted neck dissection via a retroauricular or modified facelift approach in head and neck cancer: a comparative study with conventional transcervical neck dissection. Head Neck 2015;37(2):249–254
8. Shin YS, Choi EC, Kim CH, Koh YW. Robot-assisted selective neck dissection combined with facelift parotidectomy in parotid cancer. Head Neck 2014;36:592–595
9. Byeon HK, Holsinger FC, Koh YW, et al. Endoscopic supraomohyoid neck dissection via a retroauricular or modified facelift approach: preliminary results. Head Neck 2014;36:425–430

10. Kim CH, Koh YW, Kim D, Chang JW, Choi EC, Shin YS. Robotic-assisted neck dissection in submandibular gland cancer: preliminary report. J Oral Maxillofac Surg 2013;71:1450–1457
11. Park YM, Holsinger FC, Kim WS, et al. Robot-assisted selective neck dissection of levels II to V via a modified facelift or retroauricular approach. Otolaryngol Head Neck Surg 2013;148: 778–785
12. Kim CH, Chang JW, Choi EC, Shin YS, Koh YW. Robotically assisted selective neck dissection in parotid gland cancer: preliminary report. Laryngoscope 2013;123:646–650
13. Lee HS, Kim WS, Hong HJ, et al. Robot-assisted supraomohyoid neck dissection via a modified face-lift or retroauricular approach in early-stage cN0 squamous cell carcinoma of the oral cavity: a comparative study with conventional technique. Ann Surg Oncol 2012;19:3871–3878
14. Koh YW, Chung WY, Hong HJ, et al. Robot-assisted selective neck dissection via modified face-lift approach for early oral tongue cancer: a video demonstration. Ann Surg Oncol 2012;19: 1334–1335
15. Kim WS, Lee HS, Kang SM, et al. Feasibility of robot-assisted neck dissections via a transaxillary and retroauricular ("TARA") approach in head and neck cancer: preliminary results. Ann Surg Oncol 2012;19:1009–1017
16. Shin YS, Hong HJ, Koh YW, et al. Gasless transaxillary robot-assisted neck dissection: a preclinical feasibility study in four cadavers. Yonsei Med J 2012;53:193–197
17. Byeon HK, Ban MJ, Lee JM, et al. Robot-assisted Sistrunk's operation, total thyroidectomy, and neck dissection via a transaxillary and retroauricular (TARA) approach in papillary carcinoma arising in thyroglossal duct cyst and thyroid gland. Ann Surg Oncol 2012;19:4259–4261
18. Kim WS, Koh YW, Byeon HK, et al. Robot-assisted neck dissection via a transaxillary and retroauricular approach versus a conventional transcervical approach in papillary thyroid cancer with cervical lymph node metastases. J Laparoendosc Adv Surg Tech A 2014;24:367–372
19. Singer MC, Seybt MW, Terris DJ. Robotic facelift thyroidectomy: I. Preclinical simulation and morphometric assessment. Laryngoscope 2011;121:1631–1635
20. Terris DJ, Singer MC. Qualitative and quantitative differences between 2 robotic thyroidectomy techniques. Otolaryngol Head Neck Surg 2012;147:20–25
21. Kim WS, Ban MJ, Chang JW, et al. Learning curve for robot-assisted neck dissection in head and neck cancer: a 3-year prospective case study and analysis. JAMA Otolaryngol Head Neck Surg 2014;140:1191–1197
22. Park YM, Lee WJ, Yun IS, et al. Free flap reconstruction after robot-assisted neck dissection via a modified face-lift or retroauricular approach. Ann Surg Oncol 2013;20:891–898
23. Lee HS, Kim D, Lee SY, et al. Robot-assisted versus endoscopic submandibular gland resection via retroauricular approach: a prospective nonrandomized study. Br J Oral Maxillofac Surg 2014;52:179–184
24. Lee HS, Park do Y, Hwang CS, et al. Feasibility of robot-assisted submandibular gland resection via retroauricular approach: preliminary results. Laryngoscope 2013;123:369–373
25. Johnson PJ, Rivera Serrano CM, Castro M, et al. Demonstration of transoral surgery in cadaveric specimens with the medrobotics flex system. Laryngoscope 2013;123:1168–1172
26. Mandapathil M, Greene B, Wilhelm T. Transoral surgery using a novel single-port flexible endoscope system. Eur Arch Otorhinolaryngol 2014 Jul 14 [Epub ahead of print]

15 Robotic Surgery of the Skull Base

Michael E. Kupferman and Ehab Y. Hanna

■ Description of the Clinical Problem

In the past several years, transnasal endoscopic approaches have been increasingly used for surgical access and treatment of neoplastic and benign lesions of the anterior and central skull base. Endoscopic surgery is used with increasing frequency for surgical resection of tumors of the sinonasal tract, such as inverted papilloma, angiofibroma, osteomas, and other benign fibro-osseous lesions, and in selected patients with malignant sinonasal tumors.[1,2,3,4,5] Endoscopic approaches are also becoming popular for transsphenoidal access to the sella turcica, and are considered by many centers the preferred surgical approach for treatment of pituitary adenomas.[6,7,8,9] More recently, there has been an emerging trend to expand the use of transnasal endoscopic approaches in the surgical treatment of suprasellar, petroclival, infratemporal, and other intracranial skull base tumors.[10,11,12,13,14] Extending the transnasal approach requires the surgeon to have binocular vision to appreciate the complex three-dimensional (3D) anatomy, two-handed control of the instruments to provide retraction and dissection simultaneously, and tremor-free control throughout the dissections. The clinical problem lies in that current transnasal endoscopic technology does not provide these facilities.

■ Current Standard Treatment

The current standard of treatment utilizes transnasal endoscopes that provide high resolution but are two-dimensional. This limits the surgeon's 3D perception of the surgical field. Complex dissection can benefit from a 3D perspective. The current standard transnasal approach also limits the surgeon's ability to dissect with two hands. Although the two-handed approach has been popularized and demonstrated as a useful technique for complex transnasal dissection, the instrumentation is limited in its ability to grasp and manipulate tissue. The current approach provides instrumentation that can be used for blunt and sharp dissection yet the suturing and manipulation of tissue is challenging. This limitation is highlighted by the relatively high rate of postoperative cerebrospinal fluid leaks following extensive skull base resections. Although this has improved as the transnasal technique has evolved, large skull base defects remain a challenge. A reliable dural repair is achieved with underlay grafts and cartilage bolsters; however, suturing the dural patch provides the most reliable watertight closure. Current transnasal instrumentation is limited because suturing and knot placement are difficult with the current instrumentation.

■ Benefits and Drawbacks of the Transoral Robotic Approach

The increasing popularity of these endoscopic skull base approaches may be attributed to a larger trend toward more minimally invasive techniques across all surgical disciplines. The main advantage of transnasal endoscopic skull base approaches is providing more direct access to the anterior and central skull base while avoiding craniofacial incisions and extensive bone removal commonly used in open surgical approaches. Also, the wider angle of vision and angled lenses increase the range of the endoscopic visual surgical field compared with the line of sight visual field gained by surgical loupes or microscopes.

One major disadvantage of transnasal endoscopic approaches is the inability to provide watertight dural closure and reconstruction, which limits its safety and widespread adoption in surgery for intradural skull base tumors. Current techniques of endoscopic skull base reconstruction, such as tissue grafts, mucosal flaps, and tissue sealants, provide adequate reconstruction of limited skull base defects, such as a posttraumatic cerebrospinal fluid leak.[15,16] However, for larger dural defects, these endoscopic techniques have higher cerebrospinal fluid leak rates compared with traditional reconstructive techniques used in open surgery, such as the vascularized pericranial flap.[10]

The potential advantages of a robotic approach include the 3D camera and the ability to use a two-handed single operator surgical approach. Although the standard transnasal approach provides excellent access, the robotic technology has the potential to improve outcomes through improved visual access and handedness.

■ Review of Available Data

While the application of robotic technology to surgery has rapidly expanded over the last 5 years, one of the least studied but fertile areas for application of surgical robotics in the head and neck is for minimally invasive skull base surgery. Certain advantages that these novel systems offer are the ability to perform bimanual surgery in confined cavities with instrumentation that exceeds the capabilities of the human hand, providing the surgeon with a 3D view of the surgical field. Significant advances in surgical robotics have been made,[17] although a role for robotic-based applications in skull base surgery has not been completely defined. There is a paucity of data related to the application of robotics to skull base surgery largely because the technique is in its infancy.

■ Surgical Procedure

Approach to the Anterior Cranial Fossa

The feasibility of using the surgical robot to access the anterior and central skull base has been demonstrated in a cadaver model.[18] Caldwell-Luc incisions and wide anterior maxillary antrostomies, followed by wide middle meatal antrostomies, are the entry points for the surgical arms (**Fig. 15.1a**). Sufficient access can be obtained without compromising the infraorbital nerves (**Fig. 15.1b**), and a posterior septectomy provides a common bilateral surgical field. The robotic endoscope is then placed into the patient's nares and the right and left surgical arms are introduced through the respective maxillary sinuses (**Fig. 15.1c**).

Anterior and posterior ethmoidectomies are performed, and sphenoidotomies provide exposure to the planum sphenoidale, sella turcica, and parasellar regions (**Fig. 15.2**). With current technology, this would be best performed using traditional transnasal endoscopic techniques prior to docking the robotic patient cart. In addition, current robotic instrumentation does not include a drill, although prototypes are under preclinical investigation. Therefore, removal of the anterior skull base bone would likewise be best performed without robotic assistance.

Access to the anterior cranial fossa is provided by sharp dissection of the anterior skull base and incision of the dura (**Fig. 15.3**). The dual robotic arms can be used for primary repair of the dura.[19] This approach provides excellent access to the anterior and central skull base, including the cribriform

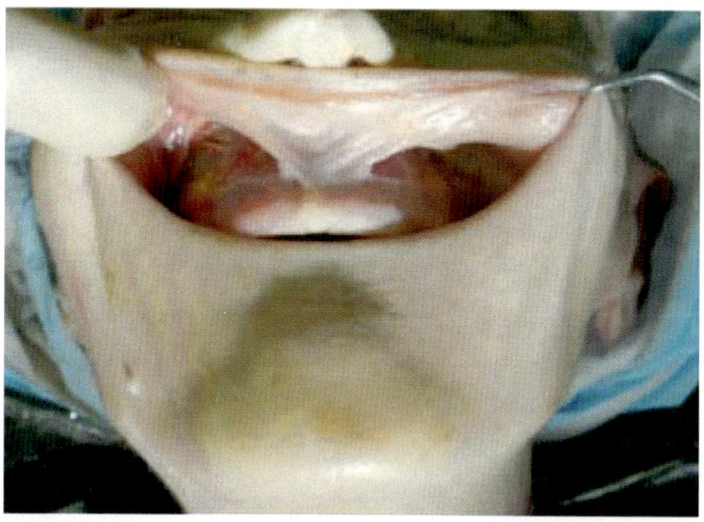

a

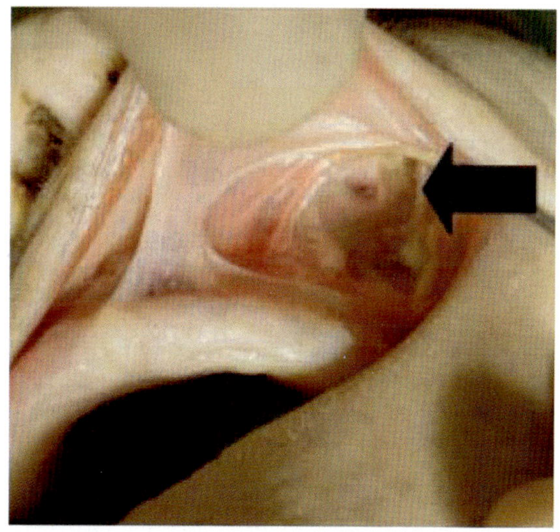

b

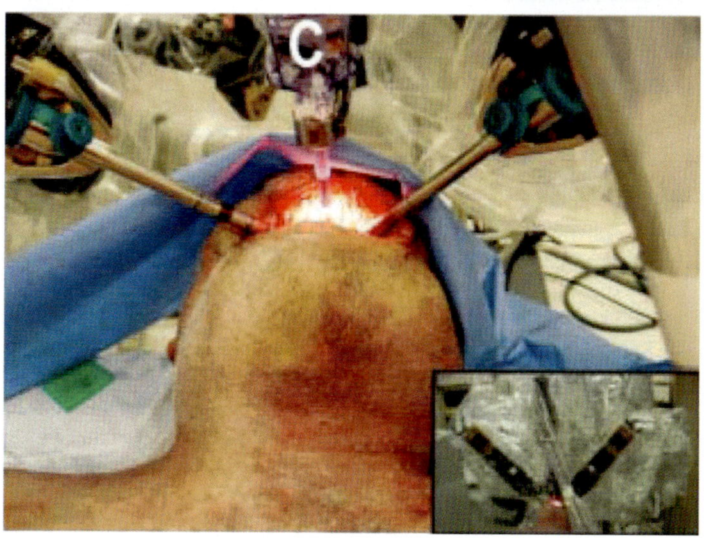

c

Fig. 15.1 (a) Sublabial incisions with bilateral exposure of the face of the maxilla. **(b)** Identification and preservation of the infraorbital nerve (*arrow*). **(c)** Docking of the camera (*C*) and the robotic arms via maxillary antrotomies.

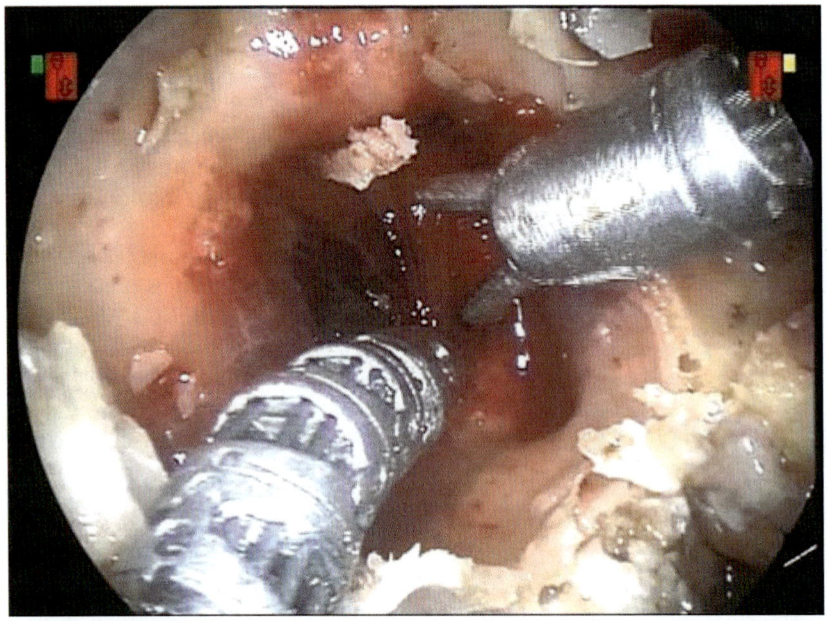

a

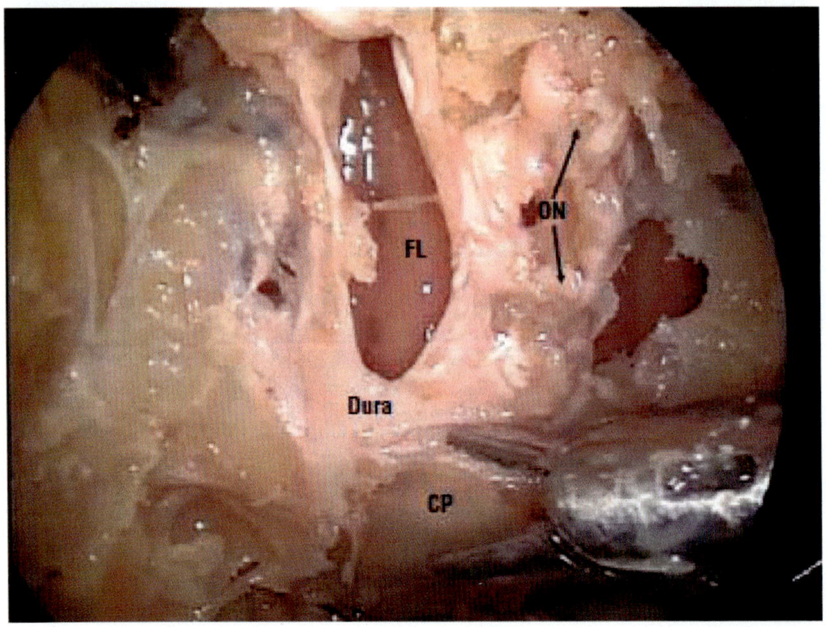

b

Fig. 15.2 **(a)** Dissection of the posterior wall of the sphenoid sinus. **(b)** The cribriform plate (CP) is removed bilaterally, and the cut edges of the olfactory nerves (ON) are shown; the dura is incised or resected to expose the inferior surface of the frontal lobes (FL) intracranially.

plate, fovea ethmoidalis, medial orbits, planum sphenoidale, nasopharynx, pterygopalatine fossa, and clivus. The most significant advantage of this approach is the ability to perform two-handed tremor-free endoscopic closure of dural defects. To date, this approach remains investigational in nature.

Approach to the Pituitary Fossa

While the transnasal endoscopic approach to the pituitary fossa has become a widely utilized technique for surgical resection,[20,21] robotic surgery in this anatomic location may provide unique advantages over the four-handed technique. The feasibility of a robotic approach to the pituitary fossa has been described by the authors, and remains investigational.[22]

Similar to the approach to the anterior cranial fossa, access involves creating bilateral maxillary antrostomies and docking the robotic arms and camera, as described above. An anterior sphenoidotomy is then performed, and the sellar floor removed to expose the dura of the pituitary fossa (**Fig. 15.4**).

The dura is opened sharply with the robotic scissors to allow for exploration of the pituitary gland (**Fig. 15.5a**). Blunt and sharp dissection may be then performed to excise the pituitary gland after the optic chiasm and hypothalamus are exposed (**Fig. 15.5b**). Dissection of the lateral wall of the sphenoid sinus may also be performed with high-speed drills and fine rongeurs

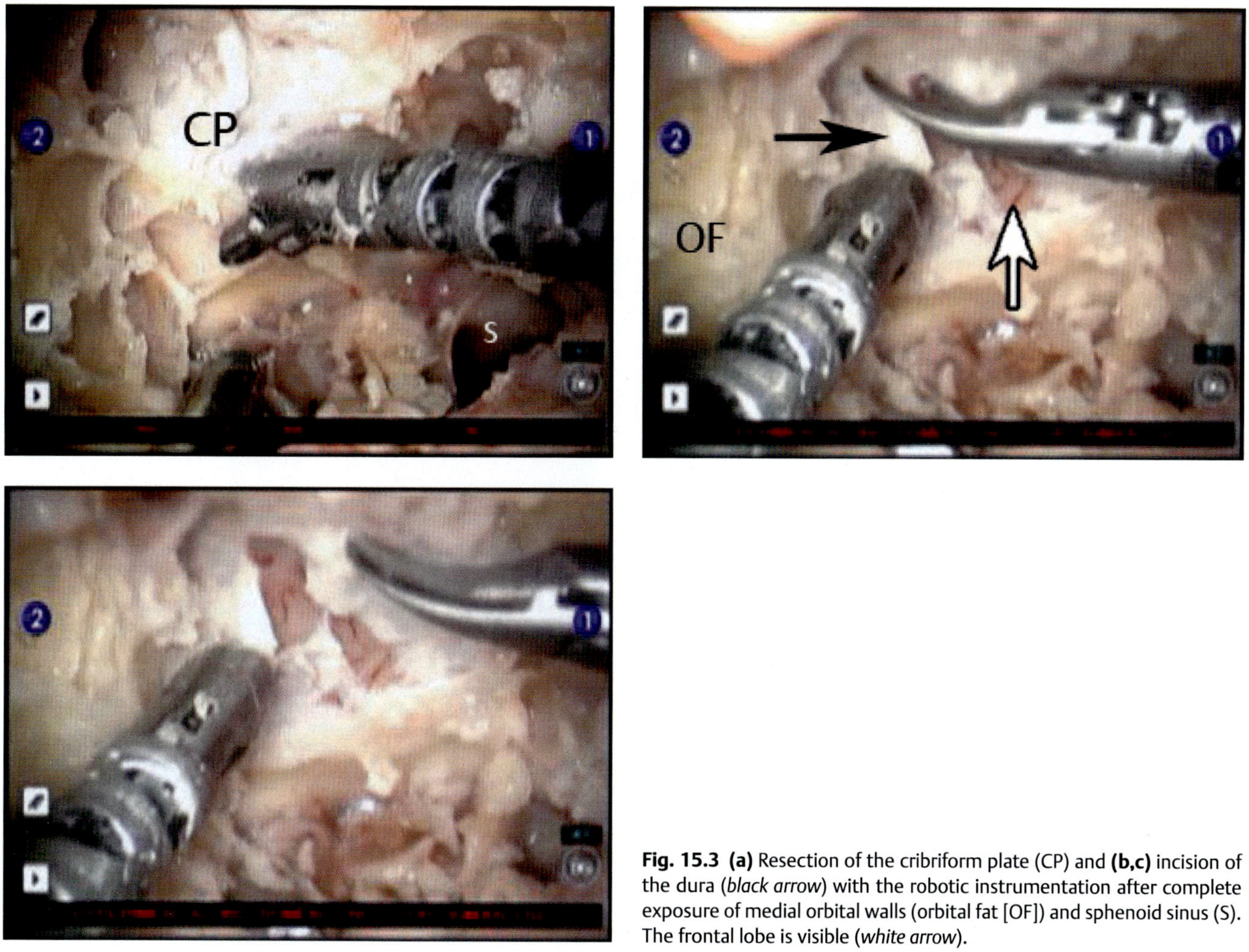

Fig. 15.3 **(a)** Resection of the cribriform plate (CP) and **(b,c)** incision of the dura (*black arrow*) with the robotic instrumentation after complete exposure of medial orbital walls (orbital fat [OF]) and sphenoid sinus (S). The frontal lobe is visible (*white arrow*).

to access the cavernous sinus. Using this technique, access to the central skull base, including the planum sphenoidale, the pituitary gland, cavernous carotid, mammillary bodies, and optic chiasm can be achieved (**Fig. 15.5c**).

A transcervical approach to the skull base in canine and cadaver models has been previously described. Access to the sphenoid, clivus, sella, and suprasellar anterior fossa can be obtained by placing a 30-degree robotic endoscope transorally and placing the right and left robotic arms through the lateral pharyngeal walls via a transcervical technique, posterior to the submandibular gland.[23]

Approach to the Nasopharynx

Robotic surgery of the nasopharynx is perhaps the only anatomic site of the skull base that is amenable to surgical dissection with current iterations of surgical robotics. The feasibility of robotic resection of nasopharyngeal lesions in a cadaver was first described in 2008,[24] and subsequent case reports of surgical management of nasopharyngeal cancers have been published in the literature.[25]

A Dingman retractor is utilized to expose the oral cavity, and the soft palate is divided under direct visualization; lateral retraction of the divided palate is achieved with Vicryl suture (**Fig. 15.6a**). The da Vinci robot (Intuitive Surgical, Inc.) is then docked at the head of the bed, and the robotic arms are positioned into the oral cavity. Typically, a 30-degree endoscope providing a superiorly oriented view of the oropharynx and nasopharynx is utilized. Using the Maryland forceps and the spatula cautery, the nasopharynx soft tissue may then be progressively degloved (**Fig. 15.6b**) between the carotid arteries and eustachian tubes (**Fig. 15.6c**) laterally and the skull base and prevertebral musculature posteriorly. Once the tumor is resected, the palate is closed in three layers with absorbable suture. The advantage of this technique is that it allows for en bloc excision of nasopharyngeal lesions, and may offer the advantage of decreased morbidity compared to either re-irradiation or open surgical approaches for recurrent nasopharyngeal carcinoma. Further study is necessary to delineate the optimal surgical indications.

Approach to the Infratemporal Fossa

Both preclinical studies and case reports addressing the infratemporal fossa and parapharyngeal space via robotic approaches have been described.[26,27] Dissection is performed

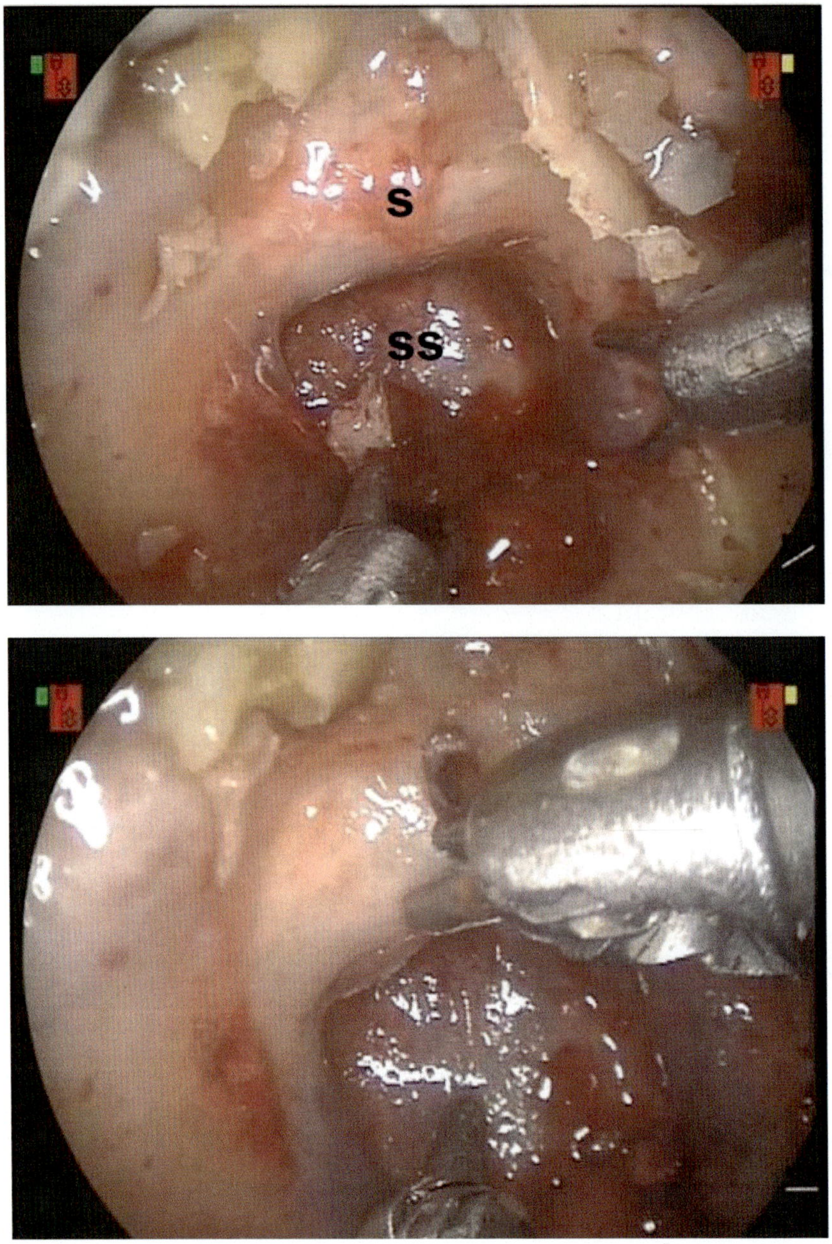

a

b

Fig. 15.4 (a) Exposure of the anterior face of the sella (*s*, sella; *ss*, sphenoid sinus). **(b)** Entry into the pituitary fossa.

through the lateral pharyngeal wall to access the parapharyngeal space. Using the 30-degree endoscope directed superiorly, the parapharyngeal space can be carefully explored to identify the neurovascular contents: jugular vein, internal carotid, and cranial nerves IX, X, XI, and XII. To gain exposure superiorly and laterally (to the infratemporal fossa), the styloid musculature can be resected and pterygoid muscles partially released. This approach may be best suited for well-circumscribed benign lesions.

Skull Base Reconstruction

Perhaps the most significant limitation of current transnasal endoscopic techniques is the inability to reconstruct dural defects with a sutured watertight dural closure. Options for repair of the skull base include: free mucosal grafts, fascia lata grafts, pedicled mucosal grafts, and biological materials.[15,16,28,29,30] While each has advantages and disadvantages, only the pedicled mucoperiosteal grafts are vascularized,[31] a necessary component of any reconstruction in patients undergoing postoperative irradiation, or in previously irradiated patients. One of the major drawbacks of the endoscopic approach is the inability to perform a suture-based reconstruction of the dura using currently available technology, an approach that is easily undertaken with a pericranial flap through the transcranial approach. We previously reported the feasibility of an endonasal robotic surgical dural reconstruction to address this problem in skull base surgery.

Repair of the skull base defect can be performed robotically with two distinct techniques. First, repair of the dura may be

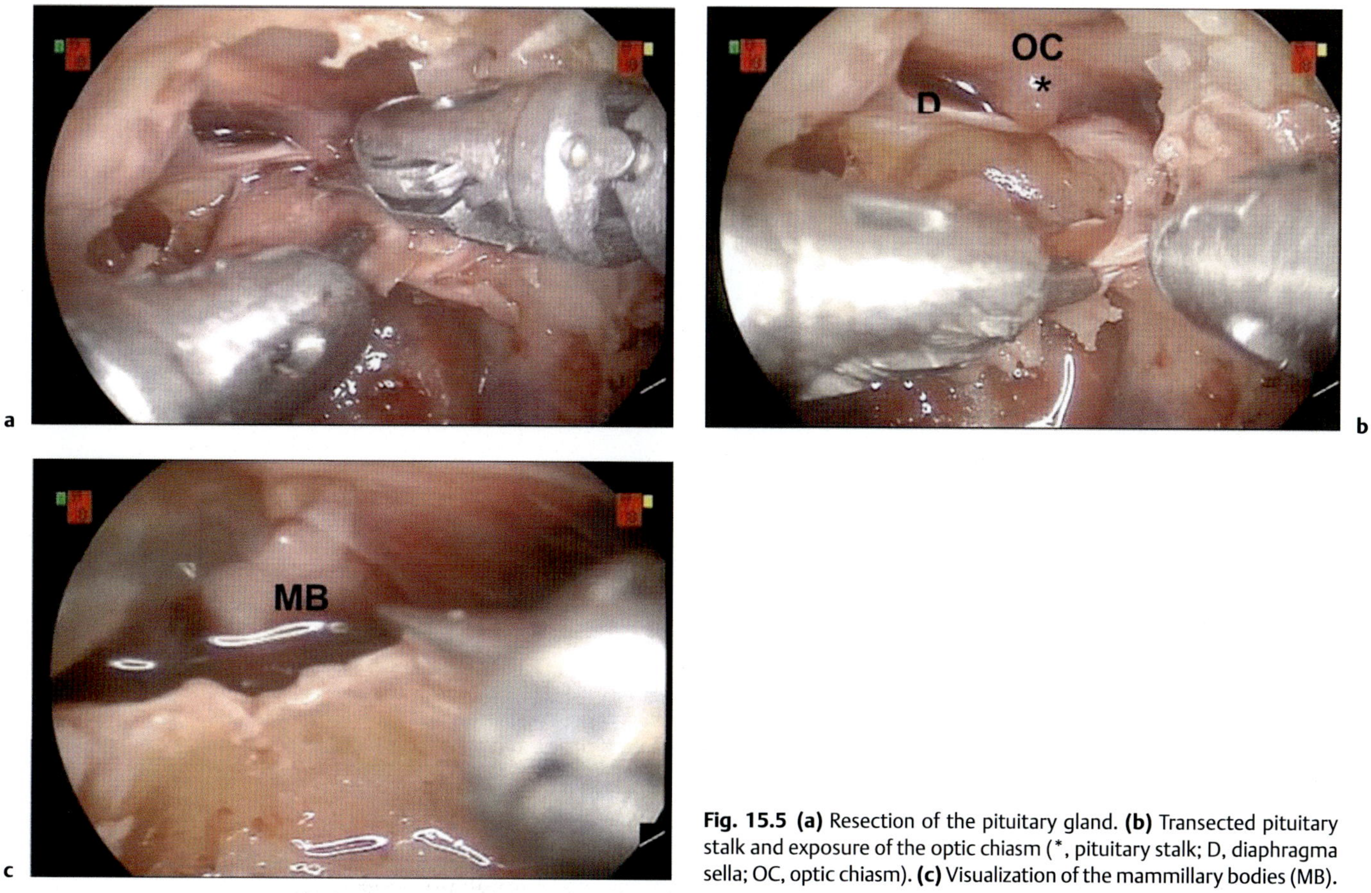

Fig. 15.5 (a) Resection of the pituitary gland. **(b)** Transected pituitary stalk and exposure of the optic chiasm (*, pituitary stalk; D, diaphragma sella; OC, optic chiasm). **(c)** Visualization of the mammillary bodies (MB).

primarily reconstructed with both continuous and interrupted suture technique (**Fig. 15.7a**). Additionally, harvested sinonasal mucoperiosteal graft can be sutured into dural defects with both running and interrupted suture techniques (**Fig. 15.7b**). While these techniques have been demonstrated in cadaver models, their application in human use has yet to be realized.

A balanced analysis of where robotic surgery may lie on the spectrum of surgical modalities suggests that robotic-assisted skull base surgery offers unique advantages that are lacking in either microscopic or transnasal endoscopic techniques. These can be divided into four major areas: optical, ergonomic, dissection, and reconstructive. The following is a discussion of how endoscopic robotic surgery can overcome some of the limitations of these other techniques, and where robotic surgery has limitations.

■ Complication Avoidance and Management

The two-dimensional visualization provided by single channel optical systems in current endoscopes of course lacks the 3D depth perception provided by the binocular optical systems used in standard microsurgery. Therefore, during endoscopic surgery, depth perception relies more on tactile than on visual cues. Visual depth perception is particularly important when operating on critical intracranial neurovascular structures, especially when working in a deep and limited space. The 5-mm robotic endoscope has a dual channel optical system coupled with a dual charge-coupled device, which allows for 3D visualization of the surgical field at the surgeon's console. This binocular endoscope allows the surgeon to have the combined benefit of a wider angle of vision and the depth perception of 3D visualization.

■ Ergonomic Limitations

Current endoscopic techniques have several ergonomic limitations. Bimanual surgery is only feasible if the endoscope is held by an assistant or a mechanical holder. A surgical assistant is preferred because of the constant need to adjust the position (depth and angle) of the endoscope during endoscopic surgery. This not only limits the direct control of the endoscope by the primary surgeon, but also requires the assistance of a relatively experienced endoscopic surgeon who can seamlessly follow the primary surgeon in every step of the operation.

Also, both surgeons have to work within the confined space provided by the nostrils, which in some cases limits ergonomic freedom. In addition, as the surgical field gets deeper, longer instruments are needed and, with lack of proper arm support, precision may be limited by fine tremor, especially when using fine instrumentation for delicate dissection of critical neurovascular structures. The robotic system has four arms, all of which are controlled by the primary surgeon sitting at the

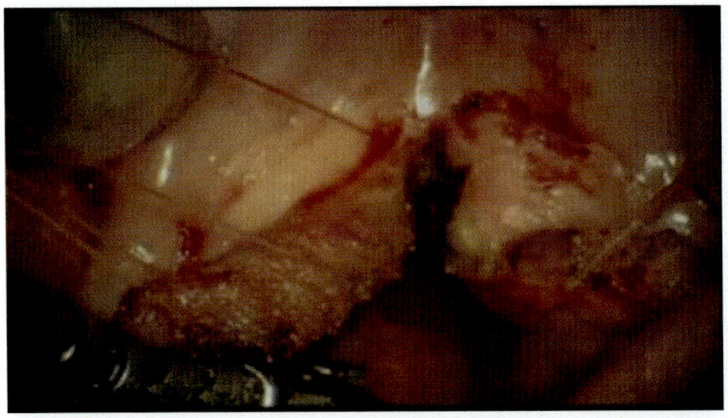
a

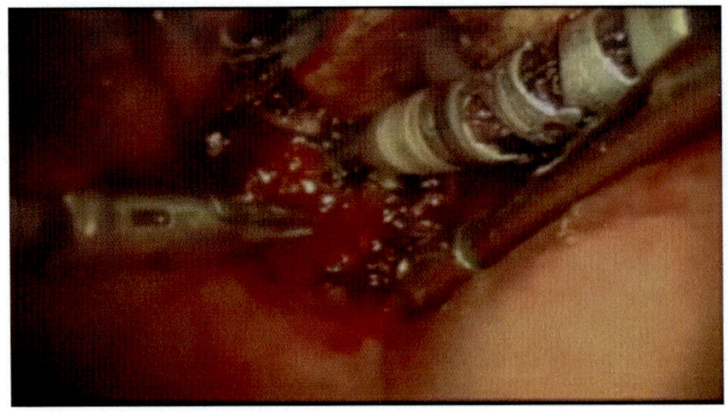
b

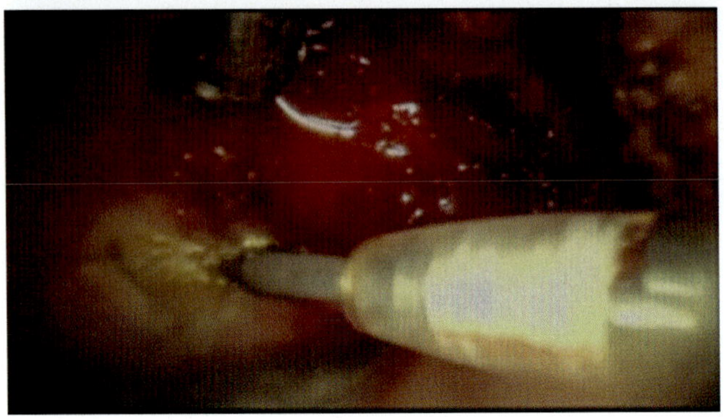
c

Fig. 15.6 (a) Exposure of the nasopharynx is achieved with a palatal-split incision. **(b)** Incisions in the superior and inferior aspects of the nasopharynx commence the posterior dissection. **(c)** Incision through the eustachian tube commences the lateral dissection.

console. One arm, the camera port, holds the endoscope; two arms hold right and left hand instruments; and a fourth, spare arm may be dedicated for retraction or a third instrument. This allows the primary surgeon simultaneous direct control of the endoscope and the instrumentation, an advantage not feasible with nonrobotic endoscopic techniques. Another advantage of the EndoWrist technology used in the da Vinci robotic instrumentation is its ability to provide movement at the instrument tip with 7 degrees of freedom and 90 degrees of articulation and motion scaling. This allows the surgeon, who sits comfortably at the console with an adjustable arm, support to perform precise tremor-free movement in a deep and confined space, with working angles usually not achievable with nonrobotic instruments.

Dissection Limitations

In its current iteration, the da Vinci robotic system is designed exclusively for soft tissue surgery, while the paranasal sinuses and skull base are bony anatomic structures. Access to tumors in these domains requires bone-cutting instrumentation, including rongeurs, osteotomes, and drills. The exquisitely tuned internal pulley system within the robotic arms is not engineered for the stress forces that bony dissection requires. In our experience, use of the robotic dissecting instruments led to rapid deterioration in the functionality and life span of the equipment (unpublished data). Further optimization of the robotic arms will be required before skull base surgery can be effectively performed with the novel technology.

Reconstructive Limitations

The most significant limitation of current transnasal endoscopic techniques is the inability to suture and provide watertight dural closure or reconstruction of dural defects. Endoscopic repair of dural defects relies on nonvascularized fat, mucosal, or allogeneic grafts, or vascularized septal or nasal rotational mucosal flaps. These reconstructions are then covered with fibrin sealants and supported by either absorbable or nonabsorbable packing. While these methods may provide adequate reconstruction of minor dural tears or defects, their ability to provide safe and reliable reconstruction of larger dural defects remains to be seen. Preliminary results suggest that these methods have a higher cerebrospinal fluid leak rate compared with the more standard dural reconstruction using pedicled (axial) flaps, such as the pericranial flap or microvascular free flaps. Adequate and reliable dural reconstruction is critical in minimizing the morbidity of skull base resections, particularly in patients who received or will undergo high-dose radiation therapy. As described above, robotic-assisted surgery allows for successful and precise endoscopic suturing of the dura. This may drastically impact the utility and safety of endoscopic surgery of intracranial intradural lesions of the skull base.

Future Directions and Conclusion

While still in the developmental stages, robotic applications to skull base surgery are forthcoming. Transantral robotic surgery

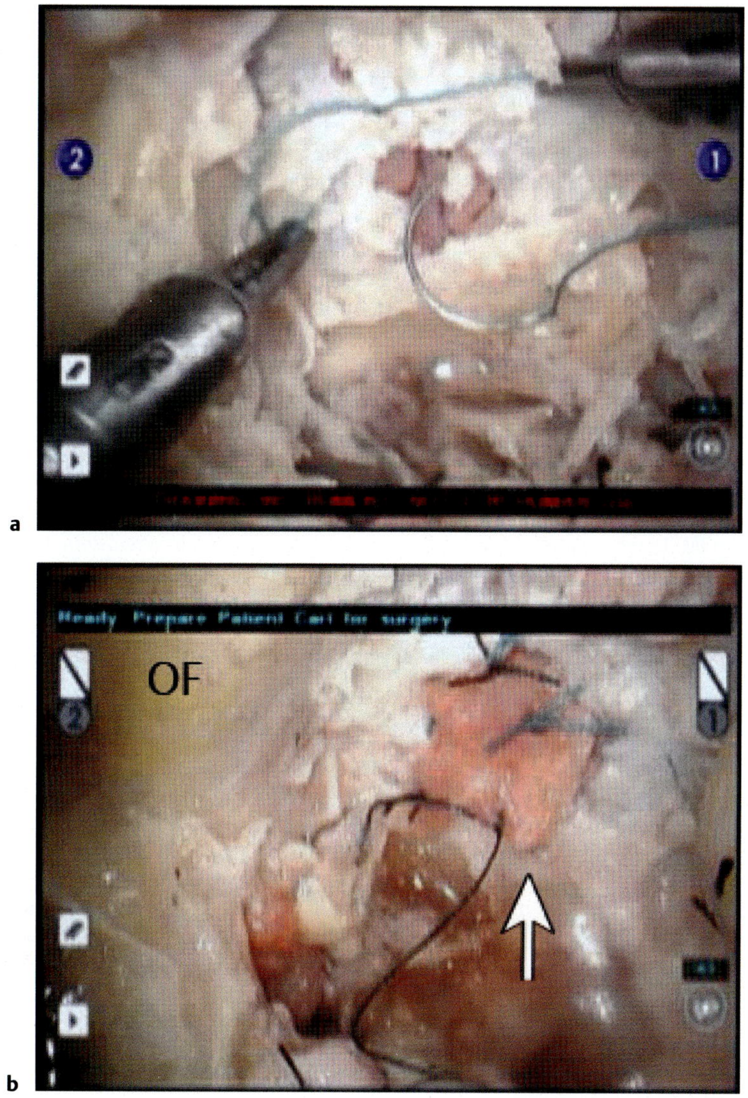

Fig. 15.7 **(a)** Primary repair of a dural defect with polyglactin suture (Ethicon). **(b)** Repair of a large dural defect with a mucosal graft (*white arrow*). OF, orbital fat.

provides stereoscopic endoscopic access to the anterior skull base and pituitary fossa, and allows for two-handed endoscopic manipulation and reconstruction. Traditional suture and reconstructive techniques can be implemented in this confined surgical site with the use of robotic technology. These advantages may expand the indications of minimally invasive endoscopic approaches to the skull base. Future development and refinement of endonasal robotic instrumentation is critical before applying these techniques in the clinical setting.

References

1. Hanna E, DeMonte F, Ibrahim S, Roberts D, Levine N, Kupferman M. Endoscopic resection of sinonasal cancers with and without craniotomy: oncologic results. Arch Otolaryngol Head Neck Surg 2009;135(12):1219–1224
2. Lund V, Howard DJ, Wei WI. Endoscopic resection of malignant tumors of the nose and sinuses. Am J Rhinol 2007;21(1):89–94
3. Nicolai P, Battaglia P, Bignami M, et al. Endoscopic surgery for malignant tumors of the sinonasal tract and adjacent skull base: a 10-year experience. Am J Rhinol 2008;22(3):308–316
4. Suriano M, De Vincentiis M, Colli A, Benfari G, Mascelli A, Gallo A. Endoscopic treatment of esthesioneuroblastoma: a minimally invasive approach combined with radiation therapy. Otolaryngol Head Neck Surg 2007;136(1):104–107
5. Shipchandler TZ, Batra PS, Citardi MJ, Bolger WE, Lanza DC. Outcomes for endoscopic resection of sinonasal squamous cell carcinoma. Laryngoscope 2005;115(11):1983–1987
6. Anand VK, Schwartz TH, Hiltzik DH, Kacker A. Endoscopic transphenoidal pituitary surgery with real-time intraoperative magnetic resonance imaging. Am J Rhinol 2006;20(4):401–405
7. Schwartz TH, Stieg PE, Anand VK. Endoscopic transsphenoidal pituitary surgery with intraoperative magnetic resonance imaging. Neurosurgery 2006;58(1 Suppl):ONS44–51; discussion ONS44–51
8. Sethi DS, Leong JL. Endoscopic pituitary surgery. Otolaryngol Clin North Am 2006;39(3):563–583, x
9. Teo C. Application of endoscopy to the surgical management of craniopharyngiomas. Childs Nerv Syst 2005;21(8-9):696–700

10. Kassam A, Carrau RL, Snyderman CH, Gardner P, Mintz A. Evolution of reconstructive techniques following endoscopic expanded endonasal approaches. Neurosurg Focus 2005;19(1):E8
11. Kassam A, Snyderman CH, Mintz A, Gardner P, Carrau RL. Expanded endonasal approach: the rostrocaudal axis. Part I. Crista galli to the sella turcica. Neurosurg Focus 2005;19(1):E3
12. Kassam AB, Gardner P, Snyderman C, Mintz A, Carrau R. Expanded endonasal approach: fully endoscopic, completely transnasal approach to the middle third of the clivus, petrous bone, middle cranial fossa, and infratemporal fossa. Neurosurg Focus 2005;19(1):E6
13. Kassam AB, Snyderman C, Gardner P, Carrau R, Spiro R. The expanded endonasal approach: a fully endoscopic transnasal approach and resection of the odontoid process: technical case report. Neurosurgery 2005;57(1 Suppl):E213; discussion E213
14. Solari D, Magro F, Cappabianca P, et al. Anatomical study of the pterygopalatine fossa using an endoscopic endonasal approach: spatial relations and distances between surgical landmarks. J Neurosurg 2007;106(1):157–163
15. Basu D, Haughey BH, Hartman JM. Determinants of success in endoscopic cerebrospinal fluid leak repair. Otolaryngol Head Neck Surg 2006;135(5):769–773
16. Locatelli D, Rampa F, Acchiardi I, Bignami M, De Bernardi F, Castelnuovo P. Endoscopic endonasal approaches for repair of cerebrospinal fluid leaks: nine-year experience. Neurosurgery 2006;58(4 Suppl 2):ONS-246-256; discussion ONS-256–247
17. Weinstein GS, O'Malley BW Jr, Snyder W, Hockstein NG. Transoral robotic surgery: supraglottic partial laryngectomy. Ann Otol Rhinol Laryngol 2007;116(1):19–23
18. Hanna EY, Holsinger C, DeMonte F, Kupferman M. Robotic endoscopic surgery of the skull base: a novel surgical approach. Arch Otolaryngol Head Neck Surg 2007;133(12):1209–1214
19. Kupferman ME, Demonte F, Levine N, Hanna E. Feasibility of a robotic surgical approach to reconstruct the skull base. Skull Base 2011;21(2):79–82
20. Cappabianca P, Cavallo LM, de Divitiis O, Solari D, Esposito F, Colao A. Endoscopic pituitary surgery. Pituitary 2008;11(4): 385–390
21. Liu JK, Weiss MH, Couldwell WT. Surgical approaches to pituitary tumors. Neurosurg Clin N Am 2003;14(1):93–107
22. Kupferman M, Demonte F, Holsinger FC, Hanna E. Transantral robotic access to the pituitary gland. Otolaryngol Head Neck Surg 2009;141(3):413–415
23. O'Malley BW Jr, Weinstein GS. Robotic anterior and midline skull base surgery: preclinical investigations. Int J Radiat Oncol Biol Phys 2007;69(2 Suppl):S125–128
24. Ozer E, Waltonen J. Transoral robotic nasopharyngectomy: a novel approach for nasopharyngeal lesions. Laryngoscope 2008;118(9):1613–1616
25. Wei WI, Ho WK. Transoral robotic resection of recurrent nasopharyngeal carcinoma. Laryngoscope 2010;120(10):2011–2014
26. McCool RR, Warren FM, Wiggins RH 3rd, Hunt JP. Robotic surgery of the infratemporal fossa utilizing novel suprahyoid port. Laryngoscope 2010;120(9):1738–1743
27. O'Malley BW Jr, Weinstein GS. Robotic skull base surgery: preclinical investigations to human clinical application. Arch Otolaryngol Head Neck Surg 2007;133(12):1215–1219
28. Hadad G, Bassagasteguy L, Carrau RL, et al. A novel reconstructive technique after endoscopic expanded endonasal approaches: vascular pedicle nasoseptal flap. Laryngoscope 2006; 116(10):1882–1886
29. Leong JL, Citardi MJ, Batra PS. Reconstruction of skull base defects after minimally invasive endoscopic resection of anterior skull base neoplasms. Am J Rhinol 2006;20(5):476–482
30. Mehta RP, Cueva RA, Brown JD, et al. What's new in skull base medicine and surgery? Skull Base Committee Report. Otolaryngol Head Neck Surg 2006;135(4):620–630
31. Kassam ABMD, Carrau RLMD, Snyderman CHMD, et al. Endoscopic reconstruction of the cranial base using a pedicled nasoseptal flap. Neurosurgery 2008;63(1 Suppl 1):ONS44–ONS53

16 The Future of Robotic Surgery

Roger Smith

■ Introduction

There has been no shortage of speculation and experimentation in extending robotic surgical systems from their current capabilities to new and innovative applications. New concepts and prototypes are described in many books on surgery and technology.[1,2,3,4,5] Advanced robots have been foreseen at least since the 1950 appearance of Isaac Asimov's hugely popular collection of stories entitled *I, Robot*.[6] Asimov painted a picture of intelligent robots with a sense of honor and a sense of self that were constantly in conflict. Machines would possess special capabilities that could improve human performance and alleviate dangerous and tedious work, freeing humans to dedicate their intelligence and creativity to higher pursuits. In the science fiction of Asimov and Arthur C. Clarke, robots possess sufficient intelligence and moral principles to create self-awareness and self-value that conflicted with their programming. This conflict was the basis for the classic struggle for survival between the astronaut and the supercomputer HAL-9000 in Clarke's novel and screenplay, *2001: A Space Odyssey*.[7] The picture painted by this book and the subsequent movie illustrated the apprehensions that still exist around robotic assistive technologies.

Asimov is most famous for inventing the Three Laws of Robotics as a moral compass for safely controlling and directing intelligent machines:

1. A robot may not injure a human being or, through inaction, allow a human being to come to harm.
2. A robot must obey orders given to it by human beings except where such orders would conflict with the First Law.
3. A robot must protect its own existence as long as such protection does not conflict with the First or Second Law.

The first law is almost a Hippocratic Oath in which the robot is programmed (pledges) not to use its intelligence or physical power to do direct harm to humans (patients) or to allow harm to come to them through inaction. The second law makes the robot subservient to its human creators, and the third law instills self-preservation into the machines within the bounds of the first two laws.

These laws assume that a robot has sufficient awareness and intelligence to make unique and deliberate contributions to the world around it. However, the surgical robots available today lack intelligence sufficient to trigger the first law, and just enough programming to bring the second and third laws into play. Robots like the da Vinci (Intuitive Surgical, Inc.) contain basic fail-safes that are designed to prevent malfunction during operations, a function similar to the first law of robotics. They act only in direct conjunction with orders from a human, the second law, and these orders are subordinate to the fail-safes (first law). The fail-safes provide some small self-preservation (third law), but do not prevent a human surgeon from damaging the arms and instruments with his/her manual commands.

The da Vinci, the Rio orthopedic robot (Mako Surgical Inc.), and the Renaissance spinal robot (Mazor Robotics Ltd.) all provide useful assistance to surgeons, but reside just at the edge of what would classically be called a robot, possessing only the most basic of programmed intelligence. But these and other devices are the necessary stepping stones to more sophisticated machines that lie in the future. These devices demonstrate and expand the current technology, but more important is the role they play in the social education and acceptance of robotic assistance.

Scientists and science fiction writers who wrestle with the integration of robots into society all come face-to-face with the human apprehensions that arise when machines and humans are working together. This apprehension is much more common than the early adopters of robots realize or are willing to admit. To lay persons, lawyers, and policymakers who are required to accept the technology, robots trigger real fear.

- What is it thinking?
- How will it malfunction?
- How can it really understand my situation?
- Will it take my job?

These fears are not new. They are not rare. They are not easily dispelled. They are as real an impediment to the success of the devices in surgery as are the technological barriers. Dealing with them will require aggressive efforts at education and socialization.

■ Bill Joy's Theory of the Human Future

Famous technologists like Bill Joy, one of the founders of the computer and Internet revolution, believe in a very different kind of future for human beings. There may be a future in which humans are not an essential part of the global ecosystem and are no longer at the top of the evolutionary food chain. Joy famously speculated that evolution had moved from biological organisms into mechanical and computer systems.[8] A human's place in the future may be somewhere slightly lower down the pyramid with new advanced systems taking over some portion of the leadership in new developments and management of society. He asked, "Does the future need us?" These kinds of theories continue to feed the fear that humans have of robotic or computer-assisted activities in society. We are probably a century or more away from this kind of turn in the power structure, but the question alone can be terrifying. Does the future need surgeons with robots, or does it just need the robot?

■ Theories of Innovation

The addition of robotic assistance to minimally invasive surgery represents a significant innovation in the tools and techniques that are most prevalent in the field. The emergence and success of these kinds of innovations have been studied and modeled by multiple authors and academics. The insights that those works provide from other industries may be very useful in understanding the most likely trajectory of this new technology in surgery.

■ Disruptive Surgical Innovation

In his research work at Harvard University, Clayton Christensen has demonstrated the existence and the powerful effects of "disruptive innovations." In *The Innovator's Dilemma* he explored multiple examples of innovative new ideas or technologies that had within them the seeds necessary to disrupt an entire market sector.[9] The dilemma that he presents is that established, market dominating companies and surgical techniques are in a very poor position to capitalize on new technologies, but small start-up enterprises and entrepreneurs are in a good position to adopt these advances and put them to use.

Existing companies, hospitals, and surgeons have built their businesses by mastering a previous set of technologies and processes. As a result they are deeply invested in these methods through investments in facilities, equipment, staff, marketing, and internal business processes. Shifting away from these cash-cow techniques and businesses is extremely risky and in the short-term would dismantle the engine of revenue that is working so well for established players. As a result, they are forced to ignore or minimize new technologies that very clearly have the potential to overturn current practices and displace them with new and better solutions.

Conversely, new start-ups are not burdened by any of the established costs and infrastructure. With sufficient financial support they are able to construct an entire system around the new technology and deliver it to the market efficiently without the burden of accumulated overhead costs and the existing "loss leaders" in their system. These new technologies need only meet the needs of a small portion of the market in order to generate enough revenue to make the start-up and its investors profitable.

In Christensen's model, start-ups begin by pursuing the low end of the market where the demands made of the new technology are easiest to meet (**Fig. 16.1**). In many cases, these customers are also a low profit margin piece of the market. So the established players see the start-up as little threat. Because they

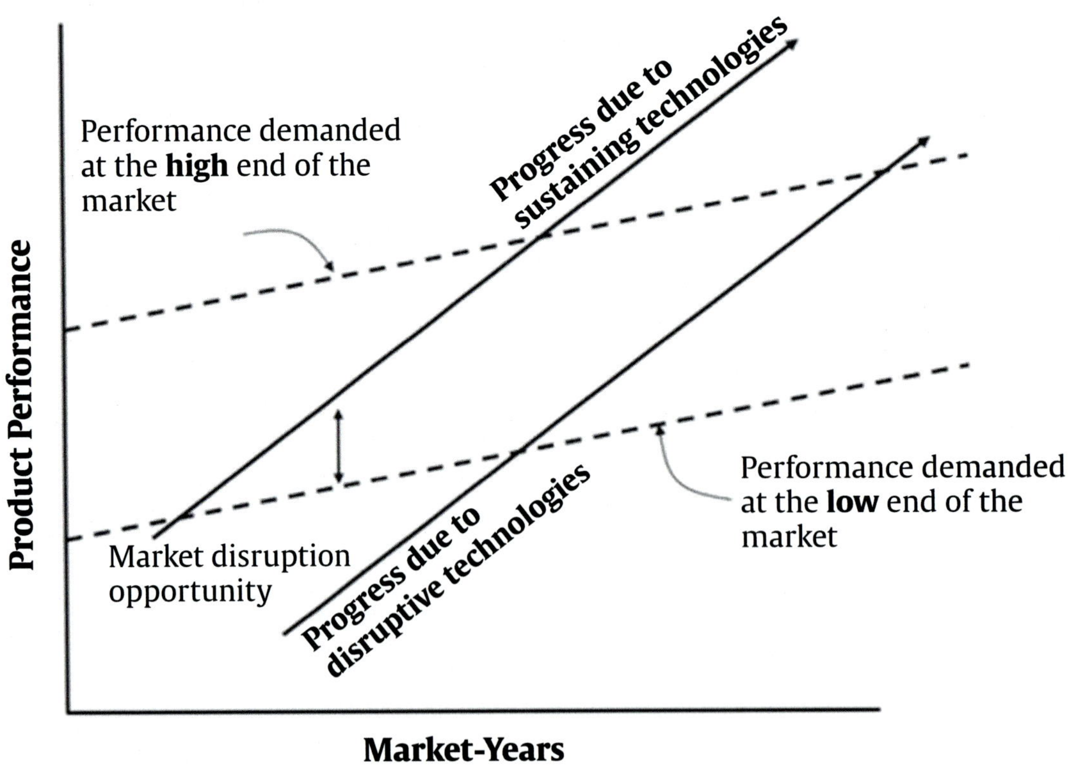

Fig. 16.1 Christensen's disruptive innovation model. (Used with permission from Christensen CM. The Innovator's Dilemma: When New Technologies Cause Great Firms to Fail. Boston, MA: Harvard Business School Press; 1997.)

are taking away business that, in many cases, the established players did not really want anyway, it frees up resources for higher margin applications. In his book, Christensen illustrates this brilliantly with examples from the steel, computer, and automotive industries. The emergence of small, specialized steel mills that converted scrap metal into new products was a disruptive innovation with the seeds to overturn the entire steel industry. In the beginning, the scrap could not be converted into the high-quality steel needed for construction I-beams. Rather it was limited to the very rough rebar that was used to reinforce concrete slabs. Since rebar was a low profit margin product, the appearance of these mini-mills allowed the large players to discontinue manufacturing rebar and redirect their capacity toward the more profitable I-beams. However, this concession created a foundation from which the new competitors could generate revenue and invest in improving the technology. In the short-term the mini-mills provided an advantage to the large manufacturers, allowing them to focus on high margin products. But, as the technologies in the mini-mills improved, they moved up the scale of quality to meet the needs of slightly more demanding customers, satisfying the market for slightly higher margin products. They disrupted the market from the low end, but moving up to progressively more difficult products. This is the progress due to disruptive technologies which Christensen showed in his model. As mini-mill technologies continued to improve, they disrupted the market for all forms of steel, challenging the largest established players and causing many of them to go out of business.

Robotic surgery technologies seem to present a similar disruptive force in health care (**Fig. 16.2**). Beginning in the 1980s, manual minimally invasive surgical tools and techniques were the disruptive innovation to open surgery. Those tools continued to advance in capabilities, reaching into more specialties. Surgeons using the tools became more proficient and eventually surpassed their own capabilities in previously open procedures. After 30 years of improvements, minimally invasive surgery tools and techniques have become an equal partner with open techniques in the surgical market. Today, robotically assisted minimally invasive surgery tools like the da Vinci, Rio, and Renaissance are the disruptors to manual minimally invasive surgery. The former disruptor is becoming the disrupted.

The current family of robots offers a very limited set of capabilities that are powerful and effective in specific situations. Each device has been designed to create very real advantages in a few specific procedures. But, beyond that niche, the technology is not sufficiently flexible to offer improvements over many of the current manual minimally invasive surgery and open techniques and tools. Additionally, the costs associated with these specialized robotic devices can only be justified for procedures that offer high volumes of cases that are very similar. For rare pathologies or procedures, there are just too few cases to justify the high initial investment required.

Once a robot has been purchased, however, the equipment cost barrier has been overcome. So a robotic system like the da Vinci may enter the hospital strictly to meet the needs of the urology or gynecology departments where case volumes are sufficient to generate the necessary revenue to achieve a positive return on investment. But, once installed, the cost barriers for other types of procedures are much lower. These are reduced to instrument costs, surgeon competence, and available capacity on the robot.

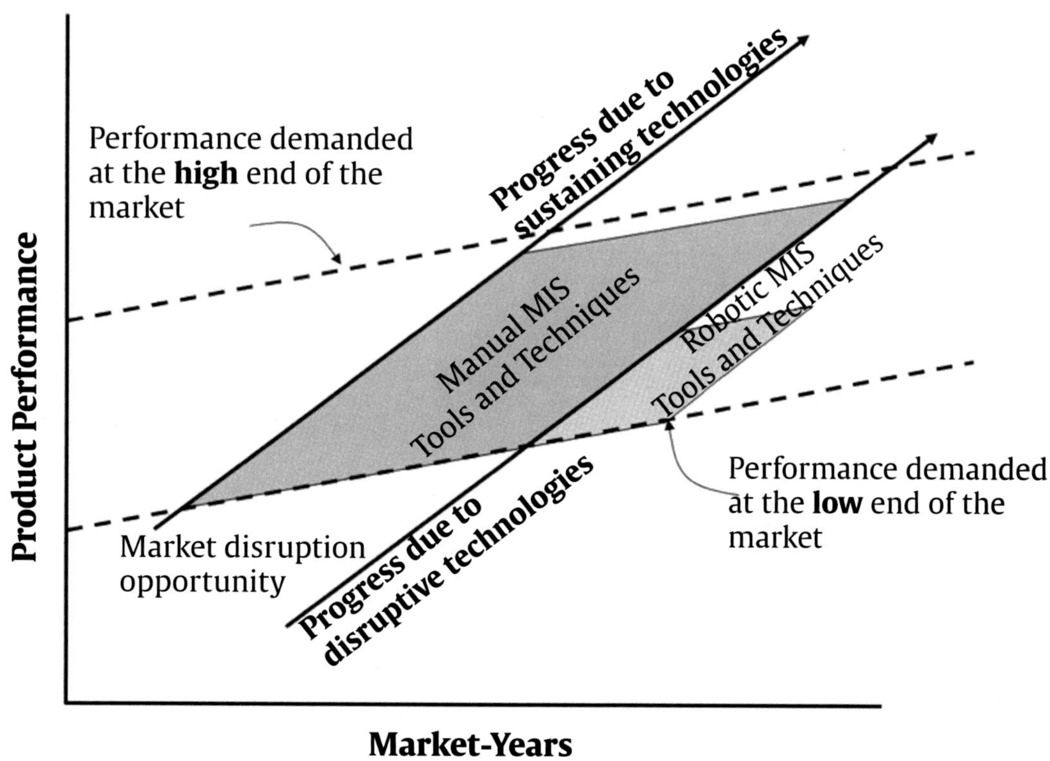

Fig. 16.2 Disruptive technologies in surgical methods. MIS, minimally invasive surgery. (Adapted with permission from Christensen CM. The Innovator's Dilemma: When New Technologies Cause Great Firms to Fail. Boston, MA: Harvard Business School Press; 1997.)

The robotics companies that we have mentioned recognize that they have a disruptive technology in their hands and are following along a path that has been clearly blazed in steel production, computer systems, and web-based services, each of which has completely transformed a market area.

Using the Christensen model as a template and examining the potential for improved applications and technologies in robotics, there are some clear indications for where this new family of surgical tools is headed:

1. Broadened application: Once purchased, robotic devices are a sunk cost. Broadening the scope of their applications is in the interest of the hospital and new surgeons who are trying to establish their expertise. The robot's use will expand to new areas for which the initial purchase could not be justified, but where the per case operational costs are affordable. ENT procedures are an excellent example of this happening with the da Vinci robot, which was originally purchased for urological applications.
2. Device adaptation: There is also motivation to create new instruments that make additional procedures possible with the robot. Hospitals and surgeons may be able to demonstrate how close the system is to supporting procedures that are just beyond its reach in the current configuration. With relatively small investments on the manufacturing side, specialized instruments or add-on devices will open additional surgical doors for its use, such as the 5-mm instruments necessary for using the da Vinci for ENT procedures.
3. Generational improvements: As with mini steel mills, computer hard drives, cellphones, and wearable sensors, the current generation of products is an expression of technologies that have only recently appeared, but that have the potential to continue to improve for many decades. There will be multiple future generations of the core technologies that will effectively lower production costs, eliminate patent barriers, reduce the size of the hardware, increase the intelligence of the device, and generally solve problems that are beyond the current generation of products. We have seen this transformation most recently in cellphones that were originally no more than untethered home telephones, but have become ubiquitous communication and computation platforms with little geographic boundary. The same is about to happen with small wearable sensors that appear in only a few specialized devices today, but that will soon be more ubiquitous than cellphones. Robotics in surgery belongs to this same family of innovation.
4. Business model adoption: The purchasing agents for robotic systems primarily reside within large hospital systems. The expense of the devices limits their use to established players in the market. Therefore, the new technology faces the resistive forces of established methods for providing surgical care. Therefore, the use of robots is somewhat dampened by its role as a new and displacing tool within these established institutions. Over time, the device and the business models that surround it will be better understood, resulting in more equal consideration in the purchasing of surgical systems.
5. Social acceptance: Finally, there is the social or patient acceptance of the devices. There is a very real fear of the complexity of any device labeled as a robot by the population of patients to be treated. Over time, with repeated exposure, more detailed media coverage, additional education, and a library of successes, this resistance will dissipate.

■ The Structure of Scientific Revolution

In his landmark book, *The Structure of Scientific Revolutions*, Thomas Kuhn explored the patterns surrounding the evolution of the theories and paradigms of science over multiple centuries.[10] However, he used the term "revolutions" in the title of his book because he was one of the first to suggest that changes within scientific disciplines occur through a violent process of revolution, not a passive process of evolution.

Scientific fields are established upon a basis of observation and experimentation that form a supportive paradigm of the world. In most cases, these theories are only partially correct. As a result, all fields face a process of maturation, adoption, abandonment, and displacement. These change processes do not occur peacefully.

Kuhn explained that research exposes anomalies that do not fit into the current paradigms that support the basis of one or more scientific fields. Such anomalies are very common and plentiful, and in most cases remain single outliers that cannot be explained. But, over time, these anomalies begin to align and support each other, suggesting that they contain clues to a different and more accurate set of theories and paradigms in the field. Eventually, these become new theories that contradict and offer to replace established theories. This creates a tension between those who would maintain the old theories and those who would replace them with the new. One of the most famous of these is the Ptolemaic Earth-centered versus the Copernican sun-centered theories of the solar system.

Scientific fields are social structures in which a hierarchy has been built based on previous discoveries. The established and respected leaders in a field arrived at their positions through important discoveries supporting the current paradigms. Therefore, new theories that would displace those pose a threat to their personal positions of power. This results in violent disagreements and ideological battles between the supporters of competing paradigms. Kuhn points out that these battles are seldom won on the basis of logical discussion and evidence. Instead, the old paradigms remain in place and the new remain at the fringes for as long as the established leaders remain in their positions of power. The new theories displace the old only as the established leaders die of old age and are replaced by a younger generation who have created the new theories or who have no personal investments in either set of theories.

The story of this revolution between factions in scientific fields appears to exist within the field of surgical care as well. Established leaders with personal reasons to maintain the current methods argue vigorously against the adoption of new technologies. For example, some surgeons would have us believe that there is no future for robotic technology, grudgingly admitting only some value for robot-assisted radical prostatectomy and hysterectomy.[11]

This division and friction is a natural and apparently unavoidable part of the change process in any field. Concerning the application of robotic tools and techniques in surgery, we should not expect anything different. It has been the process within science, a supposedly objective discipline, for centuries and will be part of the history of adoption of new medical and surgical technologies as well.

The Five Forces of Technology Adoption

New technologies constantly emerge from laboratories and garages. But, the markets are not always ready or willing to turn these new capabilities into products. There are forces at work in industry and society that create an environment of receptivity and readiness for these technologies. Without the contribution of these forces it is difficult to significantly change any part of medical or business practice to adopt the technologies. The adoption pattern of the new technology is impacted by at least five significant forces (**Fig. 16.3**).[12]

The first and most commonly examined is the device power, which refers to the raw operational capabilities of the device. Specifically, what can the surgical robot do and where can it be applied? Too many decision makers assume that this is the primary determinant of the future success of the device, and thus stop their investigations once they understand these capabilities.

The second force is device cost. Financial leaders are interested in the investment that must be made and the return that will be realized on that investment. These costs begin with the purchase price of the robot and extend to its per case instrument and operational costs.

The third force is industry success, the degree of adoption that has occurred in other industries that can make use of the technology. Throughout Kuhn's book he points out that an innovation in one field can have very significant impacts in other fields that were not originally conceived as users. The advantages, costs, and limitations of robotics are being felt in a large number of industries. Those successes and failures are instructive for predicting similar outcomes in the surgical field, since the robots are generally designed to augment or replace human actions.

Experimentation is a measure of the degree to which the technology is being applied experimentally to all types of new products and services. When affordable personal computers became available, they were originally meant to assist with accounting spreadsheets and word processing. But hobbyists, scientists, and entrepreneurs eagerly latched onto the devices and began to explore possibilities including entertainment (which launched the computer game industry), remote communication (which created networking and the Internet), computation (which became all forms of predictive modeling), and sales transactions (which became computerized cash registers). The same dispersion pattern will happen with robotic technologies.

Finally, there is the level of social acceptance of the technologies. Without a positive awareness and attitude toward the technology, it will not be accepted as an option by the customers and clients that would supposedly benefit from it. Regardless of all of the safety precautions and production advantages, the nuclear power industry was never able to overcome negative social opinion and remains a relatively small player in the power

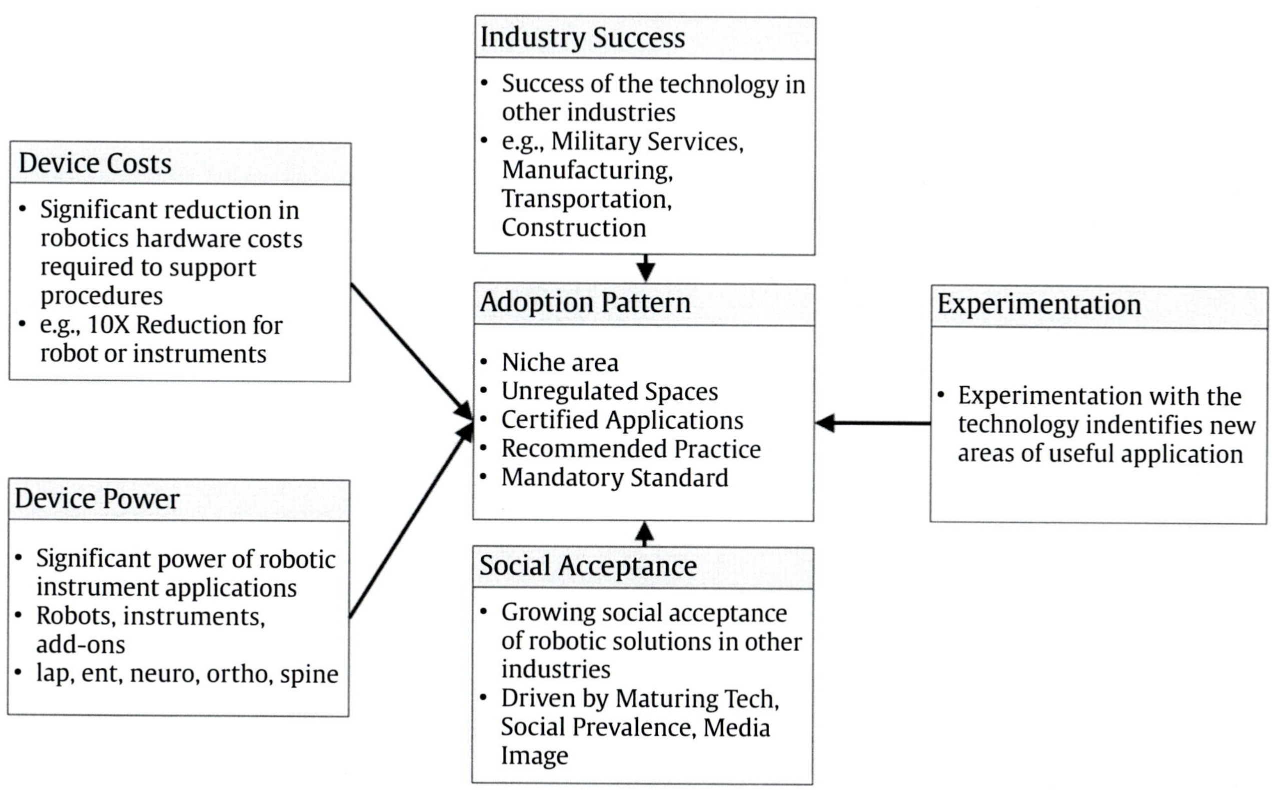

Fig. 16.3 The five forces of technology adoption.

generation industry even 50 years after it was introduced. This kind of resistance can defeat any number of positive technical attributes for robotic surgery as well.

The combination of these and other forces determines whether a new technology makes it beyond a niche application to become a certified, recommended, or mandatory tool of practice.

■ Conclusion

Robotic-assistive technologies are a disruptive innovation that has already become a permanent part of health care delivery. The current devices are impressive works of science and engineering that offer valuable new capabilities for the treatment of patients. But they are also just the tip of the iceberg of advanced technologies that will follow in coming decades. Today's devices offer only the most basic capabilities that can be classified as "robotic." The future will deliver devices that are more intelligent and autonomous than society would currently be comfortable with. Surgery, like all other professions, will evolve and change as scientists and engineers bring new technologies to maturity, and as society develops a higher level of confidence and comfort for those devices. A future in which robots perform partial procedures autonomously under the watchful eye of a human expert is coming. The most interesting question is not whether it will happen or when it will happen, but where it will first be used and which country will take the lead in embracing the devices. Who will protect the status quo and who will promote disruptive changes that will create leaders in the new paradigm of surgery?

References

1. Fujino T, ed. Simulation and Computer-Aided Surgery. New York, NY: John Wiley & Sons; 1994
2. Satava RM, ed. Cybersurgery: Advanced Technologies for Surgical Practice. New York, NY: John Wiley & Sons; 1998
3. Satava RM, Gaspari A, DiLorenzo, N, eds. Emerging Technologies in Surgery. Heidelberg, Germany: Springer-Verlag; 2007
4. Gharagozloo F, Najam, F, eds. Robotic Surgery. New York, NY: McGraw Hill; 2009
5. Patel VR, ed. Robotic Urologic Surgery. London, UK: Springer-Verlag; 2012
6. Asimov I. I, Robot. New York, NY: Spectra Books; 1950
7. Clarke AC. 2001: A Space Odyssey. New York, NY: New American Library; 1968
8. Joy B. Why the future doesn't need us. Wired Magazine. April 2000; 8(4). Accessed online, March 24, 2014 at http://www.wired.com/wired/archive/8.04/joy.html
9. Christensen CM. The Innovator's Dilemma: When New Technologies Cause Great Firms to Fail. Boston, MA: Harvard Business School Press; 1997
10. Kuhn TS. The Structure of Scientific Revolutions. Chicago, IL: University of Chicago Press; 1962
11. Heemskerk J, Bouvy ND, Baeten CG. The end of robot-assisted laparoscopy? A critical appraisal of scientific evidence on the use of robot-assisted laparoscopic surgery. Surg Endosc 2013; 28:1–11
12. Smith RD. Military simulations using virtual worlds. In: Grimshaw M, ed. Oxford Handbook of Virtuality. Oxford: Oxford University Press; 2013:666–679
13. Albala D. Single Site Robotic Systems. 2013 Annual Meeting of the Society for Robotic Surgeons. Orlando, FL; November 8, 2013

Index

Page numbers followed by *f* indicate figures; those followed by *t* indicate tables.

V

X